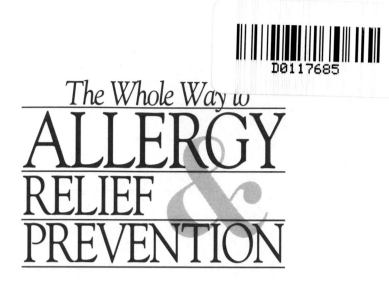

The Whole Way to
ALLERGY
RELIEF &
PREVENTION

The Whole Way to
ALLERGY
RELIEF &
PREVENTION

A DOCTOR'S COMPLETE GUIDE TO
TREATMENT & SELF-CARE

BY

Jacqueline Krohn

JACQUELINE KROHN, MD

FRANCES A. TAYLOR, MA   ERLA MAE LARSON, RN

Frances A. Taylor   *Erla Mae Larson*

Hartley & Marks
PUBLISHERS

Text © 1991 by Jacqueline A. Krohn, MD

Published in the U.S.A. by
Hartley & Marks, Inc.
Box 147
Point Roberts, Washington
98281

Published in Canada by
Hartley & Marks, Ltd.
3663 West Broadway
Vancouver, B.C.
V6R 2B8

ISBN 0-88179-036-2

LIBRARY OF CONGRESS CATALOGING-IN-PUBLICATION DATA
Krohn, Jacqueline, 1950-
The whole way to allergy relief and prevention : a doctor's complete guide to treatment and self-care / by Jacqueline Krohn, Francis A. Taylor, Erla Mae Larson.
p. cm
Includes bibliographical references and index
ISBN 0-88179-036-2 (pb.) : $19.95 ($24.95 CAN)
1. Allergy--Popular works. I. Taylor, Francis A., 1938-.II. Larson, Erla Mae, 1925- . III. Title.
RC584.K76 1991   91-35090
616.97--dc20   CIP

Printed in the U.S.A.

Typeset by The Typeworks in Goudy Oldstyle
Cover design by Elizabeth Watson
Cover illustration by Joyce Lem
U.S. portion of the pollen map on page 166 courtesy of: Meridian Bio-Medical, Inc., 1700 Royston Lane, Round Rock, Texas 78664.

If unavailable at your local bookstore, this book may be ordered from the publisher.
Send the cover price plus one dollar fifty for shipping to either of the above addresses.

This book is meant to be a source of information for those who are not enjoying the best of health because of their allergies or sensitivities. Everyone has different problems and different needs based on age, sex, lifestyle, health status, genetics, diet, psychological state, and spiritual maturity. Our intent is to share our experience and offer guidelines to help you become more informed about your health. In cooperation with your physician, you can then take the necessary steps to enjoy optimum health.

This book is not intended to be a substitute for consultation with a physician. Neither the authors nor the publisher take medical or legal responsibility for the reader who uses the contents of this book as a prescription.

CONTENTS

◆ ◆ ◆

PART 1   OUR BODY SYSTEMS AND ALLERGIES

◆ ◆ ◆

PART 2   UNDERSTANDING ALLERGIES

◆ ◆ ◆

FOREWORD

Everything you ever wanted to know about allergies is in this book.

All pediatricians have to become allergists. At least 25 percent of their phone calls and office visits are related to allergy or sensitivity problems of some sort. Even infections are frequently triggered by allergies; we know that allergic people seem to be sick more frequently. The freckle-faced, ginger-haired youth is more susceptible to strep and rheumatic fever, probably because he has milk allergies. It is well known by most children's doctors, for instance, that ear infections (*otitis media*) begin as an allergic reaction to cow's milk that closes up the eustachian tube. Germs love to grow in that walled-off phlegm. Fever, pain, and a call to the doctor soon follow.

Decades ago, colic due to cow's milk sensitivity was estimated to upset only five to 10 percent of babies. By about 1970, workers at free clinics in large cities realized they were giving soy-based milk to at least half of their clients because of sensitivities to cow's milk. Pediatricians have become adept at prescribing the usual control substances antibiotics, antihistamines, sedatives, ointments, and gas dispersers but little attention has been paid to the causes of allergies/sensitivities and their removal.

These infants do grow up, of course, but they become allergic/sensitive children and then carry their problems into adulthood. School stressors, pollutants, sugar-laced foods, accidents, divorce, or death in the family are the stressors that seem to hit almost all of our children and patients. An overlooked fact is that about 80 percent of people in North America are too alkaline to some degree. This metabolism imbalance prevents minerals from being soluble and usable by the enzymes that allow the body to function optimally.

I have formulated a rule that works for me: If you do not understand something, it is probably due to an allergy. Everywhere I go in the US and Canada, and it has also happened in Australia and New Zealand, the natives say, "This is allergy valley," or "This is hayfever hill." It seems that only a few people do not have allergies/sensitivities of some sort or another! This book by Dr. Jacqueline Krohn will help the reader sort them out. There are many positive answers in this well-researched book, so don't give up!

Lendon H. Smith, MD
Portland, Oregon

TO THE READER

The information contained in this book is based on personal experience, as well as on knowledge gained through study and clinical experience. All of the authors have experienced, in varying degrees, allergies and sensitivities to foods, chemicals, and inhalants; chronic fatigue syndrome; candidiasis; subclinical parasitic infections; mercury toxicity; and electrical imbalances. By using the treatment methods presented in this book, we have all recovered sufficiently to be able to conduct a full-time medical practice in environmental medicine.

From the beginning of our practice, we felt that an informed patient would be a more cooperative patient. We soon learned that a well-educated patient was more likely to comply with treatment, and to have a better chance of recovery. To aid in this educational process we wrote our *Allergy Patient Manual*, the nucleus from which *The Whole Way to Allergy Relief and Prevention* grew. It is our intention that this book be useful to people with only a few allergies and sensitivities as well as to those with environmental illness. Our primary goal, both in our practice and in this book, is to help people improve the quality of their lives.

We have used the most current, up-to-date information available. Although information and theories have been accumulating for many years, only recently have studies provided evidence that these theories are true. Environmental medicine is developing at a rapid pace, and is not without controversy. It remains for health practitioners to interpret and implement this information, in innovative ways, for the care of their patients.

Controversy centers around nomenclature. In some instances we have tried to avoid this conflict by using the terms "sensitivity" or "intolerance" rather than "allergy." The debate will continue for many years to come but will not solve the more important problem—the sufferer's distress. Our aim is to provide proper treatment and education to alleviate that suffering, whether symptoms are due to so-called "true" allergy or to hypersensitivity syndromes.

Jacqueline A. Krohn, MD
Frances A. Taylor, MA
Erla Mae Larson, RN
Los Alamos, New Mexico
1991

ACKNOWLEDGEMENTS

Our sincere thanks to:

Our predecessors and colleagues in the fields of science and medicine, particularly in environmental medicine, for the work, research, and publications that enabled us to write portions of this book.

Colleagues who encouraged us and provided information and guidance.

Our office staff for doing extra work to help us maintain our regular schedules while writing this book.

Sherry Francisco for the many hours she spent at the computer.

Our families, who cheerfully endured the hours we spent writing this book.

Steven Carter, our editor, and the staff of Hartley & Marks, who guided us through the maze of the publishing world.

Contributions by:

Jean Brau
Kathleen Shelton
Deborah Brandt

The Whole Way to Allergy Relief and Prevention

INTRODUCTION

A large part of the population of North America suffers from some type of allergy. (Over 13% have pollen allergies. When the number of individuals who have food and chemical sensitivities is factored in, the total of those affected is over 20% of the population.) Some people are unaware of their allergies, some view their allergies simply as a nuisance, while others have symptoms severe enough to interfere with their chosen lifestyles.

There are many clinical portraits of the person with allergies. The five main descriptions are:

- Those who have essentially only pollen allergies. They sniff and sneeze during pollen season, yet for the rest of the year feel reasonably well.
- Those who have predominantly food allergies. They have no seasonal symptoms, but have varying symptoms whenever they eat a food to which they are sensitive.
- Those who have chemical sensitivities will suffer from exposure to perfume, gasoline, fabric softener, tobacco smoke, and other chemicals, but may not have symptoms from pollen or foods.
- Those with a combination of pollen, food, and chemical allergies and sensitivities. There are infinite numbers of these combinations, varying in severity, and from person to person.

- Those with such severe allergies and sensitivities, overlaid with other health problems, that they are considered to be "universal reactors" and are described as ecologically/environmentally ill.

Ecological illness is the result of adverse reactions to substances in the air, water, food, home and work environments, and to medications. It can cause many varied, chronic symptoms, and it can involve many systems of the body, including the nervous, endocrine, immune, gastrointestinal, upper respiratory, muscular, and skeletal systems. Ecological illness often masquerades as other types of diseases and is often undiagnosed or misdiagnosed.

In this book we have endeavored to present the "whole way" to allergy relief and prevention. Anyone with allergy problems, ranging from a minor allergy to environmental illness, will find information pertinent to his or her condition. The basis from which our practice evolved and which we have utilized in this book is that of clinical ecology and environmental medicine. Clinical ecology is the study of our relationships with and adaptation to our environment (food, water, chemicals, air, inhalants, medication) and the diseases and adverse reactions resulting from these environmental sources. Environmental medicine is the practice of directly correcting or improving such environmentally caused problems with a minimal use of drugs. Its main goal is to reduce or eliminate the reactions a sensitive person experiences by using a combination of approaches, such as environmental control, immunotherapy, nutritional supplementation, and rotation diet. In many cases this comprehensive treatment enables the immune system to repair itself.

Good health and a strong immune system are our most precious possessions. Allergies are not just a nuisance to be ignored until they can no longer be denied—they constitute a health problem that must be treated. Untreated allergies can lead to more serious problems as we get older. Blood pressure problems, diabetes, cardiovascular disorders, arthritis, and other degenerative diseases can develop as a result of untreated allergies. If we do not take the time to treat allergies and to get well now, we will have to take the time to be sick later. Good health does not depend on luck; it depends on having a healthy lifestyle!

The "Tacks" of Illness

Dr. Doris Rapp of Buffalo, New York says having health problems is like having tacks in your shoe. People enjoying optimum health have shoes free of tacks; they experience no symptoms and enjoy life to its fullest. The rest of us have varying numbers of tacks in our shoes, depending on how many allergies and health problems we may have. The environmentally ill person will have the largest number of tacks.

We are born with some of our tacks, as we all have hereditary factors, both good and bad, which predispose us to some disease processes. To minimize the effect of these genetic traits, we can choose to alter our personal environ-

ment and lifestyle in order to maximize our strengths and minimize our weaknesses. We receive other tacks in our shoes as we journey through life and as our environment affects us. Infections give us one tack; the development of pollen allergy adds another. Chemicals in our environment, food sensitivities, nutritional deficiencies, electrical imbalances, and dental problems contribute still more tacks.

In order to improve our health, and reduce and eliminate the pain from these tacks, we must remove them. If we remove only a few, our pain level will be changed very little. In order to free ourselves entirely of the pain, we must remove all of the tacks—we must travel the whole way to allergy relief.

The following treatment approaches are used to remove our "tacks" of ill health, and are discussed in detail throughout the book. Some people may require the use of only one approach to return to health. Others may need to use several in order to restore health and well-being. In addition to our concern with allergy relief—with the removal of those tacks from our shoes—we are also interested in prevention and avoiding the accumulation of the tacks. Prevention can be accomplished by considering and applying the appropriate treatments before problems occur. Just as lifestyle management is the key to recovery from allergies, it is also the key to prevention.

Treatment Modalities for Allergies and Sensitivities

- *Immunotherapy:* Identifying your major allergens, and treatment with immunotherapy (with desensitizing extracts), help to control allergic reactions to foods, chemicals, and pollens.

Natural Allergy Programs Work!

In our practice, we frequently tell our patients that their health and treatment can be compared with a flower bulb, its many layers representing the different health problems they may have. These problems can be treated and corrected, layer by layer. When the center of the bulb is reached, we discover the "flower of good health."

Some people have few health problems, and thus have small flower bulbs with few layers. Others have large flower bulbs with many layers that must be peeled back, using several different facets of treatment, in order to reach the flower. Regardless of the number of layers needing treatment, we all have the capacity to heal.

SUE'S STORY OF RECOVERY

One of our patients with a very large "flower bulb" healed dramatically because of her diligent adherence to her treatment program. Sue was a 38-year-old woman who came to us complaining of severe headaches, extreme weakness, fatigue, hives and frequent rashes, colitis, intestinal cramps, nausea and vomiting, low energy, dizzy spells, arthritic symptoms, "heart cramps," sleep disturbances, bronchitis, and edema (swelling). She also experienced frequent sinus, bladder, and kidney infections.

Sue's history indicated severe allergies to pollen, dust, mold, and animal dander; acute chemical and food sensitivity; and evidence of Candida overgrowth. She had previously been given allergy shots containing formaldehyde as a preservative and, as a result, had acquired blood vessel damage.

Her daily medications, prescribed by her previous physician, included:

Lanoxin—0.25 mg, one per day
Thyrolar—one grain per day
Entracin—five grams, eight per day
Tetracycline—250 mg, two per day
Maxibolin—two mg (½ tablet), three per week

Sue also had on hand, with instructions to take as needed:

Lasix—40 mg, one every other day
Ethaquin—100 mg, one per week
Stelazine—one mg as needed, once per day
Empirin #2—as needed, three per day
Hydergine—one mg as needed, one/two per day
Bentonite liquid, as needed
Natural vegetable laxative, as needed

Other medications Sue had taken included cortisone; hormones; phenobarbital; sleeping pills; birth control pills; Inderal; Isuprel; and numerous antibiotics, nose drops, and antihistamines. She had a history of allergic reactions to drugs, including penicillin, sulfa drugs, and scopolamine, as well as reactions to bee stings.

Because Sue was suffering from

numerous severe symptoms, we suggested that she leave her job as a substitute teacher to concentrate on her health care. Fortunately, she was financially able to do so, and so she devoted her attention to taking care of her own health and that of her family. (Sue's two sons also had severe allergies.)

Sue's treatment began with allergy testing, for pollens, dust, dust mite, mold, and animal danders. She tested positive to nine trees, six grasses, 14 weeds, dust, dust mite, *Alternaria, Aspergillus, Hormodendrum (Cladosporium), Penicillium, Pullularia (Aureobasidium), Fusarium, Helminthosporium, Mucor, Rhizopus*, orris root, tobacco, histamine, cat, dog, and horse dander, and sheep's wool. Allergy extracts were made for her, based on these test results. The extracts were to be taken approximately once each week, after she determined her optimal dose.

We tested Sue for chemicals, and found her to be sensitive to phenol, ethanol, benzyl alcohol, chlorine, glycerine, formaldehyde, and auto hydrocarbon. Extracts for these chemicals were prepared, to be taken three times per day. Once Sue knew how it felt to be clear of symptoms, she began taking them once daily, repeating them as needed. Environmental cleanup was also recommended, and she followed the instructions to the last detail. Sue removed all harmful substances from her home, began using only safe products,

and purchased an air cleaner and a water filter.

Testing Sue for food sensitivities both intradermally and sublingually, we found that she was sensitive to soy, corn, wheat, egg, cane sugar, potato, banana, tomato, yeast, cow's milk, rice, pinto beans, onions, orange, chocolate, barley, peanuts, carrots, grapes, goat's milk, garlic, lemon, and spinach. This particular food grouping was consistent with the fact that Sue was an ovalacto vegetarian. She was given food extracts for all of these foods, to be taken before exposure to them. She also began rotating her foods, with a four-day rotation diet. Day 1 was Italian day, Day 2 was Oriental, Day 3 was American, and Day 4 was Mexican; Sue prepared recipes that reflected the "national flavor" of each day.

Sue's Candida questionnaire, symptoms, and culture were positive, indicating Candida overgrowth. Acidophilus and Nystatin powder were prescribed, and we recommended that she omit refined sugar from her diet. She was tested and given an extract for Candida and *T.O.E. (Trichophyton, Oidiomycetes, and Epidermophyton)*.

At one time, Sue's pollen allergies were so severe she could not go outdoors for any length of time during pollen season. Grass mowing anywhere in the neighborhood caused her to react severely. Within a short time, the pollen extracts were giving Sue enough relief for her to be able to leave her home whenever she desired. Her tolerance to molds increased, and animal danders were no longer a problem.

Chemical extracts also allowed Sue to drive her car without developing acute symptoms, and she gradually was able to shop without experiencing a reaction. Exposures to personal care products worn by other people had limited her social activities; after treatment had begun, she was able to gradually resume her social life. The "heart cramps" Sue experienced when bathing and washing her hair also disappeared.

Sue's clever rotation diet and her food extracts allowed her to eat without discomfort. Her colitis, alternating diarrhea and constipation, and headaches gradually subsided, and her rashes became a thing of the past.

One grain of thyroid was prescribed for daily use (based on basal temperature readings) to control her symptoms of hypothyroidism. Sue also used Buffered vitamin C and a heparin extract in addition to her extracts to control any allergic reactions she experienced, and took a high-quality multiple vitamin.

It was difficult for Sue to relinquish her many medications, but she gradually weaned herself from them as she began to feel better. She put the rather large sack of her medication bottles in her backyard storeroom, "just in case she needed them." She confessed that many times she was tempted to take some of them, because they provided what she felt was an easy "fix." We knew Sue was truly on the path to recovery when, after nine months on her program, she brought the sack of medications to us to throw away.

Sue experienced both ups and downs during her treatment program, but she persevered, faithfully following the prescribed treatment. Her cooperation, understanding, attention to detail, and creative spirit also contributed much to her recovery. In 18 months she was back at work full-time, in a secretarial position where she was exposed to numerous chemicals with no ill effects. She was also able to use carefully selected makeup and hair care products.

As treatment progressed, Sue's family was able to get an outside dog, and Sue was gradually able to relax her rotation diet. Over a period of time, Sue was also able to phase out her extracts, but she continued to use the air cleaner and water filter. When she occasionally became overloaded, she would increase her vitamin C intake and pay more attention to her exposures and diet. By exercising common sense, Sue was able to live a busy and healthy life. Her "flower of good health" flourished once she was able to peel back the many layers of her illness.

- *Rotation and allergen avoidance:* Improving your diet and using rotation of foods on a four- to seven-day basis help to control food sensitivities, and prevent new sensitivities from developing. Complete avoidance of some foods may also be necessary.
- *Nutritional therapy:* Some infections and disease processes create a demand for specific nutrients in amounts that cannot be obtained from food. Nutritional deficiencies resulting from poor eating habits will also contribute to the development of allergies and poor health. Vitamin and mineral therapy will give your body additional nutrients to aid in the repair process.
- *Hormonal therapy:* Appraisal of endocrine system dysfunction may be necessary. Premenstrual syndrome, low thyroid function, thyroiditis, adrenal insufficiency, and hormonal imbalance must all be considered for possible treatment.
- *Environmental clean-up:* Unwanted or xenobiotic (foreign to the body) chemicals and cleaning supplies must be removed from your home and work environments in order to reduce your body's toxic load. Air or water filtration may also benefit your health. Natural methods of pest and fungus control must be used, rather than pesticides and fungicides. Alternative methods of home heating and cooking, rather than using a natural gas source, may have to be substituted.
- *Proper exercise and rest:* Though exercise is a well known stress reducer, most people who are not feeling well believe they should not exercise. Even mild exercise has benefits for the body by increasing the excretion of chemicals and toxins. Muscular activity acts as a pump for the proper flow of body fluids; nutrients and oxygen are carried to the cells for

energy and repair; and waste products are carried to the proper organs for excretion. Then, during periods of rest, the repair processes are intensified.
- *Relaxation and meditation exercises:* Stress, regardless of its origin, adversely affects the immune system. Relaxation and meditation exercises reduce stress and calm both the mind and the body. Problems can be approached with renewed vigor and improved attitude when your body, mind, and spirit are refreshed.
- *Positive attitude and visual imagery:* Development of a positive, productive attitude aids in stress management while improving health. Humor and laughter contribute to a positive attitude. Visual imagery can be helpful: by visualizing yourself as well and healthy, and by visualizing beautiful scenes, memories, or colors, you encourage a positive response from your body.
- *Treatment for infection:* Allergies or sensitivities can develop following a severe infection. Latent infections also intensify allergies. Any viral, bacterial, fungal, or parasitic infection that you may have should be treated along with your allergies or sensitivities in order to reduce the total burden on your immune system.
- *Evaluation and treatment of digestive function:* Poor digestive function can exacerbate allergies and should be evaluated. This should include determining the level of acid in the stomach and the alkaline level in the small intestine. Any deficiencies can then be corrected through supplementation.
- *Consideration of emotional and spiritual health:* There is a crucial relationship between good health and your emotional, mental, and spiritual condition. Unresolved emo-

tional and psychological problems, trauma, or conflicts will slow down or prevent recovery.

- *Identifying electrical imbalances:* The human body is electrical as well as chemical in nature. Electrical imbalances that adversely affect healing are due to several factors: genetic predisposition, lack of essential minerals, diet, and environmental factors.
- *Evaluating dental health:* For some people, amalgam (silver) fillings in the teeth lead to health problems. The mercury leaking from these fillings is extremely toxic to the human body and can be responsible for numerous adverse symptoms. Root canals can also be a hidden source of problems as toxins from minute remaining areas of infection are released.

As you and your physician identify your particular "tacks" or problems, an individualized recovery program can be planned. You will need to be patient and consistent with your treatment until all of your symptoms are gone. For some people, treatment will be very simple, requiring only a few changes, while for others symptoms may be only a small part of the whole picture and other factors may have to be considered.

The success of your treatment and the length of your recovery period will depend on several factors: the number of allergies or sensitivities you have; the length of time you have been ill; any infections you may have; your nutritional state; and the level of exposure to environmental elements. The whole person needs to be addressed; mind, body, emotions, and spirit. This approach to good health may seem slow at times, but your body can repair itself.

As you proceed along the "whole way," you will gradually learn to "read" your body and become more aware of subtle changes that indicate problems or improvements. Our bodies are constantly sending us messages—if we listen, these messages will give us much information about how well the body is functioning. Most of us have been taught to ignore symptoms, to "grit our teeth," and to continue our daily routines. We have learned to accept less than optimum health that leads to less than optimum performance. We live in a state of "half health" much of the time and continued practice of this attitude leads to accumulated damage to the body. As you learn to read your body, you will be amazed at the volumes of information that surface.

Dr. Marshall Mandell has said that in order to treat our ills, we "look for magic, but must in the long run settle for hard work." This "hard work" can be shared through a partnership between you and your physician. Your physician can help to diagnose the problem and suggest ways for you to proceed. True healing is brought about through a consistent response from the entire person, not simply from a specific physical treatment, a new idea, or a "magic pill." Improved health is within your reach, providing you are willing to plan and work for it. As Dr. Lendon Smith remarks, "Not everyone needs to do all this: just those of us who want to stay well."

The whole way of healing is a rebalancing process. There will be a period of adjustment as you change your living habits to effect permanent benefits. It will be a time of learning and self-help as well as an opportunity to benefit from the help of caring, experienced health professionals. You will gain skills enabling you to restore and maintain an optimal level of health. It may prove to be the adventure of a lifetime!

PART 1

OUR BODY

SYSTEMS AND ALLERGIES

CHAPTER 1

OUR IMMUNE SYSTEM

The immune system is our first line of defense against substances that would otherwise harm or destroy our bodies. So important is the immune system to our survival that it is distributed throughout our bodies and functions on a 24-hour basis. It is genetically programmed to fight off diseases, from colds to cancer. The cells of the immune system communicate with each other, while acting with the endocrine and nervous systems to maintain body homeostasis and balance. Immune system functions are extremely intricate and complex—and we still do not fully understand how an organism triggers, regulates, completes, or stops an immune response. Familiarity with the workings of the immune system is important for those who want to learn to control the maverick responses of their bodies to both internal and external environments.

Organs and Lines of Defense of the Immune System

The immune system is a multifaceted composite of cells and organs that extends throughout the body. The various organ components are listed below.

• **The lymphatic system:** A complex network of vessels that move fluid (lymph) from body tissues to the bloodstream. It is a pathway for exchange of toxins, electrolytes, proteins, water, cell debris, and chemicals.

Lymph nodes are small protuberances along the lymphatic network that filter lymph and prevent foreign substances from entering the bloodstream. These nodes are located in areas such as the groin, the armpits, the covering of the intestinal tract (mesentary), the neck, between the ribs, along the spinal column, and in soft tissue in the knees and elbows. These nodes contain aggregations of lymphocytes and antigen producing cells, and become enlarged when they are actively fighting off either an infection or increased numbers of allergens.

• **The thymus gland:** The principal activator of the immune system. Known as the master gland of immunity, this gland was thought for many years to be useless after the age of puberty. However, major advances in our understanding of its role in immunity have been made in the last decade.

The thymus gland is located at the base of the neck under the sternum at the level of the second rib. Its principal function appears to be aiding the maturation of lymphocytes into T-cells. When stressed, the gland tends to shrink in size. The thymus gland is often very large in babies, and becomes smaller as a person grows older.

The primary function of the thymus gland is to produce T-cells, which are one type of lymphocyte. It also produces hormones (thymosin, thymopoetin, and interferon) that help initiate, mature, and regulate the function of the immune system.

The thymus initiates the differentiation of white blood cells into several different types. These include neutrophils, which are cell eaters; macrophages, which are giant cell eaters; two kinds of lymphocytes, known as T-cells and B-cells; and eosinophils, which regulate inflammatory processes. These are the "artillery and soldiers" responsible for eliminating unwanted chemicals, foreign protein, drugs, and organisms that make their way into the body. There are one trillion of these cells in the body.

- *The lacrimal glands:* Located at the corners of the eyes, they secrete tears, which contain white blood cells and chemicals that kill bacteria. Tears also have a mechanical flushing action to rid the body of foreign invaders, and are a route of excretion for chemicals.

- *The salivary glands:* Located in the mouth under the tongue and in the cheeks, they contain substances that resist infection. This is the first line of defense in the digestive and respiratory tract.

- *The tonsils and adenoids:* The second line of defense. They are composed of lymphoid tissue; act as a barrier to infectious organisms.

- *The stomach:* Produces hydrochloric acid that inhibits the growth of bacteria.

- *The spleen:* Largest of the lymphoid organs, it produces some of the white blood cells that ingest foreign proteins and debris, and helps resist infections of encapsulated organisms, such as pneumococcus.

- *The liver:* During an immune response, the liver is stimulated to release a large number of protein molecules known as acute phase proteins. They exert an important influence on tissue repair, immune cell functions, and the inflammatory process. The liver and spleen also affect the intake and/or release of iron and zinc during infection. Bacteria require a high iron concentration for their metabolic processes. They are not able to multiply if their iron supply is limited by this regulatory function in the liver and spleen.

- *The small intestine:* Contains collections of lymphocytes (both T- and B-cells) on the mucosal wall, known as Peyer's patches. Secretory IgA (an antibody) is produced by local plasma cells.

- *The large intestine:* Acts as a barrier to foreign organisms by harboring and colonizing bacteria that are friendly to the body. These "good" bacteria deter the colonization and entry of harmful bacteria, viruses, fungi, and/or parasites.

- *The skin:* Protects the body against the invasion of harmful organisms. There are also protective non-pathogenic bacteria that colonize the skin.

- *The bone marrow:* The production site for two types of white blood cells—B-cells, which secrete antibodies; and neutrophils, which consume foreign cells.

- *The appendix:* Also composed of lymphoid tissue. It is now considered an important part of the immune complex rather than a nonfunctional mass of tissue.

- *The mucous membrane:* Contain mast and basophil cells, T-cells, and IgA. These cells produce the chemicals that are released during an allergic reaction. They also secrete mucus that engulfs microorganisms and propels them for excretion.

The Immune System's Cellular Components

T-Cells

Mature T-cells have a number of functions and are divided into three categories. The killer T-cells recognize and destroy foreign protein, such as bacteria, viruses, cancer cells, fungi, and protozoa. When a T-cell encounters an antigen, it attaches itself to the invader and "injects" it. These T-cells also activate debris-eating phagocytes to destroy pathogens that they have absorbed. Helper T-cells interact with B-cells to help them make antibody molecules. Suppressor T-cells interact with B-cells to turn off their production of antibodies.

B-Cells

B-cells are produced in the bone marrow and spleen, and in the lymphoid tissue of the immune system (apart from the thymus gland). The B-cells have the ability to multiply rapidly when they encounter antigens. Their function is to secrete immune chemicals known as antibodies or immunoglobulins, which circulate freely in all body fluids. These cells do battle against offending organisms or antigens so they can be inactivated or eliminated. For each antigen present in the body there is a specific antibody produced by an individual B-cell. The B-cells have surface-bound immunoglobulin (IgG) receptors that are directly responsible for cell activation. However, a shortage of T-cells will prevent the activation of the B-cells.

Immunoglobulins

There are five types of immunoglobulins (antibodies): IgA, IgD, IgE, IgG, and IgM. (Tests to identify and measure immunoglobulins are discussed in *Testing and Medical Treatment*, p.

66.) Each has a different "weapon" for attack. Some neutralize antigens by covering up their active or toxic sites, while some render antigens harmless by binding or clumping them together. Some immunoglobulins "rip" open antigens, and still others prevent viruses from entering cells.

- **IgA:** Found mainly in the mucous membranes and body secretions (tears, saliva), it protects mucous membranes from invasion by microorganisms.
- **IgD:** Found in cell membranes, and involved in cell activation. It is believed to play a part in recognizing "self" and "foreign" antigens.
- **IgE:** Frequently involved in allergic reactions to pollen and food, and found in both blood and interstitial fluid (from within the organs). It attaches to the outside of basophils (white blood cells that mediate inflammatory reactions) and similar (histamine containing) mast cells. Contact with an allergen causes these cells to burst, which in turn dumps histamine or enzymes into the surrounding fluid to inactivate the allergen. The release of histamine causes either local inflammation and/or systemic (entire body) flushing and other adverse symptoms.
- **IgG:** Found in both blood and tissue fluid, it is the most abundant antibody in the body and is also involved in attacking bacteria and other antigens such as food. Both IgG and IgM coat microorganisms. High IgG levels indicate a past infection.
- **IgM:** Found mainly in the bloodstream, and most often involved in attacking bacteria and other antigens, IgM is the first antibody that the body produces against a foreign antigen. High IgM levels indicate a current or recent infection.

COMPLEMENT SYSTEM

Antibodies sometimes team up with the body's complement system in order to mount a stronger defense against immune system enemies. Complement enzymes involve at least nine complex serum protein units (C_1–C_9) that circulate in the blood in inactive form. There are approximately 20 of these protein combinations. Once activated—usually by antigen-antibody binding (immune complexes)—they join and split one another sequentially, thus producing active, but short-lived, enzymes that bind to and rupture the antigen surface. This system adds another dimension to the weapons of the immune response.

Additionally, fragments of the complement enzymes attach to the antigen itself, labelling it an enemy, or move off into the bloodstream to attract phagocytic cells. Some antibodies activate complement enzymes in a way that produces agglutination (or clumping) of cells. The sources of these proteins are not completely known, but C_1 is thought to be produced in the colon, C_2 is made by macrophages, and C_3 is found in the liver. The purpose of the complement system is the destruction of the "foreign" cells by lysis, or dissolution.

In the step-by-step progression and activation of the "complement cascade," histamine and other chemicals are released from mast cells and basophils and are increasingly recognized as contributors to hypersensitivity responses.

Complement enzymes can also destroy the body's own blood cells in some types of autoimmune disease syndromes, which can lead to anemia (subnormal levels of red blood cells) and to leukopenia (subnormal levels of white blood cells).

MAST CELLS AND BASOPHILS

Mast cells and basophils are white cells found in most tissues adjoining the blood vessels. When these cells are activated, they release histamine and other substances, causing the blood vessels to dilate.

ALLERGENS AND ANTIGENS

Antigens are any molecules that are recognized by the immune system and that induce an immune reaction. Microbial antigens prompt the production of antibodies that aid in the destruction of the organisms, and prevent reinfection with the same organism in future. Antigens are often protein, but non-proteins can also be antigens. Antigens that produce a different type of immune response, known as an allergic inflammatory response, are called allergens. Allergens can be inhalants (from weeds, molds, grasses, trees, dust, cats, and dogs), foods of all types, chemicals (either internal or external), microorganisms, or insects.

Allergens enter the body by the same routes as microorganisms. We can breathe them in through our respiratory tract; they can enter the digestive tract with our food and drink; we can contact them through the skin and mucous membrane; we can be exposed to them in sexual contact; they can be inserted into the body by injection or by insect bite; and we can even manufacture them in our bodies.

Some allergens, called haptens, are too small to elicit a reaction from the body. When these allergens couple themselves to our own protein, they are called neoantigens. The body can then set up an allergic response to this form of antigen. The ability of the immune system to remember the substance it has previously encountered can actually work against the body during an allergic response.

Chemicals Released During an Allergic Reaction

The release of chemicals from mast cells, basophils, and other cells is thought to be partially responsible for yet another function of the immune system. These chemicals may account for varying degrees of sensitivity, various symptoms associated with sensitivity, and varying time lapses between exposure to an allergen and the response.

- *Histamine:* Responsible for two main effects in an inflammatory response. It causes the blood capillaries to widen and increases their permeability so more fluid passes from the blood into the tissues. This causes local swelling, as well as generalized edema and redness. Histamine also causes contraction of the smooth (involuntary) muscles in the lungs, blood vessels, heart, stomach, intestines, and bladder.

- *Heparin:* Inhibits the action of thrombin, an enzyme essential to blood coagulation. This may lead to increased blood flow to the inflamed site. Heparin and histamine are released at the same time.

- *Platelet activating factor:* Causes aggregation of blood platelets. When this occurs, the grouped platelets release chemicals that also affect the blood vessels, either increasing or decreasing their diameter. Eventually, this action either increases or decreases blood pressure (which occurs in acute reactions). These platelets also activate other cells involved in inflammation.

- *Serotonin:* Plays a role in allergic responses, especially to foods. Ninety percent of the body's serotonin is found in the mucous membrane cells of the gastrointestinal tract. It acts differently from histamine, even though the end result of inflammation is the same. A

chemical (5-hydroxyindoleacetic acid) is released with the breakdown of serotonin in mucous membrane, and this is thought to cause irritation of surrounding cells.

- *Lymphokines:* A group of molecules, other than antibodies, produced by lymphocytes. They are involved in signalling between the cells of the immune system.

- *Leukotrienes:* Derived from a fatty acid known as arachidonic acid, leukotrienes are found in cell membranes. They cause the bronchial muscles in the lungs to contract. This action allows one to inhale adequate air, while at the same time preventing the adequate exhalation of air. This is the bronchospasm found in asthma. Leukotrienes act more slowly than histamine. A higher level of leukotrienes are present in tissues affected by inflammatory and allergic reactions. This takes place in the skin in atopic dermatitis (skin inflammation) and psoriasis; in the colon in inflammatory bowel diseases; in tears resulting from uveitis (iris inflammation); and in the nasal passages in allergic rhinitis (mucous membrane inflammation). More research is being conducted on leukotrienes and their role in inflammatory processes.

- *Prostaglandins:* Also produced from arachidonic acid in cell membranes, they are hormone-like substances and regulate cell functions in every part of the body. Prostaglandins act to dilate blood vessels, affect smooth muscle contraction, enhance the effect of other chemicals, heat inflamed tissue, and increase pain in affected areas. There are a number of prostaglandins and many have antagonistic roles. Extensive research is being conducted to further distinguish their functions.

- *Thromboxanes:* Powerful vasoconstrictors (contract blood vessels) and bronchoconstrictors (contract bronchial tubes). They also cause platelet aggregation (clumping) similar to the platelet activating factor and appear to influence the activity of leukotrienes. Like leukotrienes and prostaglandins, thromboxane is derived from arachidonic acid.

- *Bradykinin:* One of several kinins released during an inflammatory process when mast cells and basophils split open. Kinins tend to act synergistically with other chemicals to add to the inflammatory cascade. Bradykinin causes pain by stimulating nerve endings and causes blood pressure to drop by widening peripheral arteries.
- *Interleukins:* Antigens involved in activating and differentiating lymphocytes. They irritate tissues and can set up inflammatory responses.
- *Interferons:* Produced predominantly by certain stimulated lymphocytes. They act to regulate the extent and speed of other immune responses.

Immune Response in Allergy

The immune response is a stimulus-response sequence of events. The immune system protects us in two ways: one is via cell-mediated immunity, the other via antibody-mediated immunity. The work of the cell-mediated immune response is done by phagocytes, neutrophils, and macrophages (types of white blood cells). Phagocytes are nonspecific, which means they engulf and destroy a wide variety of molecules, particles, and organisms. These scavengers are found in the blood and lymphatic systems and in most other tissues in the body. They are very efficient and engulf not only foreign materials but also "self" materials, such as damaged or dead cells. When they are

busy at work they inflame localized or systemic areas. After these specialized white cells have destroyed the invader they present it to the T- and B-cells.

The T- and B-cells prepare weapons to destroy antigens. First the T-cells become sensitized and are released into the lymph system, the bloodstream, and finally to all parts of the body. When the sensitized T-cells find the antigen, they attach in a "lock and key position" and inject them with "poison." The T-cells send out chemicals that sensitize other nearby T-cells and attract macrophages. These "cell eaters" come to aid in the defense and consume dead neutrophils and antigens.

While the T-cells are fighting, the B-cells, having "studied" the antigen, begin to grow and divide into daughter cells called plasma cells. These plasma cells act like factories, manufacturing antibodies. The antibodies then seek out and destroy any antigens resembling the one for which they have been programmed. It takes time for the B-cells to produce plasma cells, and for the plasma cells to produce antibodies. The "cell eaters" (T-cells and macrophages) must continue the battle until the antibodies can come to their aid.

Many B-cells also become long-lived memory cells that retain the original specific antigen-binding information. Later re-exposure to the same microbial or other antigens stimulates these memory cells to divide and produce more cloned plasma cells, and to speed up the body's immune functions. This quick response accounts for sensitive people's instantaneous reaction to chemical, food, or inhalant antigens.

Antibodies at Work

Antibodies, which are the immunoglobulins, can rip open cell membranes and kill an antigen or can neutralize it by covering up its toxic site. Multiple antibodies can bind themselves to several antigens, rendering them harmless. About 75 percent of total immunoglobulins are IgG, which together with IgM attack bacteria and viruses.

Wherever there is antibody-antigen action in the body, there will also be an inflammatory response, accompanied by swelling (edema), redness, heat, tenderness, and impaired function. This response is the body's attempt to heal itself. The inflammation is caused by release of prostaglandins, serotonin, leukotrienes, kinins, and histamine, and by increased blood supply carrying more white blood cells to the area. Complement enzymes then line up to fight. They attach themselves, in a specified order, to the antigen to form an additional weapon.

For anyone with allergies, the most important portion of the immune response takes place after the antibodies have attached to the invaders. At this point they carry the antigen to the mast cells and basophils found in the blood, skin, and mucous membranes, causing the cells to release histamine and other chemicals. Histamine increases capillary permeability, allowing the white cells to flow freely out of the capillaries and into the tissues, where they can fight invaders. This triggers water retention and swelling.

Because the histamine and other released substances irritate normal cells, the body turns off their release when the invader has been repelled. When histamine levels around a mast cell reach a certain concentration, the mast cell releases a chemical that turns off histamine production in the releasing cell and all surrounding mast cells. In some people, however, this mechanism does not function properly and the reaction "cascades." The T-suppressor cells

then work to prevent the formation of any more antibody.

Immune System Stressors

Unfortunately, in the allergic person, the immune system is continually at work, much like a car with its engine left running. In his book, *Type 1/Type 2 Allergy Relief*, Dr. Alan Levin likens the B-cells to the car's engine and the T-cells to the brakes. Allergic individuals have high-powered engines and weak brakes, so their car—or immune system—often goes out of control. An overstimulated immune system follows the same general law that applies to other overstimulated tissues: overstimulation eventually leads to inhibition of function. This continuous assault can lead to recurrent infection and inflammatory diseases such as sinusitis, arthritis, asthma, bronchitis, colitis, myositis, migraine headaches, and ulcers. Undiagnosed or untreated allergic responses can, over a period of years, lead to degenerative diseases.

Each of us has a different level of immune competence. This level varies with hereditary factors; number and degree of our exposures to infections, chemicals, and drugs; age; nutritional status; stress level; and amount of exercise. In some cases, the allergic person is hereditarily endowed with too few T-cells or over-active B-cells, resulting in improper immune response, producing "allergic" symptoms. Others may have more sensitive mast cells and basophils and so may release excess histamine during reactions.

Stress in any form has a negative effect on our immune system. Studies have shown that surviving spouses have lowered numbers of T-cells for several months after the deaths of their partners. Hormones produced by the adrenal glands in response to stress can interfere with T-cell functions. Even positive stress, like winning a million-dollar sweepstakes, can adversely affect the immune system, which can be damaged by constant stress just as it can be impaired by chronic disease or infection. Maintaining regular sleeping habits and healthy eating routines, and pursuing gratifying work or hobbies, can help lessen the burden on mental and physical well-being after stress.

Dysfunction of the endocrine system can also alter the immune system's ability to respond. Recent research has shown that the brain and nervous system play a role in regulating our immune response. Lack of adequate nutrients can also have debilitating effects on all parts and functions of the immune system. Repeated or chronic infections have also long been known to lower immunity, but the body's ability to fight back can also be compromised when we are "overloaded" and assaulted repeatedly by food, chemical, or pollen antigens.

AUTOIMMUNITY

Recently, more intense research has been conducted on the immune system because of the spread of AIDS. One malfunction of the immune system being investigated is autoimmunity. This extremely complex syndrome takes place when the body no longer tolerates "self" molecules, producing an immune response to the self that interferes with normal cell function. Diseases such as diabetes, rheumatoid arthritis, multiple sclerosis, lupus erythematosus, myasthenia gravis, and Grave's disease (hyperthyroidism) are thought to be related to autoimmunity. Although we do not yet understand the exact mechanisms, it seems that a combination of genetic susceptibility and unknown environmental agents may trigger this malfunction.

Dr. Peter Rothschild feels that immune complexes may be involved in some of these diseases. Immune complexes are formed when antibodies and antigens bond; under normal conditions, these complexes are destroyed and eliminated shortly after their development. Sometimes they are stored in body tissues, which leads to complement activation, in turn causing inflammatory reactions, formation of fibrin, and tissue lesions. These immune complexes are evident in all diseased tissues. As long as these tissue-bound immune complexes remain, the immune system will be overstimulated and overloaded. When additional antigen loads are placed on the immune system, it is unable to respond adequately and one becomes increasingly immune deficient.

Clinicians have found that the immune system can gradually be improved and strengthened, even though it may be heavily damaged. Immunotherapy, exercise, nutritional reinforcement with therapeutic levels of nutrients, and environmental control, together with eliminating infections, using herbal preparations and free radical scavenger enzymes, improving diet, getting adequate rest, and reducing stress all help to repair the immune system.

Total Load/Overload

In order to better understand our bodies in relation to how we feel, and in terms of our general health, we need to look at the concept of total load and overload. In day-to-day living, our bodies are subjected to many stresses: physical, emotional, and environmental.

Physical stresses include infections (viral, bacterial, parasitic, and fungal); chronic disease; poor nutrition; food allergies; chemical allergies; allergies to pollens and other inhalants; pregnancy; inadequate or excessive exercise levels; insufficient fatty acids; vitamin, mineral, and amino acid imbalances; hormonal imbalance and/or sensitivity; yeast overgrowth; acid/alkaline imbalance; lowered immune system function; poor digestion, hampered by insufficient hydrochloric acid and/or pancreatic enzyme production; and insufficient sleep.

Emotional stresses come in many forms, including job frustrations, marital problems, divorce, death of a friend or relative, insufficient acknowledgment and touching, criticism, rejection, sibling rivalry, and failure to succeed. Abuse of any kind (past or present), whether it be sexual, physical, emotional, or verbal also causes emotional stress.

Environmental stresses include extremes of heat, cold, or altitude; air and water pollution; or food pollution. Other stresses in your environment can be improper lighting; high-intensity electricity sources; radiation; excess lead or heavy metal exposures; pesticides; fungicides; toxic cleaning products; tobacco and wood smoke; car and diesel exhaust; natural and propane gas; and new building materials.

Our body can adjust to perhaps a few stressors, but when there is an accumulation or repetition of stressors our metabolism loses its adaptability. Any one of these stresses can upset the normal control mechanisms of the immune, nervous, or endocrine systems. At this point we develop symptoms because our total body burden is too high. The collective response exceeds a "threshold" level that the body metabolism can tolerate. The body can then no longer maintain health and balance.

We can learn to systematically reduce the overloading stressors so that the energy that the body produces can be rerouted to perform all of its functions.

Our Immune System "Rain Barrel"

Dr. William Rea describes our immune system as a rain barrel. By visualizing this we can more easily understand the total load/overload concept. Any combination of stresses "fills up" our rain barrel. If we can keep our rain barrels emptied by controlling our allergies, cleaning up our environment, improving our nutrition, exercising regularly, and reducing other controllable stress, we can tolerate moderate life stresses without overflowing the sides of our rain barrel. If, however, our rain barrel remains full, the slightest additional stress factor will cause it to overflow, resulting in distressing symptoms.

The rain barrel concept explains why sometimes we develop symptoms from an allergen, while at other times we do not. This depends on how full our rain barrel is at the time of the additional stress. Some people have large rain barrels, while others have small ones—heredity plays a role in determining their size. We need to drain our rain barrels and keep them as empty as possible, so that our immune system will not be pushed to exceed its adaptive capacity and will begin to heal.

Preventing the Rain Barrel Effect

Evaluating the causes of each sensitive person's overload is important in planning an effective treatment plan. There are many paths to recovery that prevent the rain barrel effect:
- Treating sensitivities through immunotherapy, rotation of foods in your diet, and selective food elimination.
- Cleaning up your environment.
- Avoiding exposures to allergens.
- Treating infections.

- Alleviating stress.
- Nutritional therapy.
- Hormonal therapy.
- Adequate rest/sleep.
- Exercise.
- Relaxation and meditation exercises.
- Positive visual imagery.
- Counselling.

As you begin to identify the stresses that are causing your overload, an individualized program should be planned to help reduce your total load. You can then better tolerate those substances to which you are sensitive and work toward an optimum state of health.

OUR ENDOCRINE SYSTEM

In a diagnostic work-up of anyone who is environmentally ill, one often finds evidence of dysfunction of parts of the endocrine system. It is difficult to assess whether this is caused by hereditary factors, stress from environmental illness, or both. Endocrine dysfunction can be corrected by assessing and treating hormonal imbalance, testing for and treating allergies, taking nutritional supplements, reducing stress, and obtaining adequate exercise.

Our thyroid, parathyroid, pituitary, hypothalamus, pancreas, adrenal glands, pineal glands, and gonads (ovaries and testes) are all ductless glands that make up our endocrine system. These glands produce hormones and secrete them either directly into the bloodstream or into extracellular fluids, allowing them to reach virtually all cells of the body. The gastrointestinal tract, kidneys, liver, and placenta can also be considered part of the endocrine system because they too produce hormones that are released into the bloodstream. The endocrine system is interrelated with the immune system and the central nervous system.

The endocrine system is the body's second most important communications system, after the nervous system. Many of the glands secrete more than one hormone, and some of the endocrine glands, such as the pancreas, also have exocrine functions. These functions are the release of products through ducts that lead to the body's surface.

Our endocrine system:
- Controls the rate of chemical reactions.
- Regulates cell membrane permeability.
- Activates specific functions of cells.
- Regulates the slower metabolic reactions.
- Regulates circulation.
- Maintains water and electrolyte (e.g., sodium, potassium, magnesium) balance.
- Regulates digestion and absorption of food.
- Balances energy and metabolism.
- Regulates the reproductive cycle.
- Responds to stress stimuli.

Hormones

Hormones are chemical messengers, produced by specialized cells in the endocrine glands, that speed up or slow down our body's chemical reactions. There is a feedback mechanism between the hormones and the glands in which the hormones from one gland can stimulate the production of hormones from other glands. Hormones produced in one area of our body can have an effect elsewhere in the body. Hormone production can also be stimulated by the central nervous system, and by the concentration of available organic nutrients and mineral ions.

One particular hormone may be produced by

more than one type of endocrine gland. For example, somatostatin is secreted by endocrine cells in the intestinal tract as well as in the pancreas and in the hypothalamus of the brain. Some of the molecules classed as hormones can also be produced by other body tissues and may act as neurotransmitters by transmitting nerve impulses.

Hormones are not secreted at constant rates but rather in short bursts, depending on the amount and duration of regulatory stimuli. Some glands, like the pineal, follow circadian rhythms (based on daily alternations of darkness and light) in their hormone secretion. Others, like the adrenals, produce more hormones in response to external stimulation at irregular intervals, while still other glands like the ovaries, release hormones at regular intervals in response to levels of hormones in the blood.

Hormones would not function if there were not specific matching receptor sites on our body's cells for attachment of the hormones, similar to the lock and key mechanism of antigen/antibody binding. This binding of hormone to target cell initiates a response from the target cell.

In many cases, the secretion of a hormone can be influenced by more than one stimulus. At times the signals may be in opposition, causing erratic action of the endocrine glands and varying blood levels of hormones. Hormones are highly specific in that each one will affect only one organ or one group of cells (target cells).

Our hormone levels depend not only on amounts of secretion, but also on our body's ability to remove the excess. This is accomplished by direct excretion through the liver and kidneys, and also through metabolic transformation and degradation by enzymes. If these functions are not performed adequately, excesses of specific hormones or metabolites (products of metabolism) can continue to circulate in the body, causing hypersensitivity reactions and/or autoimmune responses, such as thyroiditis or production of anti-ovarian antibodies. It has also been suggested that incomplete unexcreted fragments of a hormone may mediate new and different effects of that hormone. These effects may be undesirable as well as unpredictable.

There are three types of hormones. One type, an amine, is derived from the amino acid known as tyrosine. It has three sub-types of hormones: thyroid hormone (produced in the thyroid), epinephrine, and norepinephrine (both produced in the adrenal gland). A second type of hormone is a peptide molecule that can range in size from a group of three amino acids to large groups of amino acids, such as insulin (produced in the pancreas). The third type of hormone is a steroid. All steroid hormones are produced by the adrenal cortex, testes, ovaries, and the placenta, and require cholesterol for their production.

After excretion by a specific endocrine gland, a hormone may undergo further metabolic steps in order to be fully effective. Some enzymes are required to activate and bond some hormones with receptor target sites on cells. Others are required to transform a stored hormone into its active state, to synthesize hormones in an endocrine gland, and to convert one hormone into another. Concentration of these key enzymes can be low or nonfunctioning because of hereditary or genetic factors, lack of proper nutrients, or damage from circulating toxins, either exogenous (originating outside the body) or endogenous (originating within the body). When this occurs, malfunction and disease processes can be set in motion, causing such ailments as hypothyroidism, dwarfism, hypoadrenal function, or hypersensitivity to one's own hormones.

An additional problem can arise if receptor sites for hormones are either nonfunctional, damaged, overloaded, unable to uncouple or transform the attached hormone, or improperly stimulated or prepared by another hormone. Such malfunction results in decreased hormone production, an excess of circulating hormones that can damage other tissues, or an inability of the receptor to accept a hormone. These malfunctions can also lead to various disease syndromes. It is possible to adjust malfunctions by using varying dosages of specific hormones, such as thyroid, cortisol, estrogen, progesterone, testosterone, and vasopressin.

Pituitary Gland

The pituitary or master gland is a small gland that lies in a pocket of bone at the base of the brain. It is integrally connected to the hypothalamus (part of the nervous system in the brain), which collects neural information about the status of body functions and conditions including: hunger; thirst; stress; emotional state; body position; internal and external temperature; talking and walking; and sleep.

After the information is collected and processed, the hypothalamus stimulates specific cells of the pituitary to produce and secrete hormones.

The pituitary gland is made up of two lobes—the posterior and anterior lobes. The posterior lobe is actually an outgrowth of the hypothalamus and is composed of neural tissue. It secretes two hormones, (vasopressin and oxytocin), which are synthesized in the neural tissue and picked up by surrounding capillaries. These

hormones are also produced by nerve tissue elsewhere in the body, where they act as neurotransmitters or neuromodulators. This is another example of the close interrelationship between the endocrine and nervous systems.

Vasopressin is also known as an antidiuretic hormone. It regulates fluid levels in the body by directing the kidneys to reabsorb sodium ions but not water. The water is then excreted. Increased amounts of vasopressin are released during stress situations. Oxytocin, the other hormone secreted by the posterior lobe, has an influence over uterine contractility and causes the contractions of the nipple in the "milk let-down" process in nursing mothers.

The anterior pituitary lobe is also regulated by the hypothalamus. While there is no important neural connection between the anterior lobe and the hypothalamus, the hormones produced by the anterior pituitary lobe act to stimulate the secretion of other hormones in a chain fashion.

Some of these hormones can influence more than one type of hormone, and can inhibit as well as stimulate. This is another example of the intricate check and balance mechanisms of our body.

If there is any malfunction of the interconnected endocrine glands, the feedback mechanism between the glands and the nervous system can ultimately affect the pituitary gland and the hypothalamus. As a result, the problem is compounded because incorrect messages are received, and then improper stimuli are sent back to the glands within the system.

If there is damage or a nutritional deficit in the hypothalamus, this leads to a disruption of signals, and wrong messages are sent to the endocrine glands. Excess sugar and alcohol disrupt hypothalamus function. If disruption takes place over a long period of time, there will be

Pituitary Hormones	Stimulates Secretion Of
Thyroid stimulating hormone (TSH)	Thyroid hormones (thyroxine, triiodothyronine, and calcitonin)
Adrenocorticotrophic hormone (ACTH)	Cortisol from adrenal cortex
Follicular stimulating hormone (FSH)	Estrogen, progesterone, and testosterone
Luteinizing hormone (LH)	Regulates the growth of sperm and ova
Growth hormone	Somatomedin (growth-promoting peptide) Has direct effect on carbohydrate, lipid, and protein metabolism
Prolactin	Stimulates the breasts to produce milk

pituitary insufficiency and inhibited function of many of the endocrine glands, with long-lasting effects. Some examples of these effects are hypo- or hyperthyroidism, dwarfism or giantism, obesity, muscular weakness, edema, PMS, infertility, fatigue, stress syndromes, depression, irregular menses, and hypoadrenalism.

Thyroid Gland

The first gland to be discovered, the thyroid, is located behind and below the larynx. The pituitary stimulates the thyroid to produce three hormones: thyroxine; triiodothyronine; and calcitonin. Thyroxine is produced from iodine and tyrosine (an amino acid). The thyroid gland can store several weeks' supply of thyroxine bound to a large protein known as thyroglobulin. Magnesium, zinc, copper, iodine, and cobalt are essential for the function of the thyroid gland. Calcitonin is released from cells in the thyroid separate from those that produce thyroxine and triiodothyronine. Calcitonin lowers plasma calcium by inhibiting its release from bone. It acts in opposition to the parathyroid hormone.

The thyroid gland:
• Regulates our metabolic rate.
• Stimulates protein metabolism in cells.
• Stimulates chemical reactions in cells.
• Stimulates glucose absorption.
• Increases the rate of absorption of nutrients in the intestinal tract.
• Increases the intestinal tract's motility.
• Controls children's growth rate.
• Affects the rate of adult metabolic repair.
• Increases heat and energy production in cells.
• Increases oxygen consumption.
• Affects our heart rate and strength; the central nervous system; muscle function; sleep quality; hormone production; and respiration rate.

Thyroid dysfunction symptoms are caused by either an acceleration of these functions (hyperthyroidism) or a slowdown (hypothyroidism).

Classic symptoms of thyroid dysfunction are:
• Increased allergic responses.
• Fatigue and waking up as tired in the morning as you were at bedtime.

- Insomnia.
- Memory loss, especially short-term memory.
- Poor thinking processes.
- Nervousness, ranging from mild anxiety to full-blown panic attacks and suicidal tendencies.
- Palpitations and heartbeat irregularities.
- Lowered sex drive.
- Digestive disorders.
- Low basal temperature readings.

Thyroid dysfunction can be caused by malfunction of the hypothalamus; infectious (parasitic, viral, bacterial, or fungal) diseases; nutritional deficiencies; hereditary factors; prolonged stress; damage from toxic materials; or tumor growths. A person may manufacture anti-thyroid antibodies as a result of immune system malfunctions following prolonged stress, as in chronic allergic states or following infections. Some people may have an over-functioning thyroid that is inflamed or enlarged and produces excess thyroid hormones. The function then reverses. The gland remains tender, but slows down the production of hormones, resulting in hypothyroidism. This fluctuation can continue, making diagnosis and treatment difficult.

TESTING THYROID FUNCTION

The following tests are used to determine thyroid function:
- Anti-thyroid Antibody Panel (includes determination of Antithyroglobulin and Antimicrosomal Antibodies);
- Serum levels of T_3, T_4, and TSH (thyroid hormones);
- Radioactive iodine uptake(RAD);
- Basal metabolic temperature readings.

The thyroid gland can function in a borderline way, creating symptoms that complicate the diagnostic picture. The problem may not be severe enough to show up in blood tests but will show low function on a basal temperature reading. Even though thyroid function may be borderline, the symptoms may be severe enough to cause distress and create changes in metabolism that may mimic allergic reactions. Low dose thyroid supplementation will significantly improve the person's health.

Thyroid support can be accomplished in a number of ways: using nutritional supplements, including iodine and tyrosine; initiating thyroid replacement with either desiccated thyroid preparations or synthetic single hormones; reducing infectious disease processes; improving diet; reducing stress; surgically removing tumors when indicated; and by using homeopathic preparations designed for thyroid support.

BASAL TEMPERATURE STUDY FOR THYROID FUNCTIONS

In spite of complex evaluation and cross-examination, the true status of the thyroid gland is elusive. Laboratory tests for thyroid evaluation are relatively inaccurate for near borderline hypothyroid function. Most of these tests indicate the levels of thyroid hormone circulating in the blood, but they do not accurately represent the amount of thyroid hormone available and being used at the cellular level.

Functional tests tell us more about a person's thyroid. Body surface temperature, measured under the arm, is an indication of thyroid function. If the temperature is consistently low, an underfunction of the thyroid is suspected. Normal values for underarm temperature are 97.4–98.2°F. If the temperature is over 98.2°F, hyperthyroidism is considered a possibility. A temperature below 97.4°F is indicative of hypothyroidism.

This basal temperature method is quite useful and accurate when done properly. There are other conditions in which basal temperature may be low, including starvation, adrenal or pituitary gland deficiency, and toxicity from microorganisms. Starvation is easily ruled out. Thyroid supplementation is useful in some deficiencies of the adrenal and pituitary glands.

Hypothyroidism is frequently found in those with allergic symptoms, and it may also be associated with fatigue, weakness, constipation, loss of hair, coldness of extremities, menstrual problems, depression, headaches, dry, coarse skin and hair, brittle nails, and pale skin.

How to Take Your Basal Temperature

- Before retiring at night, shake down a thermometer and lay it on your bedside table or nearby chair. *Be sure it is shaken down to at least 96°F.*
- The next morning, *before getting out of bed,* place the thermometer in the armpit of your bare arm. Press your arm against your body so the thermometer will not slip, making sure there is no clothing between your skin and the thermometer. An electric blanket or excess bed covers will cause the thermometer readings to be high.
- *Leave the thermometer in place for 10 minutes. Stay in bed.* Remove the thermometer, and read and record the temperature.
- Record your temperature for 14 days. Note any symptoms of illness and/or menstrual cycle next to the temperature.
- For women who are still menstruating, begin the temperature readings the second day of your period.

After recording your temperatures for two weeks, average the values. If your basal temperature average is below 97.4°F, you may want to discuss the possibility of trial thyroid supplementation with your physician.

Several types of thyroid preparations are available for supplementation. Synthetic thyroid preparations are formulated in the laboratory and contain T_3 or T_4, two of the thyroid hormones. While the dose is standardized and controlled, T_4 is not the most active thyroid hormone. Also, some people are unable to convert T_4 to T_3, which is the more potent thyroid hormone required by the body, and must take T_3.

Natural desiccated thyroid contains both T_3 and T_4, and is easily assimilated by most individuals. Newer processing methods now provide a standardized dose. Natural thyroid is processed from either beef or pork thyroid glands. Good results are achieved with both of these, but the balance of the pork thyroid hormones is closer to that of our own.

Thyroid supplementation is the treatment of choice for those who manufacture anti-thyroid antibodies, which attack their own thyroid glands. Among those with allergies to other substances, there is a significant number of individuals who also have anti-thyroid antibodies.

Adrenal Glands

The adrenals are the "fight or flight" glands stimulated by the pituitary and located above the kidneys. They are made up of the medulla, which is the inner core, and the cortex, which is the outer covering.

The medulla secretes two amine hormones, epinephrine and norepinephrine, which are released directly into the bloodstream. Under extreme stress, the adrenal glands prepare the "fight" response, increasing blood to the heart, brain, and the long muscles, while decreasing blood to the skin and intestinal tract. These changes also prepare us for the "flight" response—the skin becomes white, the hands get cold, and the mouth becomes dry during a stress situation.

Epinephrine is a dilator for the vascular (circulatory) system, and for the airways in the lungs. Also known as adrenaline and considered to be a hormone, epinephrine is involved in regulating organic metabolic processes and can function as a neurotransmitter. Calcium concentration in the muscle cells of blood vessels is regulated by epinephrine. It inhibits insulin secretion and stimulates the release of glucagon (a protein hormone), which causes increased plasma concentrations of glucose, glycerol, and fatty acids. By these functions, epinephrine is involved in the body's "fight or flight" response to stress, whether perceived or real.

Norepinephrine is epinephrine without an attached methyl group. It narrows the blood vessels and constricts peripheral circulation in the skin, eyes, and the body's mucous linings. It functions as an active neurotransmitter between the nerve fiber and the cells responsible for changes in organs. In its function as an inhibitory neurotransmitter, it is thought to decrease distracting background electrical activity in the brain so that sensory input from the body is made more clear. This results in improved information processing during directed attention or learning situations.

Enkephalin and endorphins (peptide neurotransmitters that have inhibitory dulling properties) are also released by the adrenal medulla, as well as by the pituitary. They interrupt memory formation, especially if a painful sensation is involved.

The cortex is the outer layer of the adrenal gland. This outer shell is composed of three separate layers that have opposing enzyme functions. These enzymes interrelate to produce the adrenal cortex hormones. Cortisol and aldosterone are the two most important of the hormones produced.

Cortisol release is stimulated in response to stress by the secretion of ACTH (Adrenocorticotrophic hormone) from the hypothalamus/pituitary activity. Cortisol causes the release of glycogen, which becomes glucose to provide instant energy. It also affects the breakdown (catabolism) of proteins that provide more energy and glucose, which is of major importance to brain function. With these physiological changes, the body is prepared for fight or flight in any stress situation. In today's world, a large variety of psychological events occur that our bodies perceive as stress, and respond by releasing cortisol. When the body is unable to appropriately utilize the excess cortisol through either fight or flight, the increased levels of cortisol circulate and damage body tissues. As a result, there is a profound reduction in the immune system's inflammatory response, which in turn decreases resistance to infection or effective response to allergens. A chronically high cortisol level also triggers the retention of sodium ions that can lead to hypertension. Increased cortisol reduces the stomach's ability to handle normal levels of acid, which can lead to gastritis and/or ulcers. It also inhibits secretion of growth hormones (and contributes to the breakdown of body protein during chronic illness). Cortisol released in children during the stress of infection or chronic allergic states is partially responsible for periods of retarded growth.

The chronic stress state produced by overstimulation of cortisol, followed by underfunctioning of the adrenal gland, can cause such symptoms as: chronic fatigue; hypotension (low blood pressure); dizziness; hair loss; weight loss; inability to exercise; inappropriate response to temperature changes; lack of perspiration; and depression.

Aldosterone, the other important hormone produced by the adrenal cortex, stimulates the reabsorption of sodium from the kidney in order to regulate the electrolyte balance in the body when plasma volume is decreased. Extracellular potassium concentration also works directly on the adrenal glands to stimulate aldosterone production. This helps to control arterial blood pressure and aids the body in acclimatizing to heat.

Adrenal androgens are similar to but much less potent than testosterone and are produced in small amounts. They have some effect on growth by stimulating protein synthesis, especially during puberty and are thought to contribute to sex drive in women.

Testing Adrenal Function

Adrenal function can be tested with a 24-hour urine collection that measures overall hormone production of the adrenal gland (adrenal cortex). This can be done before and after ACTH stimulation. An ACTH stimulation test can also be performed by intravenous or intramuscular injection of synthetic ACTH (Cortrosyn) and by obtaining blood cortisol levels before and after stimulation.

Avoiding stress is the most important factor in supporting the adrenal gland. For hypersensitive people, any method aimed at relieving environmental, food, or inhalant stressors is encouraged. Immunotherapy helps to relieve the chronic stress of repeated reactivity. Suitable exercise will help to reduce and eliminate excess circulating cortisol before it can damage

and alter cell function. The adrenal gland needs vitamin C, potassium, and pantothenic acid (B_5) to function properly. Physicians have found that sometimes very small amounts of adrenal cortical extract have been helpful.

Thymus Gland

The thymus gland, the master gland of immunity, is a small gland under the breast bone by the second rib, surrounded by ropes of nerves. At one time the thymus was thought to be useless because it shrinks and becomes fibrous at puberty. The adrenal glands swell under stress, whereas the thymus shrinks. It secretes thymosin, which stimulates T-cell function. Up to age seven, it regulates, through the T-cells, the amount of immunity you will have for the rest of your life. B-cells migrate from the bone marrow and undergo a differentiation process to become T-cells as they move from the outer shell of the thymus to its center. As the T-cells change, new proteins are formed on the surface of the cells.

After this differentiation, the T-cells leave the thymus and make their home in other lymph tissues throughout the body. The thymus continues to influence the T-cells and their clones by means of a hormone (thymosin) that is excreted by the cells on the inner lining of the gland. The T-cells produce interleukins and interferon, which stimulate cell division and further differentiation during an infectious or inflammatory process.

For a time, researchers were using thymosin injections (obtained from calves after slaughter) to enhance the function of the immune system, but it was an extremely expensive material to use. Although thymosin has been successfully synthesized, its availability in North

America has been restricted by health regulatory boards. Human clinical tests have been conducted on patients with immune incompetence, life-threatening asthma, some autoimmune diseases, and cancer. Animal studies are also being done to graft young thymus tissue and inject young mouse stem cells (immature T-cells) into aging mice to discover if this will enhance immunity.

Inadequate nutrition stresses the thymus. In 1983, A. Barbul and E. Seifter conducted studies on rats and reversed thymus shrinkage by administering one-percent dietary arginine or ornithine (both amino acids) in their food. (However, it is possible that the treatment affected growth hormone, rather than the thymus directly.) Vitamin A, a powerful immune stimulant, will increase the function of the thymus gland and reduce the shrinking process in the thymus during infection or inflammation. Zinc deficiency has also been found to shrink the thymus. Any of the following antioxidant vitamins and minerals are helpful for thymus gland function: zinc, vitamins A, C, and E, sulfur-based compounds (methionine, cysteine, glutathione, or taurine), and selenium. Desiccated glandular substance may also help to boost some people's immune function.

Parathyroid

The parathyroid is a butterfly-shaped organ on either side of and behind the thyroid. It is composed of four separate glands grouped together, and regulates blood calcium and phosphate metabolism.

Parathyroid hormone is controlled by the calcium concentration in the extracellular fluid surrounding the parathyroid glands. Lower levels of calcium stimulate the production of the hormone and higher levels have the opposite effect. The different functions of the hormone are:

- To stimulate the kidney to synthesize vitamin D (also a hormone). An increase in the level of vitamin D heightens intestinal absorption of calcium and phosphate.
- To increase reabsorption of calcium in the kidneys.
- To reduce reabsorption of phosphate—and thus increase phosphate excretion—which in turn increases calcium deposits on bone. This is one step in maintaining a homeostasis of extracellular calcium and phosphate.
- To increase the movement of calcium and phosphate from bone into extracellular fluids so there is an available source of extra calcium when needed throughout the body.
- To aid breast milk production.
- To increase the excretion of phosphate in the kidneys for protein balance in the body.

Pineal Gland

The pineal gland is located near the midbrain. It regulates growth and is very active until the age of seven, after which it tends to become more fibrous and atrophy. Until recently, it was thought that the gland had no further function after this age; however, it is now felt that light passing the retina of the eye stimulates the pineal gland and the hypothalamus to create a sense of well-being. For this to happen, the light must be from a natural ultraviolet source, as some artificial forms of light can actually disrupt the pineal gland's function. The pineal gland is also stimulated by adrenalin.

Production of sex hormones, growth hormones, and some liver enzymes are all influenced by the pineal gland. It produces the hormone melatonin, a metabolite of tryptophan, which is responsible for regulating circadian rhythms in the body and sleep-wake cycles. Melatonin production is suppressed during prolonged periods of stress. Winter months with shorter days and less natural light can lead to depression and lethargy. This seasonal affective disorder is thought to be caused by a disruption in melatonin production.

Melatonin level abnormalities are found in many low tryptophan diseases. Low levels of melatonin are found nocturnally in anorexia, in the depressive state of manic depressive disease, in schizophrenia, psoriasis, Cushing's disease, and hypopituitarism. High levels of melatonin are found in narcolepsy, obesity, spina bifida, sarcoidosis, and delayed puberty.

Pancreas

The pancreas, which is below and behind the stomach, has both endocrine and exocrine functions. The endocrine portion of the pancreas produces three protein hormones: insulin, glucagon, and somatostatin. All have interrelated effects.

The pancreas has the exocrine function of producing enzymes that digest fats, proteins, and nucleic acids. It also produces bicarbonates that neutralize the stomach's acid contents as they enter the small intestine. The pancreatic enzymes can function only in the alkaline medium created by the bicarbonate. Both of these secretions are emptied into ducts that join with the bile duct before entering the small intestine.

The hormone insulin acts on most of the body's tissues, except the brain. Its secretion is stimulated by eating, which increases glucose, and is inhibited by fasting, which reduces glucose. Its action is twofold: it alters both transport by cell membranes and enzyme functions.

Insulin allows an increase of glucose uptake into the cell when an increase in energy is required. It also activates the transport of amino acids across the cell membranes to provide material for the manufacture of protein. The insulin taken up at the cell's receptor sites alters the concentration and actions of intracellular enzymes involved in both anabolic (building up) and catabolic (breaking apart) functions within the cell.

If it is overstimulated, the pancreas eventually functions poorly. Addictions of all types (alcohol, food, chemical, or tobacco) lead to overstimulation, followed by pancreatic insufficiency of both exocrine and endocrine functions. This process is often seen in hypersensitive people.

Early symptoms of insufficiency are associated with hypoglycemic symptoms: loss of stamina 1 hour after meals; dizziness; cravings for sugar; sweating or chills; blurred vision; and headache. If untreated, further damage can result and may lead to diabetes mellitus.

Glucagon, a second hormone produced by the pancreas, acts in opposition to insulin. It affects metabolism by:

• Increasing breakdown of glycogen in the liver.
• Increasing production of glucose and ketone bodies in the liver. Ketone is a byproduct of fat metabolism.
• Increased breakdown of fat tissue.

The final effect of all these functions is a higher plasma concentration of glucose.

The third hormone, somatostatin, is an intercellular chemical messenger that is stimulated by increased circulating glucose and amino acids during food absorption. Somatostatin inhibits the function of the gastrointestinal tract. It slows the rate of food digestion and absorption by decreasing gastric acid secretion, and it slows stomach emptying and lessens gall bladder contraction. As a result, somatostatin prevents excess buildup of nutrients in the plasma.

Preventing damage to the pancreas is most important for hypersensitive people. Avoidance of any addictive syndrome is foremost. Following a rotary diversified diet, taking nutritional supplements, reducing sugar intake, obtaining immunotherapy for allergies to reduce stress load, making hormone adjustments, and reducing other stressors that trigger a glucose/insulin roller-coaster effect all help prevent damage to the pancreas.

Kidneys

The major function of the kidneys is excreting waste products and water, and regulating the homeostasis between sodium, potassium, calcium, hydrogen, and bicarbonate ions. The kidneys also produce the hormones known as erythropoietin, renin, and 1,25 dihydroxy-vitamin D.

Erythropoietin acts on bone marrow to stimulate the proliferation and maturation of one type of red blood cell (erythrocytes). Its secretion is stimulated by a decrease in the level of oxygen delivered to the kidneys. Testosterone, the major male sex hormone, also stimulates the release of this hormone.

Renin is a hormone with an enzyme function in the blood designed to split angiotensin from a larger protein molecule, angiotensinogen. It is a potent stimulator of aldosterone secretion from the adrenal medulla.

In the kidneys, one step in the production of vitamin D occurs when the parathyroid hormone acts on the hormone 1,25 dihydroxy-vitamin D, produced by the kidney. If the various steps are not completed, a vitamin D

deficiency occurs, and decreased amounts of calcium are absorbed from the intestinal tract.

Gastrointestinal Tract

Five hormones are secreted by cells throughout the intestinal tract.

- *Gastrin:* A peptide hormone secreted in the stomach lining. It stimulates gastric secretions and some gastric contractions.
- *Secretin:* A peptide hormone, produced in the small intestine. The presence of acid in the small intestine stimulates its release, and secretin in turn prompts bicarbonate release from the pancreas and the liver. Acid secretions and stomach motility are inhibited by the action of secretin.
- *Cholecystokinin:* Also produced in the small intestine in response to acid material. It enhances the action of secretin, stimulates pancreatic enzyme secretion, stimulates gallbladder contraction, and stimulates the bicarbonate secretion of the liver.
- *Somatostatin:* Decreases the rate at which food is digested and absorbed. It inhibits production of growth hormone and thyroid stimulating hormone from the pituitary, and is also thought to act as a neurotransmitter. Somatostatin is also secreted by the pancreas, hypothalamus, and the stomach.
- A *gastric inhibitory peptide hormone* is also released in the small intestine.

Gonads

Gonads, the testes in the male and the ovaries in the female, are our main reproductive organs. The gonads produce sex hormones that are stimulated by two gonadotrophic hormones from the pituitary: follicular stimulating hormone (FSH) and luteinizing hormone (LH).

These are steroid hormones, synthesized from cholesterol, that induce development of the sex organs and many of the sex characteristics and changes that occur throughout life. Sex hormone secretion begins around the age of eight to ten and reaches a plateau within five to ten years.

In men, the testes produce the hormone testosterone and reproductive cells (sperm) at a constant rate. The effects of testosterone are:

- Maintaining the function of male reproductive organs.
- Stimulating male secondary sex characteristics (hair growth).
- Stimulating growth and bone growth.
- Maintaining sex drive.
- Inhibiting LH production.
- Aiding sperm production.

Testosterone, which can also be produced by the adrenals, has a mild effect on the thymus. The testes also produce a small amount of estrogen, less than one-fifth of the amount produced in women. We do not know why this estrogen is produced, nor do we understand its effects.

In men, the climacteric or "menopause" occurs when there is a gradual slowing of testosterone production. The pituitary attempts to stimulate the production of testosterone, but because the testes are no longer able to produce testosterone, there is an excess of the stimulating hormone. This excess causes changes in mood and perception—effects which are more emotional than physical.

The female gonads, the ovaries, have three functions:

- Producing ova (eggs).
- Preparing the body for conception and gestation.
- Determining the length of pregnancy.

The ovaries are stimulated by luteinizing hormone (LH) and follicular stimulating hormone (FSH) to produce the two steroid hormones, estrogen and progesterone. Their rate of production is cyclic, not steady, as is testosterone production in men. This cyclic production creates a measure of stress on all of a woman's cells and systems. Estrogen creates a negative and positive feedback on the pituitary to regulate the production of LH and FSH.

Estrogen causes secondary sex characteristics. There are six different stages of estrogen production and utilization. In the liver, excess estrogen is changed to inactive estriol and is excreted. Estrogen has the following effects:

- Stimulates growth of the ovaries, follicles, and external genitalia.
- Initiates breast development.
- Causes females to have shorter bones.
- Increases protein synthesis in pregnancy.
- Increases fat deposits in the breasts, hips, and thighs.
- Softens the skin because of fat and increased vascular supply.
- Stimulates the growth and maintenance of smooth muscle and linings of the reproductive tract.
- Causes fluid retention.

Progesterone prepares the uterus for pregnancy and develops the breasts for lactation. It also provides a negative feedback control over LH and FSH, and regulates secretions in the reproductive tract. Progesterone decreases the amount of niacin converted from the amino acid tryptophan, while estrogen increases it.

Placenta

The placenta produces the hormones known as chorionic gonadotrophin, estrogen, and progesterone. All are involved in the maintenance of pregnancy.

Premenstrual Syndrome

Many hypersensitive women develop other problems as a result of prolonged allergic reactions. Because the endocrine, immune, and nervous systems are so closely interrelated, a stress on one system eventually overflows to place stress on another system. A common complaint from such women is known as premenstrual syndrome.

Premenstrual syndrome (PMS) refers to the complex of symptoms from which over 20 million North American women suffer. These symptoms include:

Psychological and Neurological Symptoms	Depression, irritability, memory loss, sleep disorders, anxiety, hostility, crying spells, lethargy, paranoia, tension, dizziness, headaches (migraines), fainting, seizures
Glandular symptoms	Swelling and tenderness of breasts and the vaginal mucosa, increased sex drive
Gastrointestinal symptoms	Aabdominal bloating, constipation, abdominal cramping, craving for sweets, lowered tolerance for alcohol
Urinary tract symptoms	Infrequent urination
Dermatological symptoms	Facial acne
Other physical symptoms	Fatigue, swelling of extremities, weight fluctuation, thirst, pelvic pain

Most women who suffer from PMS experience several of these symptoms, and suffer from the same set of symptoms with each period. We would hope that no woman suffers from all of them. Some women experience these symptoms mid-cycle, and others have them immediately before menstruation begins. The beginning of menstruation usually relieves the symptoms, although they may last as long as four days after the onset of the menses.

Treatment of PMS

There is no single "magic pill" to relieve or cure the symptoms of premenstrual syndrome. PMS involves a dysfunction of the immune and endocrine systems of the body. The best approach is to address the total load of the body. Some ways to do this are by diagnosing and treating abnormal levels of estrogen, progesterone, FSH or LH; diagnosing and treating endometriosis (dysfunction of uterine membrane); reducing and treating allergies and infections; and cleaning up the immediate environment. This will enable the endocrine and immune systems to function more efficiently.

Since many factors are involved in PMS, treating it involves a variety of therapies:

• *Treating hormonal "sensitivities":* PMS symptoms are relieved through treatment with the proper hormonal extract. Most PMS patients have normal hormone levels, but when they are tested for progesterone, estrone, or LH, they show acute sensitivities to these hormones. Treatment with a neutralizing dose of these hormones helps to relieve the symptoms of PMS.

These hormonal extracts are also useful in relieving morning sickness and menopause symptoms.

- **Treating candidiasis:** Treatment of candidiasis to relieve the symptoms associated with yeast overgrowth also helps relieve PMS symptoms. This involves the use of antifungal agents, diet control, mold control, and the use of extracts to stimulate the immune system. Progesterone release in the body may aggravate Candida overgrowth and may cause or increase some of the premenstrual symptoms. (See "*Candida Albicans*/Yeast Infection," p. 196.)

- **Treating food and chemical allergies:** Food addiction plays an important role in PMS. Control of food allergies by testing and treatment with extracts for offending foods will significantly reduce the body's total load. Cleaning up the environment and avoiding chemicals will also help.

- **Controlling diet:** Many studies have been done linking diet to PMS. Eliminating caffeine, sugars, salt, alcoholic beverages, and highly refined carbohydrates will reduce PMS symptoms. Caffeine prolongs the action of adrenalin, which affects the stimulation of other hormones. Adrenalin stimulates gastric secretion and adversely affects blood pressure, fat metabolism, and insulin requirements. Caffeine also acts as a stimulant to the central nervous system and cardiac muscle.

Sugar and highly refined carbohydrates rapidly raise blood sugar levels, forcing the hormonal system to be overworked. This may lead to shakiness, dizziness, and headaches.

Salt contains sodium and chlorides which are essential for maintaining the body's water (and acid) balance. They also affect the nerve cell excitability and muscle contraction. When sodium excretion is inhibited by hormones released in response to excess estrogen by the pituitary, women will experience monthly water retention. Excess sodium may create an imbalance with potassium, causing erratic contractions of the uterus resulting in cramping.

Alcoholic beverages affect both the absorption of many nutrients and carbohydrate metabolism. An interim step in alcohol metabolism is acetaldehyde, which is toxic to the body, causing dizziness, disorientation, headache, cloudy vision, poor concentration, and poor memory. Acetaldehyde is also one of the many toxins released by the Candida organism during its metabolic processes.

- **Nutritional supplements:** Calcium and magnesium are important to muscle and nerve function, and are involved in transmitting hormonal messages. Magnesium is known as nature's tranquillizer and muscle relaxant. It will relieve uterine and vaginal cramping and will help to moderate PMS mood changes.

Vitamin E helps maintain cell membrane integrity and aids in converting estrogen to estriol in the liver. It is vital to the proper functioning of the reproductive organs and helps reduce premenstrual edema. Vitamin E strengthens capillary walls, thereby improving the vascularity of the uterus.

B-complex, known as the anti-stress vitamins, are necessary for carbohydrate, protein, and fat metabolism, and assist in proper functioning of the nervous system.

Vitamin B_6 helps regulate the female cycle and balance sodium.

Vitamin C strengthens blood vessels, increases iron absorption and aids in the conversion of tryptophan to serotonin, which has a calming effect on metabolism. Vitamin C is necessary for maintenance and proper functioning of collagen fibers in the uterus, which provide the elastic qualities of the uterine wall.

Vitamin A helps maintain healthy epithelial tissue, which is a barrier to bacteria and infection, and it is essential for a normal estrus (fertility) cycle.

Potassium is required for proper functioning of the smooth muscle tissue of the uterus. It is also used by the adrenal glands during periods of stress.

Essential fatty acids are precursors to prostaglandins, which cause relaxation of the uterine muscle.

Nutritional programs work slowly to alleviate PMS and must be continued over a period of time before results are achieved. Consistently using nutrient therapy will gradually decrease symptoms and prevent their recurrence.

- *Exercise:* Regular exercise helps to control PMS. It tones the muscles, relieves tension, aids in food metabolism, provides extra oxygen for improved cell metabolism, and leads to improved self-image and increased well-being.
- *Water:* Increasing water intake several days premenstrually will help to flush out degraded hormones. It will also keep the electrolytes balanced in the tissues, which will reduce edema. Nutrients will be circulated more quickly to all cells.
- *Stress reduction techniques:* Management and reduction of stress help in controlling PMS. Biofeedback, relaxation therapy, and changes in lifestyle are helpful for some people.

OUR NERVOUS SYSTEM

Basic knowledge of our nervous system is important to the allergic or hypersensitive person because it will help make us aware of our internal and external surroundings. Our nervous system is directly affected by external toxins and allergens, as well as by toxins and substances produced within our body as a result of malfunctions of various systems.

Composed of the brain, spinal cord, peripheral nerves, and special sense organs, our nervous system is our body's primary communication, regulation, and coordination network. (The other system used for communication is the endocrine system.) Our nervous system is also responsible for our behavior, states of consciousness, learning, emotional responses, motivation, memory, thoughts, and reasoning.

Nutritional factors required for proper support of the nervous system include B vitamins, magnesium, calcium, sodium, potassium, zinc, oxygen, organic germanium, coenzyme Q_{10}, glucose, choline, amino acids, manganese, and copper.

The Neuron

The basic unit of our nervous system is a cell called a neuron. Neurons come in many sizes and shapes, but they all have the same parts: cell body, dendrites, axon, and axon terminals.

The dendrites are extensions (of varying complexity, length, and number) of the cell body that increase the surface areas of the nerve cell, where signals are received from other neurons. The axon or nerve fiber extends out from the cell body. Its length can vary from microscopic to as much as 30 to 40 inches. The longer axons connect with peripheral organs and limbs, while the shorter ones are found predominantly in the brain. Many axons are covered with a fatty membrane (myelin sheath) that protects and insulates. The end of the axon branches out into filament projections known as axon terminals. These extensions transmit chemical signals to the receptor sites on glands, muscles, and organs.

Receptors on the surface of cells detect environmental and/or chemical changes; as a result, some researchers use the term detector rather than receptor. These neural receptor sites are distinct from hormonal or chemical receptor sites elsewhere in the body. Each responds more readily to one type of energy than to another. For every type of sensation or stimulus there is a specific type of receptor. Candace Pert, former Chief of Brain Biochemistry at the National Institute of Mental Health in Maryland, U.S.A., describes the receptors as "buttons." Depending on the button that is "pushed," different reactions occur in our brain or body—an emotion, the release of gastric acid, a constriction of blood vessels. Even changes in our thoughts, attitudes, and perceptions of the world around us can "push the buttons" by releasing various neurochemicals.

Neurotransmitters

The neuron's axon terminals and dendrites are not joined together but rather are separated by a narrow, extracellular gap known as a synapse. The axon terminals produce and store chemical substances called neurotransmitters that are released, on signal, into the synapse. Neurotransmitters are chemical messengers that trigger a response that is built into the target or receptor cell. They are picked up and bound by the receptor sites on the membranes of dendrites and nerve cell bodies, muscle cells, secretory cells, and skin cells.

This information transfer allows us to perceive, interpret, respond to, and interact with our internal and external environment. The neurotransmitters link our metabolic (nutritional, respiratory, and excretory), neurochemical, neuromuscular, behavioral, and hormonal functions.

The chemical synapses operate in only one direction, so a signal or message is transmitted along a neural pathway only in that specified direction. The amount of time required for this is less than one-thousandth of a second.

After the release of the neurotransmitter and acceptance by the receptor site, the excess is removed from the synapse in one of three ways:

- A chemical transformation of the neurotransmitter, by enzyme action, into an ineffective substance.
- Diffusion into extracellular spaces away from the receptor site.

- Transport of the neurotransmitter back into the specific releasing axon terminal.

The release of a neurotransmitter from the axon terminals depends primarily on the concentration and movement of ions in and out of the cell membrane of the dendrites. These ions are predominantly calcium, magnesium, sodium, potassium, and chloride. This movement of ions tends to polarize or depolarize the membrane, affecting the amount of transmitter released from the axon terminal. In some cases, more than one neurotransmitter can be released from an axon terminal. One usually enhances the effectiveness of the other.

Some of the neurotransmitters are inhibitory (depress function) and some are excitatory (stimulate function). These opposing functions produce a "check and balance" mechanism in the nervous system to regulate body processes.

Neurotransmitters are formed within the nerve cell body from nutrients (proteins, fats, minerals, and vitamins) that circulate in the bloodstream and the cerebrospinal fluid. Some contain only one amino group (monoamines). Others are more complex amine structures (amino acids), and some contain up to 50 amines (peptides).

Many peptides are considered neuromodulators rather than neurotransmitters. They tend to have a biochemical effect in the nervous system rather than the electrochemical effect of the neurotransmitters. Peptides either amplify or dampen activity of the neurotransmitters by making chemical changes in the neurons. While the neurotransmitter function takes place in milliseconds, the neuromodulators tend to create long-term effects that can be measured in minutes, hours, or even days.

Common Neurotransmitters		
Neurotransmitter	*Precursor*	*Action*
Acetylcholine	Choline and Phosphatidyl Choline	Excitatory
Amines		
Serotonin	Tryptophan	Inhibitory
Dopamine	Tyrosine	Inhibitory
Epinephrine	Tyrosine	Excitatory
Norepinephrine	Tyrosine	Excitatory
Histamine	Histadine	Excitatory
Amino Acids		
Glycine	Serine, Threonine	Inhibitory
Glutamic Acid	Aspartic Acid	Excitatory
GABA	Glutamic Acid	Inhibitory
Aspartate	Aspartic Acid	Excitatory
Glutamate	Glutamine and Glutamic Acid	Excitatory
Taurine	Cysteine	Inhibitory

Some of the modulators on this list you will recognize as also having hormone function.

Histamine
Prostaglandins
Enkephalins
Endorphins
Vasopressin (anti-diuretic hormone)
Substance P
Somatostatin
Aldosterone
Angiotensin
Estrogen
Testosterone
Gastrin
Oxytocin
Vasoactive intestinal peptide
Adrenocorticotropic hormone
Thyrotropin releasing hormone
Gonadotrophin releasing hormone

Neurotransmitters are heavily affected in debilitating, toxic physical states. The following factors can affect ne37otransmitter levels:

• Allergy.
• Hypersensitivity.
• Electromagnetic impulses.
• Temperature variations.
• Hereditary factors.
• Nutritional deficiencies.

- Internal production of free radicals.
- Infections (viral, bacterial, fungal, and parasitic).
- Drugs.
- Age.
- Oxygen supply.
- Stress.
- Chemical toxicity.

Some of these factors will cause either overproduction or underproduction of neurotransmitters; blockage of receptor sites; too few or too many receptor sites; or inhibition of enzymatic degradation of excess neurotransmitters.

Electrical Functions

The functions within the nervous system are not only chemical. Each of the neurotransmitters, as well as the calcium, magnesium, sodium, and potassium ions within the nerve cell, carry specific electrical charges—positive, negative, or neutral. The electrical potential is present at the cell membrane. The charge within the cell differs from that on the cell's surface and is dependent on the ion concentration inside and outside. As a neurotransmitter is released and then accepted by a receptor site on the next cell, the electrical potential of each cell is altered and an electrical "firing" occurs. The cells then enter a resting phase when ions are returned to their original position to await the next "firing." The varying patterns of this electrical activity can be seen with the use of sophisticated electrical equipment.

Brain electrical function, for example, can be demonstrated with an electroencephalogram, which shows several types of electrical impulse. Alpha rhythms are linked with lower levels of attention, relaxation, and happiness. The beta rhythm's faster oscillation rate is associated with attention to stimuli. During sleep, the alpha rhythm is replaced with even slower frequencies that change during varying stages of sleep.

Electrical pulsing can be detected by placing electrodes on the surface of the skin at specific points on the body, known as acupressure points. Nerve pathways and endings are close enough to the skin's surface that the flow to the electrical potential can be determined.

Divisions of Our Nervous System

The nervous system is divided into the central nervous system, made up of the brain and the spinal cord, and the peripheral system, consisting of the nerves that link the central nervous system to organs or limbs.

THE CENTRAL NERVOUS SYSTEM

The spinal cord is a long, slender cylinder that extends from the brain to the sacrum in the pelvis. It is surrounded by the protective sheath of the vertebrae. The center of the spinal cord, called the grey matter, is made up of cells that communicate with one another within the nervous system. The outer portion of the cord is called the white matter and is composed of groups of axons called pathways. These pathways run the length of the spinal cord and are either ascending or descending depending on whether they are motor or sensory message carriers.

The brain and spinal cord float in a cushion of liquid known as cerebrospinal fluid, which protects the delicate tissues from sudden, jarring movements. The fluid is released through the vascular system in order to prevent a buildup of fluid pressure around the brain. Cerebrospinal fluid provides a medium of exchange for nutrients to enter the brain cells and for end products of brain metabolism to leave the cells.

The brain is the central command headquarters. Its different sections—the brainstem, the cerebellum, and the forebrain—regulate different functions of the brain and body. These portions are subdivided into areas which all communicate with one another. Communication within the brain occurs between neural cells called interneurons, which account for about 99 percent of all nerve cells.

The brainstem connects the spinal cord with the higher brain centers. The nerve tracks or pathways that run up and down the spinal cord also run through the center of the brainstem. Ten of the cranial nerves branch out from the brainstem to innervate the muscles and glands of the head and neck and many organs in the chest and abdominal region. They also supply the sensory nerves of these areas.

The cerebellum is located at the base of the posterior skull and is involved with skeletal muscle function. It helps to maintain stability of balance and position, and to provide smooth, directed movements. Loops of contact between the cerebellum and the motor portions of the forebrain smooth out the simultaneous messages of intended movements and actual movements.

The forebrain (cerebrum), the largest part of the brain, is divided into two hemispheres and a central core that contains the thalamus and the hypothalamus. The cerebrum is coated with a heavily convoluted or folded shell, called the cortex, which is about three millimeters thick. The convolutions provide a large surface area for the interplay between neurons. This area is responsible for integrating information from the sensory nerve fibers, and for processing the information into meaningful images. The refined messages are then transferred to the motor nerve fibers to initiate muscle impulse and control.

The cortex is subdivided into the temporal, frontal, parietal (side), and occipital (back) lobes. The lobes have circuitous interconnecting pathways associated with learning, emotions, pain and pleasure, sight, language, and hearing. Sensory input from all of these is then translated into motor response. The center of the brain, called the grey matter, contributes to coordination of muscle movements.

The thalamus is a control board and relay station that integrates sensory input on its way to the cortex. The information that is relayed does not always become part of conscious experience but may stimulate automatic, subconscious responses.

The hypothalamus is a tiny area in the midbrain that is responsible for unifying many homeostatic functions of our body. Homeostasis is a balanced state that all body functions work to achieve and maintain. The hypothalamus also contains endocrine cells that produce hormones to interact with the neural tissues in the hypothalamus. The hypothalamus is an important control center that regulates our body's internal environment as we respond to the external environment.

THE PERIPHERAL SYSTEM

The second division of the nervous system is composed of nerve fibers that extend from the brain and the spinal cord. These nerve fibers are classified according to two distinct functions.

The afferent fibers handle sensory information travelling from our body's periphery to the central nervous system. The nerve cell bodies of these fibers are located outside of the brain or spinal cord in structures called ganglia. One long projection of the nerve cell extends away from the ganglia out to the receptors. Another shorter process extends into the central nervous system, where it branches and synapses with the interneurons. The interneurons receive the bits of information sent to the brain or spinal cord via the afferent fibers, and then send out signals along efferent fibers of the peripheral nervous system.

The efferent (motor) division has two parts, the somatic branch and the autonomic branch. The somatic fibers run from the central nervous system to the skeletal muscles. The cell bodies of these neurons are located in groups within the brain or spinal column, and their axons extend directly to the muscle cells without joining with other neurons. The innervation signal sent along this pathway causes contraction of the skeletal muscles. This type of neuron is sometimes called a motor neuron. Efferent nerve fibers have only an excitatory function, and play no inhibitory role. The neurotransmitter released by these fibers is acetylcholine.

The autonomic branch fibers lead from the central nervous system to smooth muscle (digestive tract and internal organs), cardiac muscle, and glands. Autonomic responses usually occur without conscious awareness or control and are also called involuntary responses. This description is no longer valid, however, because mechanisms to control heart rate and other body functions can be learned through biofeedback.

The sympathetic division of the autonomic nervous system mobilizes our body's resources to respond to pain, strong emotion, or extreme temperatures. In contrast, the parasympathetic division restores and conserves body energy, overseeing digestion and absorption of nutrients.

Autonomic fibers lead to organs in the chest area (sympathetic fibers) or to the craniosacral area (parasympathetic fibers), and some organs are innervated by both types of fibers. This dual function is evident in the relaxation and contraction of the lungs, the heart muscle, and the stomach, resulting in a finer, more accurate degree of control over the organ.

Neurotransmitters released by the sympathetic and parasympathetic fibers at the junction with the receptor sites differ. The sympathetic axon terminals release epinephrine, while the parasympathetic fibers release norepinephrine.

Neurological Dysfunction

Dysfunction of any part of the nervous system can be initiated by the same factors affecting neurotransmitter levels. (See "Neurotransmitters," p.38.) Here are a few of the more common neurological dysfunctions that lead to disease.

- Immune dysfunction has been implicated in multiple sclerosis. In this disease the myelin sheath covering and insulating the nerve fiber incurs multiple scars.
- Allergens (including foods, chemicals, inhalants, and organisms) can cause inflammation of neural tissue as a result of the immune cascade. After years of a chronic inflammatory state resulting from unrecognized, untreated allergies, the nerves can become permanently damaged. Autoimmune diseases affecting the nerve tissue can also occur. Some multiple sclerosis patients have improved dramatically when their allergies have been identified and treated, and when amalgam fillings have been removed from their teeth.
- People with chronic Epstein Barr virus sometimes have symptoms caused by autoimmune dysfunction affecting the nervous system. They can experience peripheral nerve pain, numbness, seizures, paralysis, and swelling of

the brain that can be severe enough to cause blindness and deafness.

- Alzheimer's disease involves the destruction of nerve cells that synthesize acetylcholine. In this disease, availability of oxygen to the brain cells is also reduced. The person affected progressively loses memory and cognitive function, undergoes regression and personality changes, and may eventually need complete custodial care.

- In schizophrenia there is an increase in dopamine receptors, which stimulate excessive release of dopamine at the synapses. This creates a fragmentation of mental functioning with symptoms of altered motor function, perceptual distortions, altered mood, abnormal interpersonal behavior, and disturbed thinking.

- In Parkinson's syndrome the dopamine neurons degenerate. Those with Parkinson's have trouble with voluntary movements, often have tremors, and experience rigidity of the arms, legs, and facial muscles. The amino acid L-dopa has been used with some success to stimulate the activity of dopamine in the brain.

- Encephalitis is caused by infectious diseases carried by ticks or mosquitoes, or can result from diseases such as measles, mumps, or influenza. It causes inflammation of brain tissue that can lead to sleeplessness or coma, tremor, rigidity, compulsive movements, and states of immobility.

Treatment of Nervous System Disorders

Research is proceeding rapidly to discover treatments for some of the nervous system diseases and anomalies. Some of the following methods are in their infancy, but further use will no doubt uncover more applications.

- Nutritional manipulation of diet, as well as use of vitamin and mineral cofactors, and amino acid precursors, is effective in treating neurotransmitter dysfunctions.

- Immunotherapy, avoidance of allergens, and detoxification procedures are all essential in reducing recurrent immune inflammatory cascades that damage neural tissues.

- Peptide neuromodulators are being used to address some of the dysfunctions involving neurons.

- Biofeedback retraining mechanisms can control pain, reduce blood pressure, and change body temperature. This technique has the added benefit of freeing people from feelings of helplessness that can accompany chronic illness.

- Battery-operated pacemakers are very effective in regulating the nervous impulses to the heart.

- Drug therapy is used to treat the blockage of some synapses and enzymes, and to stimulate neurotransmitter precursor production. However, drug therapies have a number of potentially devastating side effects.

- TENS units (transcutaneous electrical nerve stimulation) are successful in modulating some types of pain. The low-voltage electrical shock waves are thought to stimulate the release of serotonin, a neurotransmitter that blocks pain.

- Some physicians are administering highly diluted neurotransmitters in a type of immunotherapy. This method has been successful in modulating behavioral problems in children.

PSYCHONEUROIMMUNOLOGY—
BRINGING THE SYSTEMS TOGETHER

A new field in medicine has gradually emerged since the early 1980s. Developed as an outgrowth of studies by biologists and physiologists, the discipline formed by merging immunology, neurology, and psychology is now designated as psychoneuroimmunology. Some have suggested it should be called psychoneuroendocrinimmunology because the endocrine system is also a part of the interrelationship!

For some time, the trend was for practitioners of medicine to investigate and specialize in separate organ or systems function. This was, and is, a continuing necessity, because of the vast amount of knowledge that is available and applicable in each field of medicine. However, this exclusivity created many gaps in the care of people who did not have classically defined symptoms. After all, our body does not function as separate parts but as a complete, integrated, interdependent whole.

Hippocrates, the father of medicine, was well aware of this. He insisted that medical students view the emotions as an integral part of the cause of disease, as well as a factor in recovery. Aristotle too discussed the role of emotions in both health and disease. He felt that the soul was housed in, and inseparable from, the body,

and that all parts of our body are functionally related to serve the whole. He considered the soul to be "ideas expressed in matter." Moses Maimonides, a 13th century Jewish philosopher and surgeon, thought the emotion of happiness would complete a healing process. However, with the discovery of the microscope and emergence of the germ theory, the idea developed that organisms were the sole cause of illness. That theory is now too simplistic to assign to today's multisystem image of disease.

In the past, the family doctor tried to treat illness in relation to the whole person, as well as considering the person's relationship to family and community. This attempt was limited, however, because precise biological information was missing. Then, for a period of time, the pendulum of thought shifted to viewing psychological factors as the root cause for all unknown disease syndromes. When the cause could not be determined in the laboratory, or if the symptoms did not fall into classic disease patterns, the problem was deemed psychological in origin. Fortunately, many physicians tempered this trend with a broader approach to diagnosis and treatment. Biologists and physiologists had not yet proved that cellular level function is interdependent for all of the systems of the body. But as this knowledge became available, physicians were once again able to view people in their entirety. The cooperative effort between specialists in the fields of endocrinology, neurology, biology, physiology, psychology, and immunology is to be applauded.

With this "new" approach to medicine, the experiences of allergic and hypersensitive individuals can be validated. Those people have known, without a doubt, that neurological, behavioral, immune, hormonal, and emotional changes do occur during a reactive state and contribute to the overall debilitation of their health. Perhaps now people with allergies will no longer be misunderstood, and their symptoms will no longer be classed as merely subjective, anecdotal, or psychological.

Sensitivity responses affecting the central nervous system were previously not considered allergic in origin because evidence of immune system involvement was lacking. Now these reactions are shown to stem from chemicals released and mediated from any one or all three systems: the nervous system, the endocrine system, and the immune system.

Laboratory proof of the interdependence between the systems will have tremendous impact on the maintenance of health and the treatment of illness. Physicians will be interested not only in disease, but also in wholeness and well-being; not only in methods of treating disease, but in ways of preventing it; not only in identifying harmful microorganisms, but in knowing something about the situations that lead to their development; and, finally, not only treating their patients, but in instilling self-confidence in them so they can gain knowledge for self-care. Medicine will be based on improving the quality of life rather than preventing death. Medical intervention will mean helping to explore and maximize one's

creative potential. Medical practitioners will be able to go beyond the limited tools of their profession and help the patient find rewards from an evaluation of self and lifestyle precipitated by illness.

The Interconnection of Body Systems

Dr. Blair Justice, in his book *Who Gets Sick*, states that "most of medicine continues to pretend that mind and body are separate and that pathways by which attitudes and moods physically affect our organs and tissues are really imaginary.... and that simple physical explanations will be found to account for major disorders, as if mind and brain have no physical reality." Adverse prolonged physical symptoms do have a profound effect on the emotions and the psyche, but the reverse is also true. Drugs used to treat illness not only affect the disease but change brain, immune, and endocrine function as well.

Below are some of the recent laboratory findings that support the interconnection and communication between the nervous, endocrine, and immune systems.

- Dr. Candace Pert (who was Chief of Brain Biochemistry at the National Institute of Mental Health) and Solomon Synder succeeded, in 1973, in locating and labelling receptors the brain uses for communication between cells. The brain releases neurotransmitters and hormones to communicate with these receptors throughout the body, including receptors on endocrine glands and cells of the immune system. In turn, chemicals and hormones from the immune system and the endocrine system communicate with and modulate the brain and nerve cell function.
- During the 1960s Dr. George Soloman, a

psychiatrist at Mount Sinai School of Medicine, discovered that by electrically stimulating certain parts of the brain of research animals, their ability to fight infection was improved. By damaging those same areas, the effectiveness of the immune system was impaired. It was then found that macrophages (a type of white blood cell) had specific binding sites on their cell membranes for neurochemicals, including the mood-altering endorphins.

- Lymphatic organs (parts of the immune system) such as the thymus, spleen, and lymph nodes are supplied with cholinergic (release the neurotransmitter acetylcholine) and adrenergic (release the neurotransmitter norepinephrine) nerve fibers. T-cells from the immune system have receptors for both of these neurotransmitters on their surfaces, which either stimulate or inhibit the proliferation of the T-cells.

- IgA (immunoglobulin) production in the intestinal tract has been shown to be stimulated by the neuropeptide VIP (vasoactive intestinal peptide). The B-cell lymphocytes that produce IgA have specific receptor sites for VIP. It is thought that this interrelationship may play a role in food allergy responses. VIP has also been shown to influence immune responses in lymph glands and responses in the brain tissue.

- The autonomic nervous system influences the rate at which gastrointestinal hormones are secreted, as well as the speed of glucagon release from the pancreas. Some of the gastrointestinal hormones are also produced by neurons in the brain and function there as neurotransmitters.

- Nerve fibers from the sympathetic branch of the nervous system terminate in the adrenal glands. This explains why the adrenal glands rapidly release epinephrine in response to stress, which stimulates the responses we associate with "fight or flight."

- Endorphins and enkephalins (peptide neurotransmitters) produced during acute episodes of stress tend to stimulate the production of the immune system's natural killer cells and T-cells. However, the prolonged stress of grief has been shown to inhibit production of killer cells.

- Several neuropeptides can stimulate the release of histamine from mast cells during an immune response. They also stimulate the release of leukotrienes, which initiates and modulates allergic responses.

- A peptide neurotransmitter that inhibits the release of growth hormone from the pituitary gland also inhibits the function of T-cells.

In our clinical experience we have observed that in addition to physical problems, emotional and psychological stress factors underlie some cases of environmental illness. Psychological traumas from the past that have been long suppressed and forgotten by the conscious mind can heavily influence the immune, nervous, and endocrine systems. Many people will make progress toward good health through good physical care, but then reach a plateau and are unable to improve further. With careful investigation, gentle searching, and time, concealed issues surface so they can be addressed and put in proper perspective. Some of the most common unresolved problems are:

- Early childhood feelings of fear, abandonment, and rejection.

- Emotional pain transferred or reflected by a parent through feelings alone (not necessarily through words or actions).

- Sexual, emotional, verbal, or physical abuse.

- Grief caused by the death of a loved one.

- Emotional upheaval caused by unemployment, divorce, rejection by a parent or loved one.

• Alcoholism, addiction, or dysfunction in family situations.

• Repressed anger.

• Lack of forgiveness of a personal wrong (resentment).

• Guilt or imagined guilt from a lack of proper response to a situation.

• Loss of one's dreams or goals.

A solution for such problems cannot always be found, but there is profound relief for the affected person when their existence is recognized. An assessment can then be made of the general impact of these problems on physical status and emotional well-being.

Another encouraging aspect of this investigation is that many researchers and practitioners are clinically studying and applying techniques of healing thought. A group of distinguished physicians, scientists, psychiatrists, writers, and faculty members recently joined together at UCLA to investigate and correlate laboratory evidence of the overlap between body systems, and to gather more evidence on the way emotions influence body function. Researchers like Hans Selye, Karl Menninger, and George Engel had already provided a great deal of evidence that thought, attitude, stress, feelings, and experiences all affect the body's physiological functions. Norman Cousins had shown by his own experience, recorded in *Anatomy of An Illness*, that positive attitudes could affect the body's ability to repair. He also determined that his own sedimentation rate (blood indicator of inflammation) decreased by five points when he engaged in laughter. The task force worked to gather irrefutable evidence that one's attitude toward illness can improve health and enhance treatment. The enlightening outcome of this cooperative effort was reported in Cousins' book called *Head First—The Biology of Hope*. Ongoing related studies are being conducted in many universities and laboratories as a result of the task force's effort.

Norman Cousins, Bernie Siegel, Gerald Jampolsky, Oscar and Stephanie Simonton, Robert Schuller, Norman Vincent Peale, and Ron DelBene have all paved the way in their lectures and writings for the application of positive thinking to the improvement of health, even in the presence of terminal diseases. (See also the discussion of hope in the chapter on *The Emotional and Psychological Impact of Environmental Illness*, p. 282.) They have proved that feeling love for others triggers lower levels of the stress hormone, norepinephrine, and a higher ratio of helper/suppressor T-cells in the immune function. David McClelland, a psychologist at Harvard University, discovered that higher levels of IgA antibodies and lower levels of infection are found in people with high scores on intimacy questionnaires.

We know that areas in our brain and nervous system regulate and control most of our body's functions. Our brain in turn receives messages from our body and responds with appropriate signals to all systems. It seems to follow that our minds can also be conditioned and taught to control body functions during illness to enhance healing and recovery.

CHAPTER 5

OUR DIGESTIVE
AND ABSORPTIVE SYSTEMS

The Role of Digestion and Absorption in Allergies

Proper digestion is a key factor in recovering from food sensitivity, and understanding the basic functions of the digestive system will help you in making informed food choices.

During the digestive process, food is broken down to its constituent parts. The body then extracts nutrients from these well-digested food molecules. However, when digestion is abnormal, there are many food materials that are not adequately broken down. This can lead to sensitivity to those foods. For example, if protein molecules are too large when they are absorbed into the bloodstream, the body treats them as invaders, just as it does bacteria or viruses. The immune response sends extra white blood cells to destroy the invaders and histamine, serotonin, and kinins may be released. In this way, an allergic reaction is put into motion. Food allergy reactions are not confined to proteins as originally thought, but can include all food categories and chemicals, especially those contacted most frequently.

Parts of the Digestive System

MOUTH

Digestion begins in the mouth, where food is chewed. Chewing physically breaks apart food into smaller particles so a large surface area will be available for the action of acid in the stomach and enzymes in the small intestine. Chewing also lubricates the food with saliva for ease in swallowing. Saliva is secreted by salivary and parotid glands, in response to stimuli from the brain stem, which receives signals relayed from pressure and chemical receptors in the mouth. Saliva contains the enzyme amylase, which starts carbohydrate digestion.

ESOPHAGUS

The next step is swallowing, which propels food through the esophagus and into the stomach by waves of contraction. The swallowing process is complex, involving muscles in the larynx, pharynx, tongue, respiratory tract, and esophagus. All of these muscles work to prevent food from entering the nasal passages or lungs.

STOMACH

While in the stomach, food is churned and mixed by the action of many muscle bands that alternately contract and relax. Hydrochloric acid is secreted into the stomach by parietal cells lining the stomach. The vagus nerve signals the parietal cells to begin acid production after it receives stimulus from the sight, smell, and taste of food and from the process of chewing. The higher the protein content in the meal, the greater the stimulation of gastric acid release. Caffeine also stimulates acid release. Hydrochloric acid is a strong acid material (pH of 1–1.5; pH is a measure of acidity/alkalinity); it kills bacteria entering the stomach along with food. This is not 100-percent effective, however—a few bacteria survive to take up residence and multiply in the intestinal tract.

Optimum digestive function in the stomach occurs in an acid medium of pH 1.8 to 3. Introducing food raises the pH level in the stomach. The acid mixture starts to work on the protein structure, disintegrating connective tissue and cells in the ingested food. Stomach acid has only a limited capacity to work on complex proteins or carbohydrates, and no capacity to digest fats.

Hydrochloric acid activates the secretion of the enzyme pepsin, the hormone gastrin, and additional mucus. Mucus protects the protein in the stomach wall from the effects of hydrochloric acid. Pepsin works to break down protein, while gastrin helps stimulate acid release and contractions of the stomach. Histamine, found in the mucosa of the stomach wall, also plays a role in the release of hydrochloric acid. Very little of what is eaten is absorbed through the stomach wall—only water, alcohol, and a few minerals.

Some people have excessive acid secretion, which can cause a burning sensation in the upper abdomen and in the esophagus, burping of sour-tasting liquid, and excessive gas. This condition is known as hyperchlorhydria. Anxiety, anger, stress, and caffeine will all contribute to the overproduction of acid. Taking calcium supplements with meals will help to absorb the excess acid.

Hypochlorhydria, on the other hand, occurs when secretion is diminished, resulting in inadequate amounts of hydrochloric acid. Achlorhydria is the term used when hydrochloric acid is present in extremely low amounts in the stomach. This results in improperly digested food. Symptoms of low levels of stomach acid are often the same as those experienced by people with excess acid levels.

The usual over-the-counter treatment for symptoms of low stomach acid is the wrong approach because, as advertisements tell us, antacids "absorb up to 45 percent of their weight in stomach acid." The cause of "burning stomach" should be investigated before antacids are prescribed or taken.

Symptoms accompanying hypochlorhydria can include poor nutrient absorption from either food or nutritional supplements, sensitivity to foods, longitudinal ridges on fingernails, nails that break easily, rosacea (small broken blood vessels on cheeks), belching or bloating soon after a meal, regurgitation of sour liquid, burning in the stomach area or esophagus, food "sitting in the stomach" for long periods, or hypoglycemia-like symptoms. Some people report having diarrhea, constipation, or undigested food particles in their stools.

Levels of gastric acid can be measured by radiotelemetry (Heidelberg Gastrogram), discussed on p. 53.

Allergies and Stomach Acid   Food sensitivity is frequently associated with inadequate levels of stomach acid. Those with low stomach acid have poor nutrient absorption, and supplements are usually needed. Clinical observation has shown that low stomach acid levels increase susceptibility to and severity of bacterial, fungal, and parasitic bowel infections. Stomach acid levels are found to be inadequate in 50 percent of people over the age of 60. This contributes to the poor nutritional status (especially low calcium levels) seen in many older people. Cells lining the stomach produce an "intrinsic factor" that is essential for the absorption of vitamin B_{12} in the small intestine.

To return acid secretion to normal levels in hypochlorhydric or achlorhydric individuals, hydrochloric acid supplementation is the treatment of choice, but it must be used only when indicated and with careful supervision. The acid should never be used in conjunction with anti-inflammatory medications such as aspirin or Motrin, or with corticosteroid preparations because of the risk of inducing bleeding or ulcers. Hydrochloric acid is available in tablet, capsule, or liquid form. Capsules are most convenient and effective, since tablets do not readily dissolve and the liquid hydrochloric acid can injure tooth enamel. People with low stomach acid may have difficulty dissolving capsules in the stomach. If this is a problem, small pin pricks may be made in the capsule.

The acid is available in combination with pepsin, and with betaine or glutamic acid as carriers. Gradually increased amounts of lemon juice, vinegar, and ascorbic acid (vitamin C) also provide small amounts of acid. Excess amounts of supplemental acid will cause stomach burning, which can be neutralized immediately with some form of bicarbonate. If burning occurs, the dosage of acid must be reduced.

Occasionally, people may display a sensitivity to pepsin, and preparations are available without it.

SMALL INTESTINE

The final stage of digestion takes place in the small intestine, where most of the absorption occurs. From the stomach, the partially digested food mixed with acid (called chyme) enters the small intestine. This movement occurs about 45 minutes to an hour following a meal.

Here, enzymes work to convert proteins into amino acids, fats into glycerin and fatty acids, and carbohydrates into monosaccharides (sugars). These simple molecules are then small enough to pass through the mucosal lining of the intestine into the bloodstream to form "building blocks" for the body. Water, minerals, ions, and vitamins are also absorbed.

The small intestine is nine feet long, but its absorptive surface is 600 times that length. Its inner surface is highly folded and is covered with small fingerlike projections called villi, which, in turn, are covered with microscopic projections called microvilli. This surface is where absorption and the final stage of digestion occur. Villi cells function only for a few days and then disintegrate. There is a constant renewal of the intestinal lining if proper nutrients are available.

LARGE INTESTINE

While most ingested food molecules are absorbed before reaching the large intestine, reabsorption of sodium and water takes place in this area of the gastrointestinal tract. The cells lining the large intestine are unable to absorb amino acids or glucose, but certain types of bacteria synthesize vitamins that are absorbed. The amount of vitamins produced this way, however, is far below the daily level needed for optimal body function.

Some fungal organisms also colonize areas of the large intestine, and help to disintegrate fibers in the waste material. Overgrowth of undesirable bacterial or fungal organisms will lead to production of toxins and gas. The gas (flatus) is composed of nitrogen, carbon dioxide, and small amounts of hydrogen, methane, and hydrogen sulfide. The toxins that are absorbed into the bloodstream are water-soluble.

DIGESTIVE ENZYMES

The enzymes that complete the work of digestion enter the first part of the small intestine from the pancreas and the liver. Digestion involves the exocrine, or internal, functioning of both organs. Pancreatic enzymes are manufactured and stored in the pancreas until the stomach signals for their secretion. The pancreatic enzymes can function only in an alkaline medium, which is provided by bicarbonate solutions secreted from the liver and the pancreas. The amount of bicarbonate that is secreted is normally equal to the amount of acid released by the stomach. An alkalinity of pH 8–9 is essential for proper pancreatic enzyme function.

If the alkaline (bicarbonate) level is not adequate, the pancreatic enzymes are either destroyed or inactivated. Generalized body acidosis can then occur after meals, and the intestinal mucosa can be damaged by the excess acid. The enzymes present in the pancreatic fluid digest proteins, fats, and carbohydrates, and are also essential to the processing of the fat-soluble vitamins A, D, E, and K.

Bile, from the liver, is stored in the gallbladder and is dumped into the small intestine through the same duct as the pancreatic enzymes. Bile contains six major ingredients: bile salts; cholesterol; lecithin; bile pigments; trace minerals; and inorganic minerals (sodium, potassium, and chloride). The first three ingredients help to digest fats, while trace minerals and the first two inorganic minerals provide bicarbonate ions to neutralize stomach acid.

Bile insufficiency is easy to detect because it determines the color of the stool. Normal stool is a medium to dark brown color. Stool that is predominantly clay-colored (yellow), greyish, or very light brown usually indicates low bile content. Taking supplements of taurine, an amino acid, can help to stimulate bile production and thin the consistency of the bile so it will flow more readily. Choline, inositol, methionine, or lecithin are also helpful in increasing bile production.

Bile salts are also available as a supplement. The correct dosage is indicated by a return to a normal stool color. Take care while increasing dosage because diarrhea can be easily triggered, causing greenish, unpleasant, and irritating stool. Bile salts are derived from animal sources so you should also be aware of its allergenic potential.

Irritation of the tissues surrounding the bile duct opening into the small intestine can be caused by repeated exposure to allergenic foods, candidiasis, or parasitic infections. The local irritation causes a swelling of the duct, and backs up bile into the gallbladder. This results in thickening of the bile and gallbladder pain, which can be misdiagnosed as gallstones. Eliminating offending foods and/or treating organisms will often reduce this type of pain.

Low pancreatic enzyme and bicarbonate secretion frequently occur together with low stomach acid secretion because adequate stimulation from stomach acid is essential for the production and release of pancreatic enzymes. Insufficient pancreatic enzymes result in lowered fat digestion and a subsequent rise in blood phospholipid/cholesterol ratios. One sign of inadequate pancreatic enzyme and bile function may be floating stools.

Measuring Enzyme Levels   The radiotelemetry method of diagnosis (see p. 53) is helpful in determining the levels of available bicarbonate in the small intestine. If the levels are low, pancreatic enzyme function is also reduced, since pancreatic enzymes are activated only in an alkaline medium created by bicarbonate. A blood test is also available to measure pancreatic enzyme levels.

Blood, hair, and urine analyses can help determine your nutritional status (minerals, vitamins, and amino acids). An assessment of intestinal digestion and absorption can also be made from these results. Stool examination can detect undigested protein and vegetable fibers, starch granules, and excess fat globules, all of which indicate impaired digestion.

Impaired Digestion

Improper secretion of enzymes and bicarbonate from the pancreas or liver—or impaired digestive and absorptive surfaces in the intestinal tract—can have a variety of consequences. The most important consequence of malfunction is poor nutrition. Since nutrients are the building blocks of our cells, a deficiency will mean lowered functioning of all body systems, including the immune system. Lack of adequate nutrients will cause: frequent infections; disruption of hormone levels; poor memory and decreased mental acuity; lack of cell enzyme production, resulting in fatigue; inability to cope with stress; and increased allergic inflammatory reactions.

There are other problems associated with improper digestion and absorption:

- Repeated exposure to foods that cause inflammatory reactions can lead to abrasion of the microvilli. This leaves larger openings in the intestinal wall, allowing larger molecules of food to pass into the bloodstream, where further inflammatory processes develop. This chain of events heightens food allergy.

- Excessive blood sugar fluctuations act as a stressor to the pancreas, liver, brain, and adrenals.

- Eating many times during the day (nibbling or snacking) puts an added burden on the pancreas, eventually reducing pancreatic enzyme production.

- Excessive repetition of the same food in the diet also stresses the digestive enzyme systems so that they no longer produce adequate amounts of enzymes. Foods, then, are improperly digested, causing allergic reactions. This constant irritation can lead to irritable bowel syndrome.

- Infants up to six months of age do not have adequate levels of IgA in the cells lining the intestinal tract. These cells prevent the absorption of large particles that may be allergenic. Early exposure to solid foods (before the age of six months) can initiate food sensitivities. The infant's intestinal tract is unable to properly digest the food, and the protein or carbohydrate molecules are absorbed whole into the bloodstream. The body then mounts an immune response and produces antibodies to the food molecule. Thereafter, whenever that food is encountered, an immune reaction will occur.

- Reduced acid production in the stomach and less efficient nutrient absorption from the small intestine tend to accompany the aging process.

RADIOTELEMETRY—HEIDELBERG GASTROGRAM

The gastrogram test is an important aid to investigating digestive problems so that treatment can be initiated. In the test, a miniature high-frequency transmitter is encapsulated in an easy-to-swallow capsule. The transmitter is calibrated to receive the pH values (acidity and alkalinity) from the stomach and small intestine. These frequencies are picked up by a belt antenna, worn by the person being tested, and are transmitted to a receiver. The receiver displays the information on both a meter and a graph.

During the test, the following information can be gathered:

- Acidity of the fasting stomach.
- Ability of the stomach to reacidify if challenged by sodium bicarbonate or food.
- Emptying time of the stomach into the small intestine.
- Bicarbonate levels in the small intestine (necessary to activate the pancreatic enzymes).
- Transit time of food and waste in the gastrointestinal tract.
- Presence of a mucus mass in the stomach that would interfere with the action of hydrochloric acid.
- Presence of gastric or duodenal ulcerations.

Treatment of Digestive Irregularities

Pancreatic enzyme supplements can reduce reactions, provide adequate enzymes for digestion, and allow the pancreas to repair and recover its function. Some of the available enzymes are bromelain (from pineapple), papain (from papaya), liquid aloe vera, aged garlic, unpasteurized honey, superoxide dismutase (SOD), and pancreatic enzymes (from lamb, beef, or pork). The wide variety of enzyme sources is an aid to those who use a rotation diet (see p. 111). These enzymes are taken with meals as digestive aids and between meals for their anti-inflammatory function.

Since pancreatic enzymes do not function in an acid medium, bicarbonate supplements should accompany pancreatic enzyme therapy. The alkaline material should be taken 45 minutes to an hour following a meal, when the chyme (partly digested food) from the stomach begins to enter the small intestine.

The bicarbonate may be obtained from a variety of sources: buffered forms of vitamin C; combinations of potassium, magnesium, and calcium bicarbonates; sodium and potassium bicarbonates; or ascorbates formed by combining ascorbic acid with either sodium, magnesium, or calcium. Bicarbonates also neutralize the stage of an allergic reaction when the body tends to become acidic.

One of the most important ways to treat digestive malfunction is by eliminating the offending allergenic foods, and using a rotary diversified diet. Elimination diets or rotary diets remove the stress load on the pancreas and reduce inflammatory reactions to allow repair of the pancreas and small intestine. Please see "The Rotation Diet" (p. 111) and *Recommended Books* (p. 304) for more information about this important method of treatment.

Nutrient supplements that aid function and repair of the pancreas and intestinal tract include: amino acids, zinc, manganese, potassium, calcium, magnesium, vitamin C, and vitamin A. A supplemental material (Colixen), containing mucin and sialic acid, enhances repair of the intestinal mucosa.

OUR BODY ELECTRIC

We have evolved and adapted in an environment containing a full spectrum of magnetic and electric pulsations, in all frequencies and patterns. Our body rhythms respond to and resonate with the regular rhythms of the earth, moon, sun, and major planets, whose gravitational, magnetic, and electrical variations also affect tides, radio waves, electrical transmissions, plants, and animals.

To prove the electromagnetic effects on biological systems, an interesting study was done with oysters, placed in a water tank at great distance from the ocean. The oysters continued to open and close in rhythm with the rise and fall of the ocean tides, which are governed by the magnetic energy of the moon's gravitational force fields.

The presence of electrical and magnetic forces has been documented for thousands of years. The Egyptians inscribed tombs with a description of the effects of electricity, generated by a species of fish, on the human body. Later, the Greeks described the use of electric eels to control pain. Shamans in all cultures have used the magnetic forces in stones and crystals to treat unhealthy people.

The Chinese have perfected the art of acupuncture for healing and anesthesia, based on stimulation of the body's electromagnetic pathways. Louis Pasteur observed that fermentation was speeded up by placing a magnet near fermenting fluids and wines. In 1941, Dr. Albert Szent Gyorgyi proposed that the newly discovered electrical conductivity, semi-conduction, played a role in living cell function. The space program also has added a great deal to our knowledge of the biological effects of low gravitational forces on humans.

Electromagnetic Cell Function

All chemical reactions in our body are electrical in nature, since they involve the exchange or sharing of electrons, and the formation of ions with a negative or positive charge. An electric force draws oppositely charged substances together. In contrast, like charges repel each other. Pure water is a relatively poor conductor of electricity because it contains very few charged particles. When sodium and chloride ions are added to water, the solution becomes a relatively good conductor, since the added ions carry an electrical charge.

Body fluids contain a variety of negatively and positively charged ions. In our body, the cell membranes act as electrical barriers because they have high lipid (fat) levels, providing high electrical resistance. This membrane separates intracellular from extracellular fluids, each with a different concentration of ion components. Intracellular fluid contains more potassium and magnesium, while extracellular fluid contains more sodium and calcium ions. The exchange of ions across the cell membrane is a series of complex electrical/chemical events that produces a measurable voltage charge. Chloride ions are present on either side of the cell membrane, providing a negative charge, while the mineral ions (sodium, potassium, calcium, and magnesium) provide the positive charge.

Nerve and muscle cells have the capacity to change their membrane permeability to allow variables in the exchange between sodium, potassium, magnesium, and calcium. This allows "signals," as well as nutrients, to be more readily transferred between cells. Potassium ions are the most active element in the exchange process across the membrane. Nerve and muscle cell membranes can change their electrical potential hundreds of times in a second. This capability is described as the cell's excitability.

The following examples illustrate the correlation between chemical and electrical influences on cell function:

- By lowering extracellular calcium concentrations, the cell's excitability is temporarily increased. Lowering the calcium concentration still further may cause a complete loss of membrane excitability.
- Magnesium deficiency produces electrical instability in the heart muscle and nerve cells. This can result in arrhythmias and coronary vasospasms (contraction of blood vessels). Electrocardiograph abnormalities can occur when our body is deficient in magnesium.
- Many drugs, chemicals, and toxins are capable of changing the permeability and excitability (electrical potential) of the cell membrane.

Physics tells us that any flowing electrical current produces a magnetic field in the space around it. This field, carrying energy and information, is capable of producing an action at a distance. Magnetic properties of our body have also been demonstrated. Our brain and spinal cord carry a positive magnetic pole orientation, and the peripheral tissues carry a negative orientation. Every chemical bond is characterized by an electrical vibration.

It is important to understand that our body is matter, with chemical, electrical, and magnetic properties. The pineal gland, for example, responds to light wave impulses in its production of the hormone melatonin. The gland's level of secretion also changes with geomagnetic rhythms. Quantum mechanics researchers feel biophysical elements govern biochemistry in our body rather than vice versa.

Electromagnetism Applied

Dr. Robert Becker, in his book, *The Body Electric*, shows that growth and development, metabolism, and communication between organs and between cells cannot be explained only on the biochemical level. He proved that, in the healing process, electrical currents play a decided role in cell communication and division. By applying this knowledge Dr. Becker learned to heal bone fractures by applying miniscule electric currents on either side of the fractures.

Electrosleep, used as a method for anesthesia, also developed as a result of Dr. Becker's work. He demonstrated that different frequencies of appropriate currents sent through small electrodes placed on the head can control one's state of consciousness. Research revealed that the front of the skull is negative in electrical potential, while the back of the skull is positive. When electrodes are placed on the head (negative in front and positive in back) and small voltages and currents are applied, feeling of well-being is produced. If the electrical potential is reversed, unconsciousness results.

With the development of highly sophisticated electronic and magnetic devices, much more has been learned about our body function. The production of electrical and magnetic currents in our body can be measured using an electrocardiogram (ECG), an electro-encephalogram (EEG), galvanic skin response electrodes, a binocular iriscorder, and electromyelography. The nuclear magnetic resonance instrument (MRI) is replacing the X-ray for internal body imaging.

In 1970, Brian C. Josephson completed the development of the SQUID (superconducting quantum interferometric device). Through the use of this instrument, it is now known that our body contains both AC (alternating) and DC (direct) electrical fields of current. Magnetic fields are also associated with these currents. The brain produces a steady DC magnetic field which is one-billionth the strength of the earth's geometric field.

ENERGY MEDICINE

In addition to electromagnetic procedures for imaging and diagnosis, techniques are being applied for beneficial treatments as well. The term energy medicine is used to describe this type of treatment. For example:

- Short-wave diathermy, the generation of heat in body tissues by electric current, is used for both surface and deep healing to relieve muscle and joint pain.
- Oscillators are used to disintegrate gall bladder stones so they can be excreted more readily.
- Electrocautery and electrosurgery employ a fine wire probe that produces a high frequency electric arc between the probe and the tissue to be treated.
- TENS units (transcutaneous nerve stimulation) are in widespread use for pain relief, particularly after surgery. Their use reduces the amount of analgesics needed by the patient.
- Electroacupuncture, often called Neuro Electric Therapy, is gaining favor in England. Originally used for pain relief, it is now used as treatment for drug dependency, by measurably increasing the amount of natural brain endorphins. Unfortunately, its use has not yet been approved in North America.

Effects of Electromagnetism

Our sun produces solar winds composed of high-energy atomic particles, which travel at enormous speeds and collide with the magnetic force exerted by the earth. Some of these high-energy particles are trapped in two areas, known as the Van Allen belts, encircling the earth. These belts shield the earth from solar wind effects by either absorbing some of the energy particles or by diverting them around and away from the earth. The belts also shield the earth from X-rays and other ionizing, high-energy radiation. Without this protection, life on earth could not exist. The interaction between the sun's high energy and the earth's magnetic force produces extra low frequency (ELF) electromagnetic waves (between 0–100 cycles per second) and very low frequency (VLF) waves (between 100–1,000 cycles per second).

In an 11-year cycle, solar storms erupt on the sun, thrusting energy particles of increased intensity out into space. This, in turn, affects the strength of the earth's magnetic field. These surges disrupt radio and electrical transmissions on earth. Since biological organisms, including humans, are electric in function, they too are affected by these fluctuations. Human and animal behavioral disturbances occur during magnetic storms.

We have learned to generate and manipulate electromagnetic forces, but since this is being done beneath the Van Allen belts, we are not protected from the effect of these forces. Telecommunications, electrical power plants, transmission lines, appliances, and microwave, radar, and radio transmissions have all increased at an alarming rate during the past 50 years.

Evidence of the biological effects of long-term exposure to the increased number of ELF waves is beginning to be gathered from around the world. Effects include: increased serum triglycerides (linked with high cholesterol); increased cancer cell growth; decreased production of dopamine, serotonin, and norepinephrine (neurotransmitters) in the brain; alterations in biological cycles; and increased chronic stress responses that lead to immune system deficiencies. We have a very adaptable biological system, but when faced with overwhelming insults, our normal mechanisms begin to fail. In people who already have impaired immune, endocrine, or nervous sytems, these effects are more pronounced.

Since the potential dangers of high levels of electromagnetic waves have been demonstrated, perhaps measures will soon be implemented to protect against long-term effects.

Symptoms of Electromagnetic Imbalance

The following may indicate an electromagnetic imbalance:

• Symptoms of any type that worsen before a thunderstorm or during a wind storm.
• Symptoms that improve after a storm has begun.
• An electrical discharge that occurs when touching any object after walking across a rug.
• Electrical equipment or appliance malfunctions when you are near the appliance.
• Telephone use makes you nervous, anxious, or headachy.
• Watches may stop, lose or gain time, or cause sleepiness when they are worn.
• Fluorescent lighting causes hyperactivity, headaches, or blurred vision.
• Symptoms worsen when near high-powered electric lines or transformers.
• Nervousness or headaches occur when wearing hearing aids.
• Taking a shower or bath, or standing barefoot on damp grass, relieves many adverse symptoms.

Symptoms associated with electric or magnetic field sensitivity or imbalance vary according to one's state of health and the intensity of exposure. Symptoms can be as mild as dizziness or headache, occurring only when you are exposed to an electromagnetic field. Repeated exposure can cause neurological reactions of confusion, hyperactivity, memory loss, sleep disturbance, paresthesia (tingling skin), or convulsions; chronic stress syndromes; lowered immune responses to infection; aggravated immune responses resulting in increased hypersensitivity reactions; and general debility, as in chronic fatigue syndrome.

How to Reduce Electromagnetic Effects

Our society, with its many advantages, is not risk-free. We must continually weigh the benefits derived from new materials and products against their potential hazards. Many problems arising from external sources of electromagnetic force are beyond our control—but we can make evaluations, take precautions, and exercise control over our own use of electromagnetic devices. Consider the length of time that you use appliances each day. Although the electromagnetic field generated by an electric razor or hair dryer is greater than that of a television set or computer, exposure time to these appliances is much shorter.

There are a number of simple precautions we can take to protect against low-frequency waves:

- Keep as few electrical appliances in your bedroom as possible. This will lower electrical exposure for at least eight hours of the day.
- Position the head of your bed facing north to take advantage of the earth's magnetic force.
- Do not use electric blankets or heating pads.
- Check microwave ovens for possible leaks that can occur if food or other particles are stuck to the rubber insulating gasket on the door. Inspect the gasket for cracks or nicks. Stay at least four feet away from an operating microwave.
- Use a screening shield to reduce the waves that emanate from your computer screen.
- Check all electrical cords to be sure that their insulation is intact.
- Choose a bedroom location in your home that is far removed from the entry of the main electrical source to the house.
- If possible, choose a home site that is a long distance from high-voltage wires or transformers.
- Have a satellite dish mounted away from your house rather than on top of it.
- Use the telephone as little as possible. Remote, battery-operated telephones may cause

symptoms for some hypersensitive people.

- Hearing aids contain batteries that can create electrical imbalance, causing dizziness, sinus congestion, or headaches.
- Removal of mercury amalgam fillings is advantageous for electrically sensitive people because opposing charges build up on the amalgam, causing an electrical field discharge between the fillings.
- Go barefooted or in stockings as much as possible.
- When travelling by automobile, try to get out of the car and walk around every half-hour to have ground contact.
- Air travel for extended periods may pose a problem because of lack of grounding.
- Both trace and macro minerals should be supplemented if your drinking water is filtered or distilled. The minerals are essential to proper conductivity of electricity in the body.
- Purchase an automobile that does not have computer regulated systems.
- Avoid using free-standing or individual room electric heaters.
- Negative ion generators are helpful for some people. Take care in choosing a generator because some types produce ozone.
- There is new evidence that wearing specially prepared magnets may help balance your body's electromagnetic function and reduce the effect of external electromagnetic forces.

Air particles become positively charged before a storm or during periods of high, dry winds. Water droplets change the positive ion accumulation in their immediate surroundings to negative. Once a rain or snow storm has begun, the positive ions are shifted to a negative charge.

Many people do not feel well when the air has

a high positive ion level. Teachers are well aware of discipline problems in children prior to a storm. Hospital staff see worsening of symptoms in their very ill or elderly patients during weather changes. Animals are also known to be very restless when positive ion levels are high.

If you are electrically sensitive, you will find that being near moving water is helpful when the positive ion level is high. You can find some relief if you can be near a stream, lake, or ocean. Since this is not possible for most people, an alternative is to stand in a running shower. Even running water over your lower arms and hands a number of times each day can provide relief.

Mobile homes can be problematic for people with electromagnetic imbalances because their electrical wiring runs the length of both sides of the structure. Also, the sides and roof are nearly always metal, and the home is frequently not sufficiently grounded for electrically sensitive people. Extra grounding can be accomplished by driving a copper pipe two feet into the ground and attaching a copper wire from the pipe to the metal frame or siding of the mobile home. This should be done at two different places on the mobile home.

The sensitivity of biosystems to electromagnetic fields has been known for a long time. With the increase in man-made force fields, sensitivities are becoming more evident. Intricate cell structure and functions in biosystems are being affected. We need much more research into these effects to find solutions to the associated problems. The time has also come for medical science to incorporate new knowledge from the discipline of bio-physics, and to apply a new dimension of electrical and magnetic components to clinical practice. Diagnosing and treating illness can no longer be confined strictly to biochemical functions, but must take into account bioelectrical and biomagnetic factors.

CHAPTER 7

ALLERGY AND DEGENERATIVE DISEASES

Disease seldom has a single cause. In fairly evaluating any set of symptoms, allergy or sensitivity should be considered as either the primary cause or at least a strong contributing factor.

Many degenerative and autoimmune diseases stem from the same cause—an imbalance of metabolic functions at the cellular level, or a loss of homeostasis. All degenerative diseases begin with fatigue, imbalance, and dysfunction of the biochemical and bioelectric metabolic body processes. Often this fatigue results from maladaption to the environment and loss of nutrient availability, with a subsequent increase in toxicity and deficiency. It is aggravated by genetic and hereditary factors in each person.

When these subtle early warning signs are ignored, the degenerative, inflammatory, and metabolic imbalances begin to affect single organs or entire body systems. The ensuing symptoms are then classified and treated as a specific disease.

In his book *Brain Allergies*, Dr. William Philpott describes the degenerative disease state:

The different diseases we all know are named according to the specific tissues inflamed, the particular metabolic symptoms interfered with, the secondary invading opportunitistic organisms involved, the behavioral symptoms displayed, or the specific gland which is disordered.

Common Degenerative Diseases

In a report on chemical sensitivity to the New Jersey State Department of Health prepared in 1989, Dr. Nicholas Ashford and Dr. Claudia Miller document many correlations between the allergy/sensitivity/maladaption process and subsequent degenerative or autoimmune diseases.

ABUSE OF/ADDICTION TO TOBACCO, ALCOHOL, AND FOOD

Dr. Theron Randolph in 1980 defined obesity and alcoholism as "similar illnesses, one dealing with addicting foods in their edible form and the other in their potable form."

In 1980, Dr. Philpott observed that after a two- to three-week abstinence from tobacco use, about 10 percent of his schizophrenia patients had psychotic episodes following reintroduction to tobacco smoke. Tobacco is a member of the nightshade food family along with eggplant, potato, tomato, and green peppers. Addictions are usually to the food component of the substances to which a person is allergic.

Blood Dysfunctions

A type of eosinophilia (increase in leukocytes) with accompanying muscle pain, insomnia, and fatigue is seen frequently in allergic people.

In 1962, Dr. D. Heiner reported in the *American Journal of Diseases in Children* that allergy to cow's milk resulted in anemia.

Cardiovascular Disease

Higher histamine levels have been found in the coronary arteries of cardiac patients (reported in *Science* by S. Kalsner and R. Richards, in 1984).

In clinical practice, we have observed a number of patients with arrhythmias, palpitations, edema, and increased pulse rates after exposure to foods, chemicals, inhalants, or hormone fluctuations or during testing sessions. These abnormalities dramatically subsided with neutralizing doses of the offending substance. One woman patient experienced an increase of 40–50 points in her systolic blood pressure and 10–20 points on the diastolic reading when she ingested rice. Repeated exposures and resulting inflammatory reactions like these will eventually lead to biochemical dysfunction of the cardiovascular tissue. This damage is also caused by unresolved kinin release and inflammation.

Chronic Fatigue Syndrome

Dr. Jesse Stoff, in his book *Chronic Fatigue*, implicates allergic responses as contributing factors in the baffling syndrome of chronic fatigue. In environmental clinical practices, this debilitating syndrome is a predominant complaint.

Dr. Randolph demonstrated, in 1944, many abnormal lymphocytes in the blood of chronic allergic patients, similar to white blood cells seen in mononucleosis.

Robert A. Buist recently reported that a great majority of chronic fatigue syndrome (CFS) patients had been or are being exposed to environmental pollution, causing damage to the lipid (fat) component of red blood cells and lymphocytes. S.E. Strauss and colleagues reported that up to 75 percent of CFS patients had pre-existing inhalant, food, chemical, or drug allergies.

Dermatologic Disorders

Food challenges given to patients with atopic dermatitis (eczema) not only worsened the rash but also triggered gastrointestinal and respiratory symptoms in a study done by A. Burks and colleagues.

Dermatitis herpetiformis is associated with gluten sensitivity. A number of allergists recognize that urticaria (raised, itchy skin patches) can be caused by foods and food additives, but are hesitant to accept that chemical contacts can also cause some forms of urticaria. Delayed-pressure urticaria has been seen to occur with food challenges and to clear with fasting. Secondary skin rashes have also been noted in cases of sensitivity to molds and fungi.

Ear, Eye, Nose and Throat Disorders

Repeated inflammation of throat and eustachian tube tissues because of allergenic foods, such as milk, is known to cause recurrent otitis media (middle ear inflammation) in children. Natural gas exposure can also cause this disorder.

Chronic sinusitis with accompanying debilitating headaches is caused by tissue reactivity to the presence of molds.

In a challenge study, F. LaMarte and colleagues demonstrated a six-fold increase in plasma histamine release and observed a swollen larynx in a patient exposed to the manufacture of carbonless paper.

Ear, nose and throat specialists repeatedly see chronic inflammatory tissue damage in sinusitis, as well as vertigo, hearing loss, ringing in the ears, Meniere's syndrome, nasal obstruction, adenitis (lymph gland inflammation), and salivary gland enlargement as a result of untreated allergies.

Endocrine Dysfunction

Dr. Phyllis Saifer implicated untreated allergy in autoimmune thyroiditis.

The relationship between the stress of chronic allergy states and hypoadrenalism is also well-known. Traditional allergists commonly treat this disorder by administering cortisone to boost the function of already exhausted adrenal glands. This practice is not without severe side-effects. Early, proper management of allergies would make this type of treatment unnecessary.

Doctors D. Spraque, W. Rea, and C. Mabray found that many premenstrual abnormalities improved following adequate allergy management.

Gastrointestinal Disorders

Food sensitivity has been clearly linked to enteropathy (disease of the intestinal tract), such as gluten reactivity relating to celiac disease and milk sensitivity to small, white blisters in the mouth. Dr. Ronald Finn has recently implicated sensitivity to baker's and brewer's yeast in Crohn's disease.

Dr. J. Siegel found a higher incidence of accompanying hay fever, eczema, and asthma in patients with inflammatory bowel disease. For these patients, when the other systemic allergic responses were treated, the bowel syndrome was controlled. Cortisone injections reduce the symptoms, thus indicating further that an allergic response is active. Irritable bowel syndrome will often improve when common allergenic foods, such as milk, soy, wheat, corn, or sugar, are either eliminated or rotated in the diet, and when immunotherapy is utilized.

In 1949, allergy was also implicated in chronic ulcerative colitis by A. Rowe in a report in the *Annals of Allergy*.

Gynecological Disorders

The methyl xanthine contained in coffee, colas, tea, chocolate, and Theophylline (used to treat asthmatics) causes a common sensitivity response in some women, known as fibrocystic breast disease.

Infectious Diseases

Recurrent viral, fungal, or bacterial illnesses occur more frequently in allergic persons because the chronic stress imposed by the allergy state impairs and stresses the immune function that is designed to protect the body from invasion of pathogenic organisms.

The hyperpermeable ("leaky") gut and respiratory tract, due to continual irritation from histamine, serotonin, and leukotriene production and release, allows easier entry for organisms. Damaged skin surfaces in allergic rashes and eczema also allow easier access for microorganisms.

Kidney and Urological Diseases

Cystitis and urinary bleeding often result from allergies to the more common foods, especially wheat and dairy products. Untreated wheat and milk allergies have led to irreversible glomerulonephritis (kidney disease). R. Finn, in *Clinical Nephrology* in 1980, reported renal (kidney) damage caused by occupational exposure to hydrocarbons.

METABOLIC DISORDERS

Liver dysfunction is associated with allergy, sensitivity, and intolerance to drugs, alcohol, and chemicals.

Dr. William Philpott, in his book, *Brain Allergies,* describes the progression from hypoglycemia to diabetes mellitus in the following way: (1) Acute allergic reaction involving the pancreas and/or liver, (2) several years of adaptive addictive adjustment with the consequences of episodic hypoglycemia, (3) metabolic failure by fatigue and/or exhaustion of the adaptive stage of the body resulting in a degeneration of the pancreas, and the logical onset of diabetes mellitus.

Gallbladder disease (including stones) is usually aggravated by repeated exposure to allergenic foods.

NEUROLOGICAL DYSFUNCTIONS

High levels of insulin have been shown to cause brain wave changes in electroencephalograms (EEGs), which may account for behavioral changes in some allergic persons with diabetic disorders.

In 1980, an article in *Lancet* reported that two-thirds of migraine sufferers are allergic to certain foods. Often, the implicated food relieves a headache because of the addictive response described by Dr. Theron Randolph.

Some seizure disorders, including gait changes, slurred speech, tremors, and petit mal are initiated by exposure to foods and chemicals even when minute amounts are administered during allergy testing. Dr. Marshall Mandell has videotaped these types of symptoms during allergy testing.

Symptoms of multiple sclerosis can subside after the removal of mercury amalgam fillings. Sensitivity to the amalgam stems from the mercury content as well as other metal components. Symptoms of multiple sclerosis also improve after treatment of food, chemical, and inhalant allergies.

PSYCHOLOGICAL AND BEHAVIORAL DISORDERS

Dr. Randolph clearly denotes the adaptive, stimulatory, and withdrawal effects of all allergens on psychiatric symptoms.

Dr. Philpott, a psychiatrist, described maladaptive emotional reactions to allergens ranging from "mild central nervous system symptoms such as anxiety, dizziness, weakness, and depression to dissociation, paranoid delusions, and visual and auditory hallucination."

RHEUMATOLOGIC DISORDERS

In his book *Nutritional Therapy,* Dr. Jonathan Wright includes allergy as a prominent, causative factor in rheumatoid arthritis. Some clinics have demonstrated relief of joint swelling, pain, and movement loss following carefully monitored fasts. Symptoms returned with deliberate food challenges.

Dr. Randolph also includes the inflammatory disease syndromes of ankylosing spondylitis (spinal stiffness), osteoarthritis, Reiter's syndrome, and other forms of arthritis in the same category as allergy-induced rheumatoid arthritis. Sensitivity to a variety of chemicals and foods has also been implicated in cases of lupus erythematosis.

The Goal of Treatment

The aim of this discussion is not to oversimplify complicated medical conditions, but rather to look beyond obvious symptoms and classifications, to ferret out the subtle nuances of early warning signs, and to uncover underlying causes that lead to degenerative diseases.

The goal of treatment should be diagnosing the basic biochemical and metabolic dysfunctions, and using all possible measures to restore the rhythm and balance of our body to achieve and maintain health. Dr. Philpott refers to lifestyle changes as ". . . giving promise of reducing or eliminating the disease process," rather than using only palliative measures to treat the symptoms. This approach does not diminish the science or art of healing disease, but will enhance and augment our human capacity to grow, develop, and adapt to our environment in constructive and creative ways.

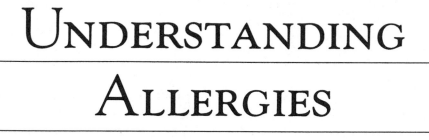

PART 2

UNDERSTANDING

ALLERGIES

TESTING AND MEDICAL TREATMENT

There are numerous methods of allergy testing. The accuracy of any test depends on the skill and competence of the technician, laboratory, or physician. Below is an overview of several commonly used tests.

Fasting and Deliberate
Food Testing

This method involves four- to seven-day fasts and then reintroducing foods, one at a time, to observe any resulting symptoms. Although this can be done at home, fasts are not safe for everyone, and withdrawal symptoms from foods can be severe. This type of food testing is best done under medical supervision if a person has multiple or incapacitating symptoms.

The foods used in the test meals must be free of chemical contaminants and prepared with no seasonings so as not to confuse results. Only one food (no mixtures) must be used at a time. Meals should be spaced three hours apart, and testing must be completed in ten days. Smoking is not allowed during the testing.

When done properly, this method gives very accurate results. The symptoms experienced when foods are reintroduced offer definite proof to the sensitive individual that a particular food is an offender. Fasting detoxifies the body, unmasks sensitivities, and makes it easier to identify an offending food. However, fasting can be a painful experience for many, and reactions to the reintroduced foods may be severe.

Deliberate food testing can be done without fasting, by eliminating only suspected foods. After four to seven days they are reintroduced one at a time, and symptoms will result if a food is an offender. However, testing foods without a fast is not as accurate, and will not identify any food combinations that are a problem. Also, suspected foods must be eliminated completely, and unless you have carefully studied all sources of a given food, you may inadvertently continue to consume it.

Fasting and deliberate food testing is sometimes performed by a physician in a hospital setting, in special environmentally controlled units. This ensures that the fast is a true one, that the food tested is in pure form, and that there is no negative environmental exposure to confuse results. Medical help is available should symptoms become overwhelming.

The treatment after this type of testing involves avoiding certain foods, or manipulating diet with such tools as a rotary diversified diet. (See "The Rotation Diet," p. 111.)

Deliberate Chemical Testing

A type of deliberate chemical testing, also called the Bronchial Inhalation Challenge, is performed in a chemical testing booth. Unlike the fasting and deliberate food testing, this test cannot be done at home. It must be supervised by a physician in a specially constructed testing booth. The person's pulse, blood pressure, and symptoms are noted before the test, and mental ability is tested.

The person is then exposed, in the booth, to the specially prepared chemical. Neither the person nor the supervisor knows which chemical is being tested. Pulse, blood pressure, and symptoms are again noted, both immediately after the test and 30 minutes later. The tests for mental ability are also repeated at these intervals.

Changes in pulse, blood pressure, symptoms, and test performance will reveal which chemicals are causing problems. Since neither the supervisor nor the person being tested know the identities of the chemicals, personal bias cannot affect the test results.

Treatment involves avoiding chemical exposures and cleaning up the person's environment. Using an air cleaner, water purifier, and charcoal mask may also be helpful.

Pulse Test

The pulse test involves taking a resting pulse, eating a certain food or being exposed to a particular substance, and then taking the pulse again after 30 minutes. An increase or decrease in pulse rate indicates a sensitivity to the substance being tested. Smoking, snacking, and chewing gum must be avoided during testing. The pulse is taken several times a day for two to three days before the test in order to establish a baseline average pulse.

Before testing, obtain a resting pulse. Sit quietly for ten minutes, then take the pulse. For the pulse test, suspected foods should be eaten singly and in pure form. Frequently eaten and favorite foods should also be tested. The pulse should have returned to normal for at least one hour before testing the next food.

One advantage of this test is that it can be done at home. Generally speaking, it is safe, and, of course, it is free. However, one must take care that physical or emotional activities and responses do not affect the results. Exposure to chemicals can also undermine its accuracy.

For some, however, the pulse test will not be helpful. Some people—those who are not "pulse changers"—will not experience significant pulse change even when exposed to substances to which they are quite sensitive. Also, those whose pulse is difficult to determine, even by trained medical personnel, will not be able to use this test. For those who are able to identify food allergies through the pulse test, treatment again involves avoidance of problem foods and diet manipulation. A rotary diversified diet may be helpful if numerous foods produce reactions.

The pulse test may also be used to identify allergies to chemicals. Problems with general chemical levels in large areas, buildings, rooms, and cars may be identified in this way. It is more difficult to discover sensitivity to a single chemical, because exposure must be limited to only one chemical.

Avoiding chemicals and cleaning up one's environment are possible treatments following this testing method. Using an air cleaner, water filters, and charcoal mask may also help.

Reactions to pollens may also be tested by the pulse method when one can be sure which pollen or group of pollens is causing the pulse change. Treatment may include the use of an air cleaner and mask to filter out the pollens.

Kinesiology Testing

Kinesiology can be applied in a form of muscle testing for allergies to foods, chemicals, inhalants, and other substances. The person being tested holds the test substance in one hand (enclosed in a container so that the identity of the substance is not known during the testing), and the tester pushes on the other outstretched arm. If the tester is able to push the arm down with less resistance while the test substance is held, the person being tested is considered to be allergic or sensitive to the substance. If the tester cannot push the arm down, or can do so only with great force, the person undergoing testing is considered not to be reactive to the substance.

The accuracy of this test depends on the skill of the tester. Some practitioners are very skilled and can obtain reproducible results, while others are unable to do so.

The treatments used with this type of testing involve avoiding the problem substance, manipulating diet, cleaning up one's environment, and taking homeopathic remedies.

Cytotoxic Testing

The cytotoxic test is a blood test for foods (and some chemicals) in which live white cells from the patient are mixed with a food antigen. The white cells will show various types of deterioration if the person is sensitive to the food being tested. If one is not sensitive or allergic to the substance, there will be no change in the white cells.

The cytotoxic test gives immediate, objective results, and detects masked sensitivities. However, it is expensive and will sometimes show a false negative result if the food has not been eaten for several months. The skill of the

person reading the slides also affects its accuracy. Cytotoxic testing has been found to be very accurate for some people, while less so for others.

Avoiding the offending food and manipulating diet are the treatments used after cytotoxic testing.

RAST

The Radioallergosorbent Test is a blood test in which IgE and IgG antibodies are labelled with a radioactive substance. The amount of antibody found in the blood in response to a given food, pollen, mold, dust/dust mite, or dander can then be measured with a Geiger-counter type of instrument. For the RAST to be accurate for foods, both IgE and IgG must be measured. Sometimes it will yield false negatives if a food has not been eaten recently.

The RAST can test for sensitivities to a large number of substances in a short period of time. Extracts for immunotherapy can be made using the testing results. The RAST is objective, and the only trauma to the patient is the taking of the blood sample. But besides being expensive, this test works only with immunological antibodies; it cannot identify problem substances for which there is no antigen-antibody response.

Antigen Leukocyte Cellular Antibody Testing (ALCAT)

This method uses a Coulter Counter to count and size white blood cells, granulocytes, lymphocytes, and platelets in blood samples. The counting is done before and after a person's serum and white cells (red cells are lysed) are incubated with a food- or mold-impregnated disc. Changes in cell size and numbers are noted, and a certain percentage of change signals a problem reaction to the food or mold.

Treatments include avoidance of problem foods and diet manipulation. Controlling all molds in their environment is the best approach for mold-sensitive people. Further testing of problem foods or molds by another method must be done if extracts are needed for immunotherapy.

Scratch or Prick Test

In this test, a drop of concentrated antigen is placed on the skin, which is then pricked or scratched so that a minute amount of antigen is absorbed. Growth of a wheal surrounded by erythema (inflammation) indicates a response to a problem substance. If a sensitive person has high IgE levels, the scratch or prick test will accurately determine allergy to pollens, molds, dust, dust mite, and animal dander. However, if IgE levels are low, there may not be a wheal—indicating an allergy—even if the person tested is sensitive to these inhalants.

Extracts may be made for immunotherapy from test results obtained by this method. However, the doses are chosen arbitrarily by the physician. Immunotherapy begins with a small dose, building up over a period of time until a protective dose is reached. It often takes a year to reach protective doses, and many individuals become sensitive to the glycerine and phenol that may be used as a stabilizer and preservative in these extracts.

When the scratch test is used for food testing, only food allergies for which the person has an extremely high IgE level will be uncovered by this test. Since over 85 percent of food allergy is non-IgE mediated, this type of testing cannot give an accurate picture of a person's food problems. The scratch test also cannot be used for testing chemicals, since most chemical reactions are not IgE mediated.

Patch Test

This test is used to diagnose contact allergies. A patch with an antigen on it is applied to the skin and is left in place for 24–48 hours. If lesions, a rash, erythema (inflammation), or hardness of the skin under the patch occur, this shows a problem reaction. Avoiding problem substances and topical palliative treatment are considered the best treatment possibilities with this method of testing.

EAV Testing

While electroacupuncture testing is being used extensively and successfully in Europe, it is conducted on only a limited and experimental basis in North America. Testing is done on an instrument (such as Vega, Dermatron, or Vitel) that measures galvanic skin response. A vial containing a suspected allergen is placed in a receptacle in the instrument. The person being tested then holds a probe from the instrument in one hand while the tester uses a second probe to touch acupuncture points on the fingers of the person's other hand. An electrical circuit is thus completed between the person being tested and the measuring device. Any change from the calibration number on the meter indicates a problem reaction.

The accuracy of this test depends on the skill of the tester. Foods, chemicals, inhalants, and many other substances can be tested in this way, and it is a rapid, painless method of diagnosis. Extracts for immunotherapy can be made based on the results of EAV testing, or homeopathic extracts can be used.

Serial Dilution Endpoint Titration

This test is similar to traditional skin testing but goes a step further. Antigens diluted serially (1:5, 1:25, 1:125, and so on) are used for this test. First, a weak antigen dose is injected under the skin. If the wheal grows two millimeters or more, it is considered a problem reaction. More injections are given (of either weaker or stronger dilutions, depending on the size of the first wheal) until a whealing pattern is obtained. This pattern is called progressive whealing. The lowest concentration that produces a two-millimeter wheal growth is considered the treatment dose (endpoint). The wheal produced by the next stronger dilution must be two millimeters or more larger than the first positive wheal. The wheal produced by the next weaker dilution should not grow.

Treatment extracts can be made based on this accurately determined treatment dose. Relief from symptoms is immediate when the extract is administered because of its precise dose. We have found this method to be very accurate for testing inhalants in those individuals with high IgE levels. However, results for food and chemical allergies tested by this method are not accurate.

Provocative Neutralization Testing

This test may be performed either intradermally (under the skin) or sublingually (under the tongue) to identify problem foods, chemicals, and inhalants. Each involves the use of antigens serially diluted at a 1:5 ratio.

In intradermal provocative tests, baseline symptoms are noted, and an antigen is injected under the skin. The wheal is measured immediately after injection and again in ten minutes,

when symptoms are again noted. A problem reaction is recognized where there is wheal growth and/or symptom change. Progressively weaker dilutions are then injected to discover a dose that relieves the symptoms and produces a negative wheal. The relieving dose is called a neutralizing dose, and treatment extracts are based on this amount. Taking the extracts on a regular basis prevents, blocks, or neutralizes reactions to the problem substance.

For sublingual provocative tests, the pulse is taken and baseline symptoms are also noted. The test antigen is then placed behind the teeth, under the tongue, where it is rapidly absorbed by the sublingual blood vessels. In ten minutes the pulse is measured again and symptoms are recorded. A problem reaction is noted if there are symptom changes and/or a change in the pulse. Progressively weaker dilutions are given until the pulse returns to its original level, or stabilizes, and the provoked symptoms clear. Again, the relieving dose is called a neutralizing dose, and extracts can be made and used to control problem reactions.

When this test is used (intradermally or sublingually) to determine sensitivity to foods, the food should be eaten within 48 hours of the testing session. Chemicals may also be tested in this way. Intradermal provocative neutralization is also very effective for testing inhalants on those with pollen reactivity symptoms and low IgE levels.

The challenge dose for provocative testing may be given nasally. Here a minute amount of powdered antigen is inhaled from the end of a toothpick in order to provoke symptoms. The neutralizing dose is then found by completing the test with intradermal injections, and extracts are made and used in the same way as for the intradermal test.

In our own clinical experience, we have found provocative neutralization to be a very useful test. Because there is usually more than one test factor—either a wheal and symptoms or the pulse and symptoms—the results are more accurately determined. Vivid symptoms produced help to convince the more reluctant that the test substance is indeed a problem. While some of these symptoms are uncomfortable, even children do well with this method of testing. It is, however, a time-consuming process, and only a few substances can be tested during each session.

Immunotherapy Treatment

Because it is so difficult for the sensitive person to avoid or control exposures to all allergens, we have found immunotherapy treatment using extracts to be very helpful. They are not a panacea to be used instead of diet control and environmental clean-up and control, but rather they are additional aids in the treatment and control of symptoms. Symptom control is desirable, not only from the standpoint of the allergic person's comfort, but also to protect the immune system. If the immune system is constantly stressed by adverse reactions to foods, chemicals, or inhalants, its efficiency decreases over a period of time, and target organ damage can occur. Also, if the immune cascade is allowed to proceed unchecked, tissue damage will follow. Protecting our immune system by the use of extracts allows it to repair and heal.

The following description of immunotherapy assumes the use of extracts based on results from either serial dilution endpoint titration or provocative neutralization tests. In immunotherapy for inhalant allergies, the extracts contain small amounts of antigen, which will cause the body to produce IgG or blocking antibodies. These antibodies block the allergic reactions when the person is exposed to the offending substance. If a person has been tested by serial dilution endpoint titration, the exact treatment dose (endpoint) is found, and relief will be immediate.

Inhalant extracts may be given either by injection or sublingually. There are some for whom greater relief is felt when the extracts are administered by injection. However, most people obtain good relief from and prefer sublingual use of extracts. Adequate control of symptoms is usually achieved by taking the extracts weekly. In the height of pollen season, however, those who are acutely sensitive to pollen may have to take extracts more often. While pollen extracts are generally necessary only during pollen season, some people have better symptom control if they take them year-round.

Because exposures to animals, dust and dust mites, and molds occur throughout the year, extracts for these substances should be taken continually. When the mold count is extremely high, or when molds are sporing, extracts may have to be used more frequently.

If testing has been done by serial dilution endpoint titration, extracts may be taken at home, as needed. This is possible because the exact treatment dose has already been determined, and there is no danger of anaphylactic shock. Over a period of time desensitization to inhalants will take place regardless of whether the extracts are taken by injection or sublingually.

The mechanism behind the neutralizing dose in food and chemical extracts has not yet been determined but several theories exist:

• Blocking antibodies are produced to prevent the reaction.

- T-cells are stimulated to stop B-cells from producing antibodies to the offending substance.
- T-cell levels are increased, thus increasing resistance to various substances.
- Immune complexes are bound so a reaction cannot take place.

Food extracts may be taken either by injection or sublingually. Injections are required every four days, while sublingual doses are usually given before exposure to the offending food. If foods are rotated in the diet, then each sublingual food extract would be needed every four days. If foods are not rotated, food extracts may be required more frequently. Taking food extracts allows individuals to eat problem foods without having symptoms, as well as relieving acute food reactions.

Chemical extracts also may be used either sublingually or by injection. Taking chemical extracts will prevent reactions to chemical exposures, as well as relieving acute reactions. The number and levels of exposure to chemicals determines the frequency with which chemical extracts must be taken.

Those who have low IgE levels and who have been tested for inhalants by provocative neutralization may take their extracts either sub-lingually or by injection. Extracts may be repeated as needed for symptom control. Extracts for foods, chemicals, and inhalants tested by provocative neutralization may also be self-administered. There is no danger of anaphylactic shock with this type of extract.

Regardless of how they work, extracts for food, chemical, and inhalant allergies offer protection and relief from unwanted symptoms. The extracts are not physiologically addictive, as are some medications. Over a period of time, the frequency of use can gradually be reduced if symptoms do not occur. Some people can eventually remain symptom-free on one or two doses per week. Others heal sufficiently to stop treatment altogether.

Food extracts allow those who would be severely nutritionally deprived because of numerous food sensitivities or allergies to have a more varied diet. People who would be confined to their homes in order to avoid chemical exposures can, with chemical extracts and a common-sense approach to exposures, lead normal lives. Inhalant extracts allow individuals to be comfortable during pollen season and to endure exposures to animal dander, dust, and mold without symptoms.

CHAPTER 9

FOOD ALLERGIES

What is Food Allergy?

Food allergy and intolerance to food are not new phenomena. Over 2,000 years ago, Hippocrates described food allergy: "To me it appears...that nobody would have sought for medicine at all, provided the same kind of diet had suited men in sickness and in health." (Hippocrates then described different responses to eating cheese.) He further stated, "Let thy food be thy medicine and thy medicine be thy food." During the same time, Lucretius wrote: "What is food for one, is to others bitter poison." Moses Maimonides (1135–1204) said, "No illness which can be treated by diet should be treated by any other means."

FOOD ALLERGY PIONEERS

In 1905, Francis Hare, an Australian physician, described many aspects of food allergy, including food addiction, obesity, and alcoholism, in his book *The Food Factor in Disease*. However, Hare's interest in the clinical effects of different food groups began earlier, in 1889. Although he did not recognize sensitization to specific foods, his description of allergic manifestations is an important contribution to the concept of food allergy or intolerance.

Dr. Arthur Coca formulated the concept of hypersensitivity, in which an antigen-antibody response does not play a role. He also coined the word "atopy," used to describe reactions mediated by antigens and antibodies. Dr. Coca founded and was the first editor of *The Journal of Immunology*, and he wrote *Familial Nonreaginic Food Allergy*. The layman's version of his concepts was published in *The Pulse Test*. In the 1930s, Dr. Coca discovered that a person's pulse will go up after exposure to an allergenic substance. While not perfect, the pulse test is helpful in determining problem substances.

Dr. Albert Rowe, the father of food allergy, is best known for his elimination diets, which are still important in identifying and treating food allergy. He developed two standardized versions of the elimination diet: the cereal-free elimination diet; and the fruit-free, cereal-free elimination diet. Dr. Rowe wrote six books; the longest, *Clinical Allergy Due to Foods, Inhalants, Contaminants, Fungi, Bacteria and Other Causes*, was published in 1937. His last publication, co-authored with his son, was in 1972.

The phenomenon known as "dumb Monday" was described by Dr. Walter Alvarez when traditional, often repeated, Sunday menus cause symptoms on Monday. Allergic reactions to the foods consumed can cause cerebral edema, headache, mental confusion, and malaise, all of which cause one to feel "dumb" and to function poorly afterwards.

The concepts of masked and unmasked food allergy, cyclic versus fixed food allergy, the deliberate feeding test, and the rotary diversified diet were all developed by Dr. Herbert Rinkel. *Food Allergy*, by Rinkel, Randolph, and Zeller, describes these ideas in detail.

Dr. Theron Randolph, of Chicago, Illinois, was the first to begin taking a detailed, ecologically oriented history, and he initiated the practice of fasting followed by controlled feeding in a hospital setting. Dr. Randolph also developed the concept of allergy/addiction, which can apply to foods, chemicals, or drugs. He proposed the following stages of addiction:

Maladapted	+ + + +	Manic, with or without convulsions
	+ + +	Hypomanic, toxic, anxious, and egocentric
Adapted	+ +	Hyperactive, irritable, hungry, and thirsty
	+	Stimulated but relatively symptom-free
	o	Behavior on an even keel, as in homeostasis
Maladapted localized response	–	Localized allergic responses
Maladapted systemic response	– –	Systemic allergic reponses
Maladapted advanced stimulatory response	– – –	Brain fag, mild depression, and disturbed thinking
	– – – –	Severe depression with or without altered consciousness

(Adapted from *An Alternative Approach to Allergies* by Theron Randolph, MD)

Dr. Randolph believes that food allergy is one of the greatest health problems in North America, and that food/drug combinations are even more addictive than foods alone. Alcoholic beverages are a prime example of the potential for allergy and addiction to a substance that has both food and chemical content. Dr. Randolph also maintains that two-thirds of symptoms diagnosed as psychosomatic are undiagnosed maladaptive reactions to foods, chemicals, and inhalants.

ALLERGY VS SENSITIVITY

Food allergy has traditionally been defined as an antigen-antibody response, or a cell-mediated reaction to food. Food hypersensitivity, on the other hand, occurs when there is an adverse reaction to food but no antigen-antibody response. In this book and in our clinical practice, we consider any adverse response to food to be an equal problem, regardless of whether it is "true allergy" (IgE-mediated) or a hypersensitivity reaction. A sensitive person cannot wait until all of the immunological mechanisms have been determined in laboratory analysis and double-blind studies before receiving treatment.

FACTORS IN FOOD ALLERGY

Over the last few decades, food allergy has become an increasing problem in North America. Not long ago, food variety was limited for most families, with the usual exposure being about 40 different items. Today, with refrigeration, quick freezing, and other food preserving techniques, our food choices are almost unlimited. Some people eat a wide variety of foods, while others limit themselves to 10 to 15 recipes which they use repeatedly.

The discouraging of breast feeding and the substitution of cow's milk or commercial formulas has fostered several generations of food allergic people. Dr. Coca believed that 90 percent of the population had food allergies, while others estimate the number of food intolerant people in North America at 60 percent of the population. The belief that children outgrow their allergies is untrue—food sensitivity in adults occurs in direct proportion to age. There are more multiple food allergies in boys than in girls. This pattern reverses in adulthood, when multiple food allergy becomes more common in women than men.

Other factors that affect both the incidence and severity of food allergies include altitude, emotional stress, hormonal imbalances, infections, metabolic diseases, seasons, and nutritional imbalances. Heredity and race also play a role in food allergy. Dr. John Gerrard of Canada has traced milk allergy through five generations; Blacks, American Indians, and Orientals have a higher incidence of milk intolerance.

TYPES OF FOOD ALLERGIES AND REACTIONS

Food allergy may be classified in several different ways. Rinkel used the terms cyclic and fixed in relation to food allergy. A cyclic food allergy is one that worsens with repeated exposure; total avoidance reinstates tolerance. For some, it will take only a few months to reestablish tolerance to a problem food; for others it may take years. Most food allergies are cyclic— once the food can again be tolerated, resensi-

tization can be prevented by avoiding overexposure to the food as it is added back into the diet. New sensitivities can be prevented by spacing exposures to all foods.

If reexposure to a food still provokes symptoms after it has been totally avoided for two years, the food allergy is considered to be fixed or permanent. Eating the food will always cause a reaction unless food extracts are taken to prevent or block the symptoms.

Food reactions are also classified as:

- *Occult* (hidden): Pathology (damage) is caused, but no symptoms are obvious.
- *Immediate*: Symptoms are obvious within minutes.
- *Delayed*: Symptoms may not appear until the next day, or several days later.
- *Thermal*: Symptoms occur after ingestion of a specific food followed by exposure to cold, heat, or light.

Immediate reactions are generally mediated by an antibody known as IgE. Food particles, either proteins or peptides (parts of protein) are absorbed through the wall of the gastrointestinal tract, unaffected by digestion. The body recognizes these undigested food particles as foreign molecules and so produces antibodies (immunoglobulin IgE). When these antibodies combine with the antigen, allergy mediators such as histamine are released from the mast cells, producing immediate symptoms.

Immediate symptoms include urticaria (hives), wheezing, eczema, rhinitis, swelling of the lips and face, or anaphylactic shock. These reactions are easily recognized as being precipitated by a specific food, since they are acute, obvious and sometimes dramatic. Every year deaths are attributed to anaphylactic shock stemming from food reactions. However, these reactions are usually to foods such as peanuts or shellfish, and are the exception rather than the rule. Food reactions are generally uncomfortable but not fatal.

A delayed food reaction is usually mediated by IgG antibodies, and the majority of food allergies fall into this category. IgG antibodies against protein can usually be detected in the blood during a delayed food reaction. Symptoms include: chronic headaches (frequently migraine); chronic indigestion or heartburn; fatigue; depression; failure to thrive; joint pain or arthritic-type symptoms; recurrent abdominal pain; canker sores; chronic respiratory symptoms, like wheezing or bronchitis; nocturnal enuresis (bedwetting); and bowel problems such as colitis, diarrhea, or constipation. This type of food reaction is frequently misdiagnosed and often untreated, because it is difficult to link the symptoms with any event or food. Food testing is imperative in order to diagnose this type of food allergy.

Adverse food reactions can also be caused by small molecules other than proteins or peptides, which form free radicals or act directly on tissues as though they were drugs.

When a person experiences symptoms from an offending food, partial relief may be obtained by eating the same food again. Many are surprised to learn they are sensitive to common foods like coffee, sugar, wheat, eggs, corn, or milk. They may insist that the physician or test results are wrong, because the substance in question is the one they use to ease their worst symptoms whenever they occur. Many report cravings for problem foods, and say they always feel better when they eat it. They experience withdrawal symptoms if they stop eating the food regularly.

This phenomenon is an allergy/addiction combined with a masked food allergy. One is unaware of the sensitivity because eating the problem food makes one feel better. When the food is eaten regularly, masking occurs, with chronic and low-grade symptoms. Constant postnasal drip, afternoon headaches or sleepy spells, or "spaciness" may be the only evidence of the problem. Avoiding the food (or chemical) for four to 10 days will unmask the allergy, and subsequent reexposure to the food will cause acute symptoms.

Allergic responses can be unpredictable, however; a person may sometimes tolerate a food that at other times would provoke symptoms. Total load is the determining factor in this case. When allergens, stress factors, or infection have created an overload, the person will be unable to tolerate the problem food. When the body's total load is small, the food can be consumed with no reaction. Low-sensitivity foods can sometimes be tolerated separately, but not when eaten together.

ALLERGENICITY OF FOODS

All foods can cause reactions, but some are more potent allergens than others. Protein foods are more allergenic than nonprotein foods, as proteins are more difficult to digest than fats or carbohydrates. If digestion of proteins is not complete, the molecule absorbed into the bloodstream is too large. The immune system recognizes the large molecule as a foreign substance rather than a nutrient and sets up a chain reaction to destroy the supposed invader. An allergic person must determine the cause of incomplete or disrupted digestion and absorption of food. Common causes include:

- Low stomach acid.
- Insufficient pancreatic enzyme production.
- Improper levels of bicarbonate in the small intestine.
- Infections of parasitic, bacterial, fungal, or

viral organisms.
- Irritation of intestinal lining as a result of long-term untreated food sensitivities.
- Stomach or duodenal ulcerations.
- Nutritional imbalances.
- Disordered amino acid metabolism as in the case of candidiasis.

If breakdown of ingested protein is inadequate, an amino acid deficiency can result, despite adequate levels of high-quality protein in our diet. The consequences may be difficulty or inability of our body to produce adequate levels of enzymes, hormones, antibodies, and immune factors. This becomes a vicious circle because adequate enzymes will not be available to digest the next ingested protein.

Meats, grains, vegetables, and fruits, in this decreasing order, tend to be fixed allergies. The allergenicity of foods is affected by the following:
- *Cooking*: Will reduce allergenicity by half.
- *Heating foods in oils*: Slows their absorption rate and reduces reactions.
- *Purity*: Foods contaminated by additives, pesticides, antibiotics, bacteria, and hormones can cause problems, while pure foods do not.
- *Prescription drugs*: Can provoke reactions to normally "safe" foods.

Cross-reactivity between foods and pollens can heighten symptoms for some people. Bananas, watermelon, zucchini, honeydew, cucumber, and other members of the gourd family cross-react with ragweed pollen, which means their allergy-producing proteins are identical. As a result, a person who is sensitive to ragweed could react with symptoms the first time he or she consumes watermelon, cucumber, or bananas. Birch pollen cross-reacts with potatoes, carrots, celery, hazelnuts and apples.

CONCOMITANT AND SYNERGISTIC FOODS

A concomitant food is one that causes reactions when another allergen, such as a chemical or a particulate inhalant (pollen, dust, or mold) is present. For example, if milk, milk products, or mint are consumed while ragweed is pollinating, one may experience an allergic reaction. However, the person may not react to any of these foods when ragweed is not in season. Reactions to a concomitant food can occur up to six weeks after the pollen season is over.

A synergistic reaction is one that occurs to two foods eaten within the same meal. For example, a person may experience an allergic reaction when corn and banana are eaten together, but not when they are eaten separately. Often, when people who are careful with their diets still have reactions, it is because they are eating synergistic foods.

Proven Synergistic Foods

Corn and banana
Beef and yeast (baker's, brewer's, malt)
Cane sugar and orange
Milk and mint
Egg and apple
Pork and black pepper

Possible Synergistic Foods
(identified but not verified)

Wheat and tea
Pork and chicken
Milk and chocolate
Cola and chocolate
Coffee and cola
Coffee and chocolate

Substance or Condition	Proven Concomitant Foods
Trees	
Cedar, juniper	Beef, yeasts (baker's, brewer's, malt)
Cottonwood	Lettuce
Elm	Milk, mint
Oak	Egg, apple
Pecan, hickory	Corn, banana
Mesquite	Cane sugar, orange
Grasses: All	Legumes: beans, peas, soybean, cottonseed oil
	Grains: wheat, corn, rye, barley, oats, rice, millet
Weeds	
Ragweed, short and western	Egg
Ragweed, giant	Milk, mint
Sage	Potato, tomato
Amaranth family (pigweed, carelessweed)	Pork, black pepper
Marshelder	Wheat
Dust	Oysters, clams, scallops
Candida	Cheeses, mushrooms, vinegar and other fermented or molded foods
Cystic breast disease	Coffee, chocolate, cola
Poison ivy	Pork, black pepper
Viral infection	Milk, mint, onion, chocolate, nuts

Substance	Possible Concomitant Foods (identified but not verified)
Weeds	
Marshelder	Tea
Chenopods (goosefoot family, such as lamb's quarters, firebush, Russian thistle, shadscale, and winterfat)	Egg, corn
Dust	Nuts
Influenza vaccine	Onion

(Adapted from a compilation by Dr. Dor W. Brown, Jr., Fredericksburg, Texas.)

DISEASE SYMPTOMS ASSOCIATED WITH FOODS

There are many symptoms that are linked to specific foods.

- *Asthma:* Can be triggered by almost any food allergen. Egg, milk, seafood, peanuts, chocolate, corn, and nuts are common offenders.
- *Colitis:* Most frequently linked to milk, although it can be caused by wheat, corn, egg, chocolate, and nuts. Dr. Abram Ber of Phoenix, Arizona, believes that next to milk, tomatoes are the most important food to eliminate from the diets of those with colitis.
- *Nocturnal enuresis (bedwetting):* Again, milk is the most frequent offender, followed by wheat, corn, egg, orange, and chocolate. Constipation also plays a role in bedwetting.
- *Duodenal ulcer:* Milk is the major cause. Unfortunately, in the past, the most common treatment for ulcers was to drink milk, which only exacerbates the problem.
- *Arthritis:* Arthritic pain and joint involvement are linked to sugar, wheat, pork, and the nightshade family, including tomatoes, potatoes, bell pepper, eggplant, chili pepper, tobacco, and pimentos. According to Dr. Jonathan Wright of Kent, Washington, the nightshade family must be avoided for six to nine months in order to determine the role of these foods in arthritis.
- *Recurrent upper respiratory infections:* Linked to food allergy, which causes the mucus membranes to become swollen. This makes it easy for microorganisms to begin colonizing the damaged mucus membranes. The offending foods can be many and varied, but milk, egg, corn, and wheat are common.
- *Recurrent ear infections:* Many children have recurrent ear infections, which begin with an allergic response very similar to that in upper respiratory infections. Almost any frequently eaten food, or a natural gas exposure, can trigger this reaction but milk is the prime culprit.
- *Bulemia:* Certain foods have been found to cause cravings in bulemic individuals.
- *Bad breath:* Can be caused by an allergy to any food. Candidiasis is also suspect in cases of chronic bad breath.
- *Eczema:* Frequently due to a food allergy. In children, milk should be suspected first, although eczema can be triggered by many other foods.
- *Hives:* May be caused by reactions to chemicals or foods. Peanuts, eggs, shellfish, tomatoes, chocolate, nuts, spices, milk, and food additives are frequently to blame.
- *Hyperactivity:* Due to food or food additive allergy. Sugars are a major cause.
- *Headaches and migraines:* May be triggered by foods or chemicals. Allergy to almost any food can cause a migraine; eggs, wheat, milk, chocolate, corn, cinnamon, wine, pork, and nuts are common offenders.
- *Obesity:* Hypoglycemia often occurs after food allergens are consumed, triggering uncontrollable hunger and eating to stop the hypoglycemia. Frequent overeating causes weight gain. Any food can trigger hypoglycemic symptoms.
- Other symptoms of food allergy include acne, eye pain, conjunctivitis, restless legs, fatigue, excessive perspiration, abnormal body odor, learning disorders, and depression.

The symptoms of food reactions are many and varied. This list includes only a few of the possibilities. While any system in the body can be affected, most sensitive people have a target organ that is usually stricken when an allergic

Relative Degrees of Allergenicity of Foods

Foods Causing Reactions:

Most commonly	*Often*	*Sometimes*	*Seldom*
corn	alcohol	alfalfa	apricot
eggs	apple	amaranth	beet
milk	bacon	banana	carrot
soy	bean, dried	barley (malt)	cranberry
sugar	beef	celery	grape
wheat	berries	cherry	honey
yeast	buckwheat	chicken	lamb
	cheese	chiles	peach
	chocolate	cloves	rabbit
	cinnamon	cottonseed	salmon
	coconut	garlic	salt
	coffee	lobster	squash
	fish	melon	sweet potato
	lettuce	mushroom	tapioca
	mustard	oat	taro root
	nuts	oysters	tea
	onion	pear	vanilla
	orange (citrus)	peppers	
	peanut	pineapple	
	peas	plums/prunes	
	pork	quinoa	
	potato	rice	
	raisin	sesame seed	
	rye	spices	
	shrimp	spinach	
	tomato	strawberry	
		sunflower	
		turkey	
		vinegar	

Odors and handling of any food material can also cause symptoms.
(Adapted from Dr. Doris Rapp and Dr. Del Stigler.)

reaction takes place. For some, there may be itching in the eyes. The stomach may be a target organ for others with nausea, belching, heartburn, or vomiting accompanying their reactions. The intestinal tract may also be a target organ, with symptoms of abdominal pain, diarrhea, or mucus in the stool. Cerebral symptoms include confusion, stupor, anger, or depression. Some will experience the same symptoms each time they have a food reaction, regardless of which food is eaten. Others will report different symptoms for each allergenic food.

Common Allergenic Foods

Testing for problem foods is an important part of allergy diagnosis for all sensitive individuals. The foods listed below are so common that it is almost impossible to avoid them completely. One may control exposures to these foods when eating at home, but when dining out it is *very* difficult to avoid them.

As a first priority, the seven basic foods for which all sensitive persons should be tested are: wheat, yeast, corn, soy, eggs, milk, and sugar.

The following foods should be tested as a secondary priority: beef, pork, chicken, tomato, and potato.

Testing for foods other than those mentioned above is recommended if they cause symptoms, or if they are eaten more than twice per week. A food which is seldom or never eaten generally does not need to be tested.

The following section lists the various possible exposures to common allergens. As you will see, food allergens occur not only in the foods we eat but also in soaps, medications, nutritional supplements, cosmetics, cookware, glues, toothpaste, alcoholic beverages, paper, paints, printing inks, and many plastics. Therefore, simply limiting exposures to foods by "rotating" them (eating a food or any form of that food only once every four days) may not be enough protection for a hypersensitive person. Food extracts provide needed protection against unavoidable and accidental exposures to these foods.

Wheat

Wheat is the staple grain in North America. While there are over 30,000 varieties of wheat, only one is grown for consumption here, referred to as spring wheat or winter wheat, depending on when the seed is planted. Wheat is classified as hard or soft, depending on the amount of gluten in the grain. Hard common wheat is ten to thirteen percent gluten and is difficult to mill. Soft common wheat is six to ten percent gluten, contains more starch, and is more easily milled. Hard durum wheat, also called semolina, is the hardest wheat of all. It represents only five percent of the total wheat

crop of North America.

Wheat contains more gluten than any other grain. Gluten is a water-soluble mixture of sticky proteins. When wheat is made into a dough, the sticky property of gluten traps gas bubbles from the leavening agents and causes the dough to rise. Rye, barley, and oats contain some gluten, while corn, rice, and millet contain none.

Gluten intolerance is known as celiac disease or non-tropical sprue. Various theories exist to explain its cause, including missing enzymes to process gluten, a metabolic error, or an immunological disorder. Gluten intolerance can appear at any age and is a lifetime disorder.

Total avoidance of gluten is necessary for the control of gluten intolerance. Unfortunately, gluten is difficult to avoid in processed foods. It is used as a starch, binder, formulation aid, emulsific filler, bulking agent, stabilizer, shaper, thickener, and glaze, and as an aid for forming tablets. Because of these uses, even foods labeled "wheat-free" may contain gluten. (Some celiacs do not tolerate millet.) Symp-toms of gluten intolerance are malabsorption, irritable bowel syndrome, diarrhea, pale malodorous stool, nausea, vomiting, poor appetite, headache, pallor, anemia, weight loss, skin rash or scaling, muscle spasms, and joint pain.

The following is a partial list of sources of wheat/gluten. It is best to read labels carefully before purchasing an item and to inquire about food content in restaurants when you are in doubt.

Food Sources of Wheat

Alcoholic beverages (including beer, gin, whiskey)
Baby foods (some)
Barley malt
Batter-fried foods
Biscuits
Bisquick
Bologna
Bouillon
Bran
Bread, unless labelled wheat-free
Bread crumbs
"Breaded" products
Bread stuffings
Bulgur
Buns (hot dog and hamburger)
Cakes
Candy
Cereals
Chocolate
Cocoa
Cold cuts
Cookies
Cornbread
Cracker crumbs
Crackers
Cream of wheat

Croutons
Doughnuts
Dumplings
Farina
Flours (wheat flour can be bleached, unbleached, enriched, or unenriched)
Fried food coating
Gluten
Graham crackers and flour
Granola (many contain wheat bran)
Gravies
Hamburger mix
Hamburgers (fast food restaurants may add wheat)
Hot dogs with wheat filler
Ice cream (thickening agents)
Ice cream cones
Liverwurst
Macaroni
Malt products
Malted milk
Matzos
Mayonnaise
Monosodium glutamate (MSG)
Muffins
Noodles
Ovaltine, Postum

Pancake mixes
Pasta
Pastries
Pepper, synthetic
Pies
Pita pockets
Pizza
Popovers
Pretzels
Puddings
Pumpernickel bread
Rolls
Rye bread
Sauces
Sausages
Soups

Soy sauce, tamari
Spaghetti noodles
Tortillas
Vermicelli
Waffles
Wheat germ
Yeasts (some)

Other Sources
Garlic capsules
Hand creams and lotions
Lip gloss
Make-up (many contain wheat germ oil)
Shampoos
Vitamin E
Vitamins

YEAST

Yeast is a widely used ingredient in many foods, medications, and vitamins. Yeast (a one-celled fungus), converts sugars to alcohol and carbon dioxide in a fermentation process. This property of yeast is essential to both bakers and brewers in manufacturing their products. The carbon dioxide causes dough containing gluten to rise; the alcoholic content of beers and liquors results from the fermentation of grains and other substances. Yeasts and molds have common carbohydrates in their cells that may cause cross-reactivity in some hypersensitive people.

Food Sources of Yeast

The following foods contain naturally occurring yeast or yeast-like substances. Yeast may also be added in the manufacturing or preparing process—always be sure to read labels!

Barbecue sauce
Black tea
Bread crumbs
Breads
Bread stuffings

Buns (hot dog and hamburger)
Buttermilk
Cakes and cake mixes
Canned refrigerated biscuits and rolls
Catsup
Cheese (all types, including cottage cheese)
Citric acid (almost always a yeast derivative)
Coffee (regular and instant)
Cookies
Crackers

Doughnuts

Dried fruits of all kinds (dates, figs, prunes, raisins)

Dried roasted nuts

Enriched farina, cornmeal, and corn grits

Fermented beverages of all types:
  Beer
  Brandy
  Gin
  Ginger ale
  Root beer
  Rum
  Whiskey
  Wine
  Vodka

Flour ("enriched" with vitamins made from yeast)

Fruit juices of all types, whether frozen or canned (only homemade are yeast-free)

Grapes (The mold on grapes and thus in grape products may sometimes bother a person allergic to yeast)

Herb teas

Malted products of all types (candy, cereals, malted milk drinks)

Meat, fish, or fowl fried in cracker crumbs or breading

Melons (watermelon, honeydew melon, and especially cantaloupe have mold on the skin surface)

Milk fortified with vitamins

Monosodium glutamate (may be a yeast derivative)

Morels

Mushrooms

Pastries

Peanuts, peanut products

Pistachios

Pizza

Prepared foods containing cheese (such as macaroni and cheese)

Pretzels

Rolls (homemade or canned)

Salt-rising bread

Sour cream

Soy sauce

Spices

Sprouts

Tamari

Torula (a type of yeast used in health foods)

Truffles

Vinegars of all types (apple, distilled, grape, pear)
  Vinegar may also be used in the preparation of the following foods and may not be included on the label.

Baby cereals

Barbecue sauce

Barley cereal

Catsup

Chili and peppers

Horseradish

Mayonnaise

Mincemeat

Mustard

Olives

Pickles

Salad dressings

Sauerkraut

Spices (cinnamon, pepper)

Tomato sauce

Other Sources:

The following items contain substances that are derived from yeast or have yeast as their source.

Antibiotics:
  Chloromycetin
  Lincocin
  Mycin drugs

Penicillin
Tetracyclines
Any others derived from mold cultures
Vitamins (unless otherwise stated on label):

All multiple vitamin capsules, powders
All vitamin B capsules
Tablets containing vitamin B made from yeast

Corn

Corn and maize (the corn species of maize, as distinct from the cattle feed crop called maize) are found in a large variety of foods. Because corn is used in many forms in the preparation of many types of foods, it is the most difficult of common allergenic foods to eliminate from the diet.

Corn may cause allergic symptoms as a contactant (talcs, bath oils and powders, starched clothing, and corn adhesives); as an inhalant (fumes from vegetable forms of corn as they cook); and as an ingestant (corn and corn products that are eaten). Some people can tolerate processed forms of corn such as corn flakes, corn meal, and cornstarch without noticeable symptoms even though they cannot tolerate fresh forms of corn (corn on the cob, canned, frozen). However, it is best for those sensitive to corn to completely avoid all of its forms.

Treating corn allergy by avoidance requires the complete elimination of corn, maize products and all foods containing any form or amount of corn. Continuing to use forms of corn that produce only negligible or subclinical reactions tends to maintain a high degree of corn sensitivity. This reduces the possibility of a sensitive person ever being able to eat corn without experiencing symptoms.

Always read labels. When inquiring whether a product contains corn, ask about each item by name. For example, when checking a bakery product, ask if the product contains any corn flour, corn meal, cornstarch, corn oil, corn sugar (dextrose), or corn syrup. Do not accept the word of untrained personnel until you have inquired using every specific name of the different forms of corn.

Vegetable oils need not be identified on commercial labels, so one must assume that commercial products containing vegetable oil will contain some amount of inexpensive corn oil. Sugars also do not have to be labelled as derived from corn, cane, or beet, which means avoiding all commercially sweetened products in order to totally eliminate corn from your diet.

The simplest way to avoid corn is to eat only fresh foods (other than corn) without any additives. Fresh meat, fruit, and vegetables are free of corn. Unsweetened, uncreamed, diet products packed in water are also usually free of corn.

Common Forms and Uses of Corn

- **Alcoholic beverages:** All ale, beer, brandy, gin, whiskey, and vodka manufactured in North America are usually fortified with corn. Most domestic wines contain corn except California wines with 13 percent alcohol content or less. California sparkling wines and California wines above 13 percent alcohol can be fortified with corn. Imported wines and brandies are usually corn-free.
- **Corn meal:** Buckwheat, oatmeal, or corn meal is commonly scattered on the hearth before panless loaves of bread are baked. Remove this layer by cutting a quarter of an inch

off the bottom of the loaf (do not scrape it off). Corn meal is also used in cereals, scrapple, mush, johnny cake, Indian pudding, and other recipes, as well as in batter for deep-frying.

- **Corn oil:** Corn oil, which is comparatively inexpensive, is used for deep-frying, in salad dressings, and in some margarines.
- **Cornstarch:** Cornstarch is used as a thickening agent in gravies, icings and frostings, pies, sauces, and many other items. Many baking powders contain cornstarch as a filler. Starched clothing and bedding and adhesives in shoes may contain cornstarch and cause contact allergic symptoms. Cornstarch is also dusted on many brands of paper cups and plates, waxed and plastic containers, and plastic bags to prevent foods from sticking to them. There are also aerosol starch preparations for home laundry use that contain cornstarch. When sprayed, these preparations may be inhaled as well as contacted by the skin. Sterile gloves are coated with talc, which contains cornstarch.

- **Corn sugar (dextrose) and corn syrup (glucose):** Corn sugar and syrup are derivatives of cornstarch. Corn sugar does not become sticky and imparts a smooth texture to candies. It is used in nearly all commercial chocolates and caramels, cough drops, hard candies, lozenges, and suckers. The malted preparations used in ice cream, candies, and cereals are also derived from corn and wheat. Most bacon, canned fruits, ham, ice cream, Jell-O, jams, preserves, processed cheese, and soft drinks contain corn sugar or corn syrup. Dextrose is the most common sugar used for intravenous feeding. Synthetic vitamin C, commercial citric acid, sorbitol, and mannitol are derived from corn sugar. Corn dextrins and adhesives are used on stamps and envelopes and many other products, and some cigarettes are blended with corn sugar.
- **Vinegar:** White or acetic acid vinegar, usually derived from corn, is used commercially in salad dressings, pickles, sauerkraut, and sauces.

Food Sources of Corn

Ale
American brandies (both apple and grape)
Aspartame (NutraSweet)
Baby foods (most)
Baby formulas:
   Prosobee
   Similac
   Nutramigen
Bacon
Baking mixes:
   Biscuits
   Doughnuts
   Pancakes
   Pie crusts

Baking powders
Batters for frying
Beers
Beets (Harvard)
Beverages (carbonated)
Bleached wheat flours
Bourbon and other whiskies
Breads and pastries
Cakes
Candy:
   Box candies (all grades)
   Candy bars
   Commercial candies
Carbonated beverages

Catsups
Cereals
Confectioner's sugar
Cookies (some)
Corn chips and other appetizers
Corn syrup
Crackers (some)
Cream pies
Cream puffs
Dates (confection)
Deep-fat frying mixtures
Dextrin
Dextrose
Flour (bleached)
French dressing
Fresh corn (canned, frozen)
Fried foods
Fritters
Frostings
Fruit juices
Fruits and fruit pies (canned and frozen)
Fructose
Frying fats
Gelatin desserts
Gin
Glucose products
Graham crackers
Grape juice
Gravies
Grits
Gum (chewing)
Ham (cured, tenderized)
High-fructose corn syrup
Hominy
Hydrolyzed vegetable oil
Ice cream (some)
Ices
Inhalants (cooking fumes from fresh corn, popcorn)
Jams
Jellies

Jell-O
Juices (vitamin C "enriched")
Karo
Leavening agents (baking powders, yeasts)
Liquors (all American and imported):
   Ale
   Beer
   Brandy
   Gin
   Vodka
   Whiskey
Maize
Mannitol
Margarine
Meats:
   All meats cooked with gravies
   All processed luncheon meats
   Bacon
   Bologna
   Ham (cured or tenderized)
   Sausages (cooked)
   Wieners (frankfurters)
Milk (in paper cartons)
Monosodium glutamate
Mull-soy
Nescafe
NutraSweet
Pablum
Pancake syrup
Parched corn
Pastries (cakes, cupcakes)
Peanut butters
Peas (canned)
Pedialyte
Pickles
Pies (cream or fruit)
Popped corn
Posole
Powdered sugar
Preserves
Puddings:

Blancmange
Custards
"Royal" pudding
Rice (coated)
Rice Krispies
Saccharin
Salad dressings
Salt:
  All iodized salt
  Salt cellars in restaurants
Sandwich spreads and meats
Sauces for:
  Fish
  Meats
  Sundaes
  Vegetables
Sauerkraut
Sausages (cooked or table-ready)
Seasonings (some)
Sherbets
Sorbitol
Soup:
  Creamed
  Thickened
  Vegetable
Soybean milks
String beans (canned, frozen)
Succotash
Sugar (powdered)
Syrups (commercially prepared glucose and
  Karo)
Tacos
Teas (instant)
Tortillas
Vanillin
Vegetables:
  Canned
  Creamed
  Frozen
Vinegar (distilled)
Vitamin C "enriched" foods and juices

Whiskies (Scotch, bourbon)
Wieners
Wines (American):
  Dessert
  Fortified
  Sparkling
Xanthan gum
Yogurt
Zein
Other Sources
Adhesives on:
  Envelopes
  Labels
  Stamps
  Stickers
  Tape
Aspirin and other tablets
Cough drops
Cough syrups
Cups (paper)
Dentifrices
Envelopes (gum on)
Excipients or diluents in:
  Capsules
  Lozenges
  Ointments
  Suppositories
  Tablets
  Vitamins
Gelatin capsules
Gloves (powdered with talc)
Inhalants:
  Bath powders
  Body powders
  Starch (while spraying, ironing)
  Talcums
Linit (starch)
Medication (tablet form)
Paper containers:
  Boxes (containing moist products)
  Cups

Plates

Plastic food wrappers (inside may be coated with cornstarch)

Talcums

Toothpaste

Vitamins

Soy

Soybeans have been grown in Asia for centuries, especially in China, where they have provided the bread, protein, and oil. Since the beginning of the 19th century, American farmers have grown soybeans for livestock, feed, or for fertilizer.

Chemists have also found many uses for soybeans, which are proving to be a bonanza. Ford Motor Company uses them to make plastic window frames, steering wheels, gearshift knobs, distributors, upholstery fabric, and other parts. Rubber substitutes and lecithin in leaded gasoline are also made from soybeans.

Many new food and industrial uses of soy can be expected. If you remember that soybeans are used as flour, oil, milk, nuts, and meat extenders, it will be possible to anticipate most new food contacts. When purchasing prepared foods, consider soy as a possible ingredient if the label says vegetable oil, vegetable broth, or textured vegetable protein.

Eating in restaurants almost always means a soy exposure, as most restaurants and fast-food chains cook with soy oil or flour. Soybean flour containing only one percent oil is now used by many bakers in dough mixtures for breads, cakes, rolls, and pastries, to keep them moist and fresh several days longer. The roasted beans are often used in place of peanuts on breakfast rolls. Some biscuits and several crisp crackers also contain soybean flour.

Food Sources of Soy

Artificial meats and nuts

Baby foods (some)

Bakery goods

Cake mixes (may contain artificial fruit made from soy)

Candies:

    Caramels

    Carob chips

    Chocolate chips

    Hard candies

    Nut candies

    (Lecithin, derived from soy, is used in candies to prevent drying and to emulsify fats.)

Cereals

Fried products:

    Corn chips

    Potato chips

    Tortilla chips

Ice cream (dairy and tofu)

Margarine and butter substitutes

Meats:

    Canned meats and fish

    Hamburgers (fast food)

    Luncheon meats

    Pork-link sausages

Milk substitutes:

    Infant formulas

    Non-dairy creamers

    Soy milk

Nuts:

    Any roasted in soy oil

    Soy (formed to look like other nuts)

    Soybeans (toasted, salted, and used as nuts)

Oils (Crisco, Spry solid or liquid)

Pastas:
  Macaroni
  Noodles
  Spaghetti
Peanut butter (some)
Processed cheeses (some)
Salad dressings (may contain soy oil, but list
  only vegetable oil on the label)
Sauces:
  Lea & Perrins
  Soy sauce
  Steak sauce
  Tamari
  Teriyaki sauce
  Worcestershire sauce
Soups (may contain soy oil and/or lecithin)
Tofu:
  Miso
  Natto
  Tempeh
Tuna (packed in vegetable oil)
Vegetables:
  Margarine or oil on vegetables
  Soy sprouts

Other Sources:
Adhesives
Automobile parts
Blankets
Candles

Celluloid
Cloth
Clothing
Coffee substitute
Cosmetics
Custards
Diet aids
Dog food
Enamels
Fertilizer
Fish food
Fodder
Glycerine
Illuminating oil
Lecithin
Linoleum
Lubricating oil
Make-up
Massage creams
Nitroglycerine
Paints
Paper finishes
Paper sizing
Printing ink
Soap
Telephones
Textile finishings
Toys
Varnish
Vitamins

Eggs

Chicken eggs are the most commonly consumed eggs in North America. Raw shell eggs purchased at a store should be displayed in a refrigerated case, as cold temperatures help maintain egg quality by slowing the loss of moisture and carbon dioxide. Upon arriving home, refrigerate eggs as soon as possible. Egg quality will decline more during one day at room temperature than during one week in the refrigerator. Raw shell eggs will keep in the refrigerator for at least three weeks after leaving the supermarket.

Refrigerator temperatures also inhibit further growth of bacteria. Each pore of an eggshell is 100 times larger than salmonella bacteria, allowing them to enter the egg easily. Dr. Robert V. Tauxe of the Center for Disease Control warns that the world supply of eggs is contaminated with salmonella. The rate of salmonella infection is escalating, causing an increase in cases of reactive arthritis (even mild cases of salmonella poisoning cause sore joints). Immunocompromised people and infants just starting on solid foods are especially high-risk groups.

Most of the contamination problems with eggs have been traced to powdered and frozen eggs, which are derived from cracked eggs of insufficient quality to be sold as raw shell eggs. If you are using powdered eggs, be certain that they have been pasteurized. Purchase only clean, raw eggs with uncracked shells, and do not use an egg if it is stuck to the carton or if the shell is dirty, stained, or spotted with foreign material.

Because of the problem with salmonella contamination, raw eggs should not be eaten. You also risk becoming ill if you eat lightly cooked eggs, including soft cooked, soft poached, soft scrambled, sunny-side up, and French toast. To be safe, eggs and egg dishes must be heated throughout to 160°F.

It is also possible for eggs to contain other contaminants. Pesticide residues, antibiotics from feed, and drugs given to chickens to boost laying can be found in eggs.

Although some people react to both the egg yolk and egg white, those sensitive to eggs are frequently allergic to the egg white. Symptoms in response to eating egg yolk may indicate a fat-intolerant disorder. The method of cooking sometimes determines whether eggs can be tolerated. When reading labels, albumin, livetin, ovomucin, ovomucoid, and vitellin indicate the presence of egg or egg components. When inquiring about egg content of food items, do not overlook the possibility of powdered eggs.

Eggs from other fowl (ducks, geese, and turkeys) and even turtle eggs may be substituted for chicken eggs in recipes. (Adjustments will have to be made to compensate for differences in the size of eggs.)

Food Sources of Egg

Baby foods
Baked goods
Baking powder
Batters for fried foods
Bavarian cream
Boiled dressings
Bouillons
Bread
Bread crumbs
Breaded foods
Cake flours
Cakes
Candies
Coddled eggs
Consommés
Cookies

Creamed eggs
Cream pies
Croquettes
Custards
Dessert powders and whips
Devilled eggs
Doughnuts
Dried eggs
Egg albumin (ovalbumin)
Eggnog
Egg substitutes (Egg Beaters)
Egg whites
Egg white solids
Egg yolk solids
Egg yolks
Escalloped eggs

French toast
Fried eggs
Fritters
Frostings
Fruit pies
Glazed rolls
Griddle cakes
Hamburger mix
Hard-boiled eggs
Hollandaise sauce
Ice cream
Ices
Icings
Lecithin
Macaroni
Macaroons
Malted cocoa drinks
Marshmallows
Mayonnaise
Meat jellies
Meatloaf
Meringues
Muffins
Noodles
Omelets
Ovaltine
Ovomalt

Pancake flour
Pancakes
Pastas
Pastries
Poached eggs
Pretzels
Puddings
Quiche
Salad dressings
Sauces
Sausages
Sherbets
Shirred eggs
Soda (root beer)
Soft-cooked eggs
Soufflés
Soups
Spaghetti noodles
Spanish creams
Syrups
Tartar sauce
Waffles
Wines (may be cleared with egg white)

Other Sources:
Laxatives

MILK

The major components of milk are lactalbumin, casein, lactose (milk sugar), and cream. It is the lactalbumin component that varies from species to species. For example, the lactalbumin of human milk is different from that of cow's milk, and both are different from the lactalbumin of goat's milk. For this reason, some people who react allergically to the lactalbumin component of cow's milk may be able to drink goat's milk without difficulty. People who are sensitive to all components of milk will be unable to tolerate milk from any animal source.

Any product containing milk, milk by-products, or milk proteins and sugars will cause the same symptoms as milk, and should be avoided. Watch for these ingredients when reading product labels or checking contents of food served to you: butter, cream, butterfat, whipped cream, skim milk, powdered milk, condensed milk, evaporated milk, milk solids, whey, yogurt, casein, caseinate, sodium or calcium caseinate, lactose, sodium or calcium lactate, non-fat milk solids, or lactalbumin.

Food Sources of Milk

Au gratin dishes
Baby foods (some)
Baked goods
Batters
Butter
Buttermilk
Cakes
Calcium caseinate
Canned milk
Carob chips
Carob coatings
Casein
Cheeses (all)
Chocolate beverages
Chocolate creams
Cocomalt
Condensed milk
Cookies
Cottage cheese
Cream
Cream sauces
Creamed soups
Curds
Custard
Doughnuts
Dried milk
Evaporated milk
Filled candy bars
Flours (prepared, such as Bisquick)
Fritters
Gravies
Hot cereals (some)
Hot dogs

Ice cream
Ice milk
Kefir
Lactalbumin
Lactate
Lactoglobulin
Lactose
Malted milk
Margarines
Milk chocolate candy
Milk puddings
Non-dairy products (some)
Nougat candy
Omelets
Ovaltine
Pancakes
Powdered milk
Pudding mixes
Rarebits
Salad dressings
Sausages
Sherbet
Skim milk
Sodium caseinate
Soufflés
Sour cream
Stroganoff
Timbales
Waffles
Whey
Whipped cream
Wiener schnitzel
Yogurt

Non-Dairy Sources of Calcium and Magnesium   Most people believe they will not get enough calcium unless milk is part of their diet. However, humans are the only species of mammal (other than some cats) who drink milk after being weaned from the breast. The majority of the world's population receives less than half the calcium that North Americans are told they need and, on the whole, has strong bones and healthy teeth.

Dairy councils constantly extol the virtues of milk. These nonprofit, promotional, and educational organizations publicize the supposed nutritional benefits of milk and milk products. However, milk is not the "perfect food," as it is frequently advertised.

PROBLEMS WITH MILK   Many people have difficulty drinking milk because it contains lactose, known as milk sugar. An enzyme, lactase, is needed to digest the lactose. Many children gradually lose the lactase enzyme, usually between the ages of one and four, and so are no longer able to digest milk sugar. Eight percent of North American caucasians lose the lactase enzyme, and other specific racial groups lose between 50 to 70 percent of their lactase enzyme. Symptoms of lactase deficiency, which may show up after milk is consumed, include cramps and diarrhea. However, lactase-deficient people can usually eat yogurt and cheese, which contain enzymes that help digest the lactose. A commercial product called Lactaid is available to aid in the digestion of dairy products.

Milk can cause other problems. Some people become constipated when they consume milk. In one study of 100 children, half stopped bedwetting when milk was removed from their diets. Milk is a poor source of iron, and is a common cause of iron-deficiency anemia in children. In babies, milk can cause a microscopic loss of blood in the stools. In addition, children will often fill up with milk and then will not eat solid foods.

There is evidence to suggest a link between high milk intake and cardiovascular disease. Cow's milk is high in saturated fats and fatty acids. Ice cream and some cheeses are even higher in fat content. For example, whole milk contains about one gram of fat per ounce, while cheddar cheese contains about 10 grams of fat per ounce.

Cow's milk is a common food allergen; people may be sensitive to all milk components. Symptoms of this allergy include vomiting, diarrhea, bloody diarrhea, asthma, runny or stuffy nose, recurrent ear infections, rashes, hives, and hyperactive behavior. Studies have linked delinquency and behavior disorders to high milk intake. Infant colic is related to cow's milk formula or milk that a breast-feeding mother may be drinking. People with Crohn's disease improve after milk is eliminated from their diets.

CALCIUM REQUIREMENTS   The Recommended Daily Allowance for calcium for growing children is 500 mg for infants up to one year; 800 mg for children up to age 10; 1,200 mg for children up to 18; and 1,000 mg for people over 18. However, these figures were derived from experiments utilizing diets high in phosphorus. Phosphorus binds to calcium in the intestine, preventing its absorption. It also leaches calcium from the body.

The ratio of calcium to phosphorus in cow's milk is 1.2:1.0. If your diet is low in phosphorus, you should take only about one-tenth the recommended amount of calcium, or 100 mg. Breast milk contains 300 mg of calcium per quart and cow's milk has 1,200 mg of calcium per quart, yet infants absorb more calcium from breast milk. The calcium to phosphorus ratio in breast milk. The calcium to phosphorus ratio in breast milk is 2:1, which emphasizes the importance of this ratio for proper calcium absorption. Milk and dairy products, poultry, some fish, whole wheat, cereal products, peas, sunflower seeds, meats, and dark green leafy vegetables have a low calcium to phosphorus ratio.

Cow's milk has a high phosphorus content, which interferes with adequate absorption and use of calcium. Meat also has a high phosphorus content. Increased phosphate (a form of phosphorus) intake has been noted to adversely affect the behavior of hyperkinetic and learning-disabled children. Phosphates are found in large quantities in processed foods, including some soda pops.

Acid-forming diets increase calcium excretion. Meats, other high-protein foods, and most cereal grains, including wheat, are acid-forming; most vegetables and fruits do not have this effect. Nutrients necessary for the proper absorption and utilization of calcium include magnesium, manganese, potassium, zinc, and vitamin D.

SOURCES OF CALCIUM There are many sources of calcium other than cow's milk. Good food sources of calcium are spinach, sardines, kidney beans, broccoli, almonds, fish, seaweed, and soybeans. Other foods with high calcium content are listed below. The indicated calcium content is for 100-gram edible portions, or 3½ ounces.

Food	Calcium (mg)
Milk	117
Raw broccoli	103
Cooked broccoli	88
Pinto beans	135
White beans	144
Salmon (canned in oil)	119
Swiss cheese	925
Cheddar cheese	750
Carob flour	352
Almonds	234
Corn tortillas (lime added)	200
Brazil nuts	186
Goat's milk	129
Tofu	128
Dried figs	126
Sunflower seeds	120
Sesame seeds (hulled)	110
Spinach	93
Peanuts	69
Raisins	62
Sardines	332
Dandelion greens	187
Turnip greens	246

Giving up milk defies our traditional training. We are conditioned to drink milk, but taste is acquired, and conditioning can be changed. Try using soy milk, goat's milk, nut milk, apple juice, or other juices on cereal. You will be pleasantly surprised. Soy milk, goat's milk, or water can be used as a substitute in cooking. (See "But the Recipe Says...," p. 113, for milk substitutions.) Goat's milk should not be used for babies under four months old because of immaturity of their kidneys. If goat's milk is used as the sole source of milk for an infant (and this is rarely recommended), it must be supplemented with folic acid and vitamin B_6 (pyridoxine).

Calcium may also be obtained by taking a calcium supplement. The best calcium supplement is one in which calcium is chelated (bound) to an amino acid to enhance absorption. The supplement should contain both calcium and magnesium in a ratio of 2 to 1, which is best for absorption and utilization. (Some magnesium-deficient people, however, require a supplement containing equal amounts of calcium and magnesium.) If you are allergic to milk, avoid calcium lactate, which is milk-based. Dolomite is poorly absorbed as a source of calcium and may contain a high lead content. Bone meal sources of calcium are also not recommended because they are difficult to digest.

See additional information on calcium and magnesium on p. 237 and p. 238.

Beef

Beef is the most common meat consumed in North America. There are more than 30 registered breeds of beef cattle. Beef is the muscle meat from steers (castrated males) 18 months old or older, and from heifers (young females which have not calved). Veal is meat from young calves between one week and 26 weeks old.

Those who eat beef can suffer from allergy to the beef itself, or to the grains fed to the animals. Insecticides found in feed grains, antibiotics given to cattle to prevent infection, and steroids injected to increase fluid weight can also cause allergic reactions. Most organic beef comes from grain-fed cattle, and will have white fat rather than the yellow fat characteristic of grass-fed cattle. However, some drugs given to cattle to change metabolism and increase fat create hard, white fat that is totally saturated.

Food Sources of Beef

Baby foods (some)
Gelatin products:
  Cakes
  Candies
  Ice cream
  Jell-O
  Pastries
  Puddings
  Pies
  Sherbets
Gravies and sauces
Meats:
  Brains
  Hamburger
  Heart
  Kidneys
  Liver
  Ribs
  Roast

Steak
Suet
Tallow
Tongue
Tripe
MSG (Monosodium glutamate)
Processed beef (products that contain beef or beef products, or those processed in the same machine as beef):
  Liverwurst
  Sandwich meats
  Sausages
  Wieners
Soups and bouillon

Other Sources:
Capsules (gelatin, all types; nutritional supplements in capsules)
Cattle dander

Drugs (injectable, processed from beef or
   containing beef fractions):
   Adrenal cortical extract
   Heparin
   Insulin
Glandulars and enzymes (read labels carefully
   or contact the manufacturer):
   Adrenal
   Heart

Liver
Pancreas
Pancreatin
Pituitary
Spleen
Thyroid
Glue
Vitamins containing liver as a base

PORK

Pork, the muscle meat from mature hogs, is sold fresh, cured, or processed. It is the most frequently processed of all meats. Severely pork-sensitive people must avoid all forms of pork.

Organic pork is frequently grain-fed, which can be a problem for those with grain allergies. Hogs fed on garbage (boiled for safety) are the best source of pork for grain-sensitive individuals. However, the practice of garbage feeding is suspected of spreading trichinosis, cholera, and brucellosis. Pretreating garbage to destroy the organisms also destroys the necessary nutrient content. Pigs that are fed cooked garbage tend to be anemic and have stomach ulcers.

The quality of pork can be affected by antibiotics in feed, inferior feed quality, drugs, vaccines, overfattening, artificial environments, and poor management. The practice of administering drugs to pigs before slaughter slows muscle changes after death and keeps the flesh red.

Trichinosis, an infection of *Trichinella spiralis* worms, was once prevalent in the United States, and was spread through infected pork. However, with the advent of cooked garbage feed, better freezing procedures, improved hog-raising methods, and more stringent pork inspection, the occurrence of trichinosis in the U.S. is down to 4 percent. These infections result from consuming raw or undercooked pork or pork products, or improperly cooked ground beef that has been adulterated with pork. Symptoms of trichinosis include submucosal inflammatory reactions, nausea, vomiting, diarrhea, fever, edema, hemorrhages under the fingernails, muscular pain, and congestive heart failure.

Food Sources of Pork

Fresh pork:
   Brains
   Chops
   Cracklings or chitterlings
   Kidneys
   Liver

Ribs
Roast
Sausage
Souse (head cheese)
Cured pork:
   Bacon

Ham
Pickled pig's feet
Pork rinds
Salt pork
Sausage
Processed pork:
   Canned meats ("potted" meats)
   Luncheon meats
   Mincemeat
   Spam
   Vienna sausage
   Wieners
Baby foods (some)
Baked beans
Bakery products
Candy bars
Chinese and Polynesian foods
Cocktail dips
Fried foods in restaurants
Fritos
Frosting mixes
Gelatin
Ice cream
Instant foods (such as mashed potatoes)
Jell-O
Lard
Margarine
Mayonnaise
Mexican foods
Non-dairy creamer
Potato chips

Pre-breaded frozen foods
Prepared cake and pancake mixes
Processed cheeses (in jars and cartons)
Puddings
Salad dressings
Shortening
Soups with pork
Vegetables seasoned with salt pork
Vegetable stock

Other Sources:
Drugs:
   Calcium and magnesium stearates
   Capsules
   Heparin
   Tonics and pills for anemia (hog stomach
contains an intrinsic factor)
Glandulars and enzymes (read labels carefully
   or contact the manufacturer):
   Adrenal
   Mixed enzyme products
   Pancreas
   Pancreatin
   Pituitary
   Thymus
   Thyroid
Glue
Glycerine (soaps, cosmetics)
Iron skillets and Dutch ovens that have not
   been thoroughly scoured after being used
   to cook pork

SUGAR AND ALL THINGS SWEET

North America has turned into a land of "sugarholics." The average North American consumes approximately his or her own weight in sugar each year, the national average being over 130 pounds of sugar per person. This amount consists of the refined sugar added to foods we choose to eat in addition to the naturally occurring sugars in fruits and vegetables. Much of the sugar we eat is "hidden" sugar—we are unaware that we are consuming it. Foods that were once unsweetened are now sweetened, and others that previously were sweet have been elevated to higher levels of sweetness.

Hidden sugars are largely the result of industrial practices that are largely unfamiliar to the public. For example, sugar content of meat is increased by feeding it to animals before slaughter to improve the flavor and color of the meat, and by adding it to the meat itself as it is prepared in packing houses and restaurants. Any dish prepared with ground meat may contain added syrups to help minimize shrinkage and to improve flavor, juiciness, and texture.

The presence of hidden sugars should be suspected in the following items, either because their manufacturers are not required to list the sugar content, or because the sugars are listed in such a fashion that the consumer does not recognize them as sugars.

Bouillon cubes
Breadings for fried or baked poultry and meats
Canned and frozen vegetables
Catsup
Cigarettes
Convenience foods
Cottage cheese
Dry roasted nuts
Frozen and canned entrées
Gravies
Instant coffee
Instant tea
Iodized salt
Luncheon meats
Mixes to stretch chopped beef
Peanut butter
Potato chips
Salad dressings
Soups
Wieners (frankfurters)

When sugar is listed, the exact percentage is difficult to determine. Sugar appears on labels under many names; the "ose" ending of words indicates a sugar. All of the following items are sugars:

Brown sugar
Corn syrup
Corn syrup solids
Dextrose
Fructose
Glucose
High-fructose corn syrup
Honey
Malt syrup
Maltodextrin
Mannitol
Maple syrup
Molasses
Raw sugar
Sorbitol
Sorghum
Sucrose
Turbinado
Xylitol

Sugar, like alcohol, is rapidly absorbed and floods the system, predisposing the sensitive person to severe reactions and addictions. High sugar intake has been linked to dental caries, obesity, diabetes, coronary heart disease, hypoglycemia, and behavioral problems. Sugar depletes the body of specific nutrients, including the B vitamins, magnesium, chromium, manganese, and other minerals. Ingesting sugar also destroys the germ-killing ability of the white blood cells for four hours.

Our body machinery is designed to cope with about two teaspoons of sugar per day. If we eat additional amounts of sugar—such as a piece of apple pie, with 19 teaspoons of sugar—it disrupts our body's "sugar equilibrium." These disruptions stress our body and overload the adrenal gland and pancreas, which are critical to allergy control.

In a study done by Dr. Timothy Jones of Yale University, adults and children were given proportionately equal doses of glucose, the form of sugar to which all carbohydrates in blood are metabolized. The children received 20 teaspoons of glucose, the sugar equivalent of two 12-ounce colas. The blood glucose levels in both the adults and children recorded similar highs and lows, but the adrenalin levels of the children were twice as high as those of the adults. More of the children felt weak and shaky. As a result of this study, Dr. Jones advises that children not be given sweets on an empty stomach. He also suggests that the increase in adrenalin could be linked to the hyperactivity some children display after eating sweets.

Young children eat small amounts of food and are dependent on this food to obtain the nutrients they need. Eating sugar, which has little nutritional value, adversely affects their appetites, thus decreasing their intake of nutrients. Sweets should also never be used as a reward food.

The following sweeteners are in common use in North America.

Sucrose Sucrose is the most commonly used sugar in our food supply. It can be refined from both sugar cane and sugar beets, and the resulting sugars have identical structures. However, many hypersensitive people can distinguish one from the other by their reaction to the small residues of the source plants.

Sucrose stimulates the production of fat in the body, particularly in women using contraceptive drugs.

Beet and cane sugars are used as:

- Fermentation mediums in baked goods, contributing to the color, flavor, and quality of the crust; retention of moisture; and extension of shelf life.
- Curing agents for processed meats.
- Preservatives in fruits, jellies, jams, and preserves.
- Sweeteners in canned goods.
- Bulking agents in ice cream, baked goods, and confections.
- "Bodying" agents in soft drinks.
- Preservatives in medications.
- Ointments.

Corn Sweeteners Over half of the cornstarch milled in North America is used to produce corn sweeteners. They are used extensively by the food industry because of their low cost and because a sweeter mix is obtained when they are combined with sucrose.

Corn sugar carries all of the allergenicity of corn, and many corn-sensitive people react to it more quickly than to other components of corn. As the food industry has stepped up its use of corn sweeteners and cornstarch, sensitivities to corn have risen. Corn-sensitive people must avoid products containing dextrose, glucose, sorbitol, and mannitol (generally made from dextrose).

Corn sugar found in infant formulas can produce eczema and gastrointestinal upsets in corn-sensitive babies, and diarrhea in all infants.

Corn sweeteners:

- Add body and texture to soft drinks.
- Add chewiness to confections and chewing gums.
- Are used in maple, nut, and root beer flavoring for beverages, ice creams, candy, and baked goods.
- Are used in processed meats, hams, bacon,

fish products, and sausages.

• Help retain bright colors in preserves, cured meats, and catsup.
• Absorb moisture to keep hard candy from becoming sticky.
• Inhibit crystallization of other sugars.
• Ferment easily, which aids brewers and distillers.

DEXTROSE Dextrose, maltose, corn syrup, and corn sugar are derivatives of cornstarch. Dextrose, in addition to the uses listed above, is an ingredient in intravenous solutions commonly used in hospitals. Many corn-sensitive patients react to these IVs, experiencing problems that are commonly attributed to "surgical complications." For example, Dr. Kendall Gerdes, of Denver, Colorado, reported a case of a woman who developed bronchospasm after receiving IV dextrose.

GLUCOSE Glucose is a commercially processed sugar derived from cornstarch, occurring naturally in grape and corn sugar. Its name can be misleading, since blood sugar is also referred to as glucose. It is frequently labelled as corn syrup because the public at one time thought it was a sugar derived from glue.

Glucose is a dangerous sweetener because of its low sweetness level. It is only one-fifth as sweet as sucrose, and so large quantities can be absorbed without a person being aware of its presence in food.

Glucose is frequently used to flavor ground meat dishes, luncheon meats, and hams, as well as to extend maple syrup.

HIGH-FRUCTOSE CORN SYRUP High-fructose corn syrup is commercially produced from dextrose. A 42 percent solution of this syrup is as sweet as sucrose. Because it is considerably cheaper than sucrose—and because supply is not subject to the fluctuations of the sugar market—the use of high-fructose corn syrup

has increased drastically since the 1970s. In 1980, two major cola companies switched to high-fructose corn syrup. Now, it is an ingredient in all soda pops.

High-fructose corn syrup is not safe for corn-sensitive individuals or for diabetics. High-fructose corn syrup contains some glucose, the amount varying from product to product, and glucose is the sugar diabetics are least able to utilize.

It is sometimes very difficult to identify the source of the fructose in a given food item because of the confusion between crystalline fructose and high-fructose corn syrups.

Processors use high-fructose corn syrup in:

Baked goods and icings
Carbonated and non-carbonated beverages
Cereals
Chocolate milk, eggnog, yogurt, ice cream, and sherbet
Diabetic and reduced-calorie foods
Jams, jellies, and preserves
Salad dressings, pickles, and catsups
Table syrups and liquid table sweeteners
Wines

Fructose Fructose or levulose is the natural sugar found in fruits, vegetables, berries, and honey. The fructose commonly found in stores is usually processed from cane or beet sugar, not from fruits. Fructose is twice as sweet as sucrose and it dissolves readily in water. It also absorbs water, which helps to keep baked goods and confections from drying out. It does not crystallize during storage and shipment, and is an excellent masking agent for the bitterness of saccharin.

Fructose is slowly metabolized in the liver into glucose, which then requires insulin for use in the body. Although the glucose is released slowly, it does not represent any particular advantage for diabetics, as has been claimed. Metabolic disturbances occur in both normal and diabetic individuals when fructose is used in intravenous solutions. It also matches sucrose in contributing to tooth decay.

Fructose is used in many processed foods, including:

Breakfast cereals
Cake and cookie mixes
Candies and chewing gums
Gelatin and frozen desserts
Jams and preserves
Jellies
Lemonade and tea mixes
Peanut butter
Protein supplements and other beverage
    powders
Puddings
Salad dressings and mayonnaise

Raw Sugar, Brown Sugar, Turbinado Sugar, & Molasses   To make sugar, juice is squeezed from sugar cane with rollers and then boiled in a vacuum pan until the sugar crystallizes. The liquid that does not crystallize becomes molasses, and the newly formed crystals (still coated with molasses) are raw sugar. When the molasses is removed from these crystals and they are refined, they become table sugar.

Raw sugar may be contaminated with insecticides, smoke residue, bacteria, dirt, fibers, lints, mold, sand, lice, waxes, and yeast. If the raw sugar is washed and centrifuged, some but not all dirt will be removed, along with some solid materials and bacteria. The resulting product is marketed as turbinado sugar if it meets the minimum sanitary level set by the government.

Raw sugar produced in North America is usually white sugar with traces of cane or beet pulp replaced. "Unrefined" or "natural" on labels is meaningless, as the raw sugar has gone through several refining processes.

When molasses is further processed, more crystals form; they are yellow to brown in color. This is "brown sugar," which tends to clump because it still has a molasses covering. However, brown sugar is often more refined than white sugar. Its deep color frequently has been added, rather than being from molasses residue.

The molasses is processed numerous times to extract all possible sugar. The remaining syrup is blackstrap molasses, the waste product of sugar manufacturing. It carries most of the mineral matter and all of the gum, ash, dirt, and indigestible matter present in the unprocessed sugar. Molasses, which is 30 percent sucrose, is not a source of natural sugar, nor is it a good source of iron. True blackstrap molasses is not sold for human consumption.

The quality of molasses depends on the maturity of the sugar cane, and on whether the processor intends that molasses or sugar should be the primary product. Many food processors use molasses blends that may also contain corn, wheat, or soy constituents. Read labels carefully when purchasing molasses.

Unsulfured molasses is made from the juice of sun-ripened West Indian cane. Blending of products from various places produces a uniform molasses, which is aged for a year or two. Sulfured molasses is a byproduct of sugar refining made from immature cane. The cane is treated with sulfur during the sugar extraction process, and a sulfur residue remains in the molasses.

Honey   Bees gather nectar, which is 80 percent sucrose. By using a digestive enzyme, invertase, they convert the nectar to two simple sugars: glucose and fructose. This mixture is called invert sugar and requires no digestion by humans. The ratio of fructose to glucose varies for different honeys.

Dissolved aromatics give each honey its own distinctive flavor and appearance. The remaining components in honey are water, a small amount of bee pollen, sucrose, dextrin, gums, and a few minerals, vitamins, and enzymes.

Honey ripened in the hive will have a smooth mellow flavor and a moisture content of less than 17 percent. Green honey, which has been removed from the hives too early, has a moisture content of over 20 percent, a bitter flavor, and will ferment easily. If honey is extracted from the hive with mild heat, it will retain some of its nutrients. Prolonged heat exposure breaks down enzymes and proteins and impairs color and flavor.

Honey is graded by clarity; the greater the clarity, the higher the grade. This grading has no significance other than measuring the size of particles filtered out. It bears no relation to quality.

Honey labelling is a neglected problem. Terms such as natural, old-fashioned, country style, organic, or undiluted are meaningless. Labels citing the source of honey are not accurate because honey is frequently blended, and bees do not visit just one type of plant. The problem that blended honey poses for the allergic person is the possibility of hidden, unlabelled allergens, not its quality or taste. Honey may also be adulterated with corn syrup or cheap sugars.

Honey may also contain some contaminants, such as traces of sulfa drugs and antibiotics used to control bee diseases. Empty combs may be fumigated with mothballs. Honey from certain plants can also be poisonous. However, these problems are not widespread—generally,

honey is a safe food. As a nutrient source, however, it is grossly overrated. Raw honey may be hazardous to infants under one year of age because it may contain botulism spores, which have caused the death of some babies.

Maple Syrup   Maple syrup is processed from maple tree sap. Maple trees are tapped by scoring the bark, and the sap is collected in buckets that hang beneath the scar. The syrup must be collected when the tree chemistry is in the "sweet water" stage. If it is collected when the tree is producing substances used for tree growth, the sap becomes "buddy" and is useless for table-grade syrup. After collection, the liquid is filtered and concentrated for marketing.

Paraformaldehyde pellets are used to kill bacteria to help keep the tap holes open. The pellets increase both production and profits by allowing the trees to be tapped earlier and permitting the sap to run for longer periods of time. The formaldehyde from the pellets supposedly evaporates during processing.

Maple syrup grading is based on appearance rather than taste, with color as the prime factor. Many households use pure maple products. However, many products thought to be pure are actually blends. Generally, most people prefer the taste of the blends. Beware of maple syrup blends that may contain corn, cane, or beet components, which may be allergenic for you. Many products contain only imitation maple flavor and none of the real thing.

The predominant sugar in maple syrup is sucrose. While maple syrup does contain some nutrients, they are not present in sufficient amounts to be nutritionally advantageous. As with molasses and honey, maple syrup should be considered to be a flavoring agent rather than a food.

Sorghum   Sorghum is a grain that is cultivated for human food and animal feed. It can be processed into sugar, syrup, and starch. In North America only 23 percent of the sorghum crop is used for human food, whereas in Asia and Africa the majority of the crop is consumed by humans. It is now possible to separate the sugar from the sorghum starch so it can be crystallized. While this crystalline sugar could help reduce our dependency on foreign sweetener sources, it is a moral question as to whether a crop traditionally earmarked for human nourishment and animal feed should be used to satisfy our cravings for sweets.

Malt   Malt is a sprouted grain, usually barley, although malts can be made from other grains. The grain is roasted under low heat, and then ground and made into either syrup or powder. Bakers use malt extract to impart flavor and color to baked goods, as well as barley malt syrup, which has a dark color and a strong flavor. Some malt is used in dough; its enzymes break down the flour starches to become sugars, which serve as yeast food. These same enzymes play comparable roles in fermenting beer and other malt beverages.

Maltodextrins   Maltodextrins are degraded carbohydrates. They are less sweet than dextrose, and are processed either from corn or maize. Maltodextrins are used to convert liquid flavors into dry powders. They are found in many dehydrated products, such as:

Doughnut, cake, cookie, and icing mixes
Instant coffee, tea, and cocktail mixes
Powdered citrus drinks
Soup and gravy mixes
Spice blends, seasonings, and salad dressing
   mixes

Maltodextrins are also used in:

Frozen desserts
Frozen eggs
Infant foods
Jelly beans
Marshmallows
Peanut butter
Sausages
Soup and gravy mixes
Spice blends, seasonings, and salad dressing
   mixes
Whipped toppings

Grain Syrups   Wheat, rye, and rice syrups are used to reduce the necessity for other sugars and colors. They are alternatives to malted barley syrups and blends, and add sweetness, enhance flavor and color, and add body and sheen to such cereal-based products as baked goods, snacks, breakfast cereals, and pet foods.

Rare Sugars: Sorbitol, Mannitol, and Xylitol
   Rare sugars are non-glucose carbohydrates called sugar alcohols. While they are initially metabolized in the liver, independent of insulin, they are eventually converted to glucose, which does require insulin. In limited amounts, rare sugars are safe for diabetics. They are absorbed poorly because we do not have the proper enzymes to process them.
   Sorbitol is found in berries, apples, pears, cherries, plums, seaweed, and algae. It can be used to mask the bitter aftertaste of saccharin and to provide the illusion of body in low-calorie drinks. Sorbitol itself, however, is not low-calorie as frequently advertised, and it can affect our body's ability to absorb and utilize certain drugs and nutrients, particularly B vitamins. Sorbitol can also cause diarrhea if consumed in large amounts, either in one large

dose or slowly over the course of a day. Commercial sorbitol is made from dextrose (corn). It is used in:

Alcoholic and nonalcoholic beverages
Baked goods, frostings, and gelatin puddings
Fats and oils
Frozen dairy products
Poultry, fish, meat, and nut products
Processed fruits
Snack foods
Sweet sauces, seasonings, and flavorings

Mannitol is found in many plants and plant extracts, but is usually derived from seaweed. Mannitol is poorly digested by our body, and in relatively small amounts can cause diarrhea. In intravenous feedings, it has been associated with a wide range of problems. Mannitol can also induce or worsen kidney diseases. It leaves a cool sweet taste in the mouth and is used in:

Antacid tablets
Breath fresheners
Chewing gum
Children's aspirin tablets
Cough and cold tablets
Sugarless candies

Xylitol is made from xylose, a wood sugar. It can also be obtained from corn cobs, peanut shells, wheat straw, cotton seed hulls, and coconut shells. Xylitol has the same sweetness as sucrose and leaves a pleasant, cool taste in the mouth, but can cause diarrhea if consumed at high levels. Intravenous xylitol infusions have been prohibited in other countries and tests of this material have produced some alarming results. It is still used in North America in chewing gum. Xylitol is also marketed as a crystalline sugar, but its cost—around $17 per pound—should keep its usage low.

Artificial Sweeteners Artificial sweeteners are non-nutritive, non-caloric sweeteners that have been synthesized in a lab. They are intended to help decrease sugar and calorie intake, and to be safe for diabetics. However, artificial sweeteners increase appetite in general and interfere with the taste, enjoyment, and satisfaction obtained from eating foods high in complex carbohydrates. They also increase preference for fat intake and interfere with our body's ability to select foods containing the nutrients it needs.

POLYDEXTROSE Artificial sweeteners add sweetness to products, but not bulk. This is a problem in the manufacture of frozen desserts, instant puddings, cakes, and hard candies. Polydextrose is a bulking agent consisting of dextrose, sorbitol, and citric acid. It is a suitable replacement for sucrose, carbohydrates, and fats in many food products. However, the sorbitol content of polydextrose can cause a laxative effect if more than 50 grams a day are consumed.

ASPARTAME Aspartame is about 200 times sweeter than sucrose and can intensify the taste of other flavors and sweeteners. It cannot be used in heated products, however, since high temperatures cause aspartame to break down. It also loses its sweetness after long storage.

Aspartame is composed of two amino acids, phenylalanine and aspartic acid, which are linked together with a molecule of methanol. When aspartame is broken down in our bodies, this molecule of methanol is released by the small intestine into the bloodstream. The methanol is converted to formaldehyde and is further degraded. In sufficient amounts, methanol and formaldehyde can cause neurological damage, eye damage, or blindness. The phenylalanine in aspartame is not safe for those with phenylketonuria (inability to oxidize a metabolic product of phenylalanine).

Taking large amounts of aspartame over time can upset the amino acid and neurotransmitter balance in our bodies. Thousands of side effects have been documented after aspartame use. Among the reported symptoms are headaches, dizziness, confusion, depression, blindness, tinnitus (ringing in the ears), nausea, diarrhea, urticaria, frequent urination, tremors, abdominal pain, shortness of breath, chest pain, convulsions, slurring of speech, and many others.

Aspartame is marketed as NutraSweet and Equal.

There is concern about the amount of aspartame being consumed by children. Research has shown that aspartame can slow neurological response to the point where a child will begin to miss a baseball that previously would have been hit.

The Food and Drug Administration (FDA) and G.D. Searle (its chief manufacturer) still maintain that aspartame is safe. However, the circumstances under which aspartame was approved by the FDA are at best open to question.

SACCHARIN   Saccharin is a non-nutritive, synthesized sweetener that is 300–500 times sweeter than sugar. Its commercial fate is uncertain, however, because of cancer found in animals that were fed saccharin. It is a weak carcinogen, but more importantly, saccharin is a co-carcinogen (a substance which assists the progress of cancer). Because of conflicting studies, a ban on saccharin has been delayed to provide additional time to gather data and study new evidence.

Saccharin frequently contains other sweeteners to mask its bitter aftertaste. These masking sweeteners are important to allergic people because, frequently, they are derived from corn. Saccharin is also an appetite stimulant because of its capacity to lower blood sugar.

Sweet and Low is one example of a saccharin sweetener.

There is no completely safe sweetener—all have drawbacks or side effects. While honey or maple syrup used in small amounts are better than refined sugars, fruit juices are probably the best choice for sweeteners. While allergy extracts are available for sugar, it is healthier to avoid it.

Reading Labels

The safest foods for allergic people to eat are fresh, organically grown fruits, vegetables, and meats. However, because many of us are unable to grow our own food, and because top-quality food is not always available, we are forced to buy commercial and some processed foods. It is important to learn to read food labels intelligently, to recognize food additives, and to use this information to make wise food purchases.

RECOGNIZING ALLERGENS AND ADDITIVES

The first aim in reading labels is to identify any food which is an allergen. Foods may be listed by their common, usual names, or they may be described by their "food component" names. For example, zein, which is corn protein, appears on labels, as does whey, which is a milk component. Familiarize yourself with the food lists (pp. 81–106) to learn the various ways common food allergens are listed on labels.

Reading labels can also help to determine the presence of food additives that may cause reactions. A food additive is a substance or mixture that has been added to aid in production, processing, packaging, or storing the food. Chance contaminants are not considered food additives. Contrary to popular belief, food additives are not a modern invention. Adding chemicals to food began when it was first discovered that salting meat would make it last longer.

Over 10,000 intentional additives are currently used in foods. Many people are allergic to even the smallest amounts of these compounds. Inconsistent labelling makes it difficult to determine whether the offending substances have been added to food. If in doubt, always write to the packer or manufacturer. Explain that you have allergies and must know more about the product in order to be able to use it.

The laws governing packaging and food processing state that labels must:

- Identify the product in a language the consumer can understand.
- Identify the manufacturer, packer, or distributor.
- Declare the quantity of contents, either in net weight or volume.
- List the ingredients in order of predominance. An item that lists sugar first or second will have a very high sugar content.
- Accurately represent the contents of the container, if a picture of the product is used on the label.

In some cases, relatively few food additives need to be listed on labels. For over 300 "standard" foods (those for which the government has written chemical recipes), *no ingredients need be listed*. Manufacturers can choose among many alternative standard chemicals without having to indicate on the label which is used. Only if the processor substitutes or adds a nonstandard chemical must they indicate that fact on the label. Ice cream, considered a standard food, can have up to 30 additives that do not have to be indicated on the label. Similarly, if monosodium glutamate is used in canned vegetables, it must appear on the label, but it may be added to mayonnaise and salad dressings without being listed if a standard recipe is followed. It is impossible for consumers to know whether the absence of additives on a label means that none are present, or whether it means the food is covered by a standard recipe and contains numerous additives.

Consumer demand for uniform appearance and flavor in food products has played a large role in increased use of food additives in recent years. To meet this demand, food processors and manufacturers are using increasingly more additives. Most are unfamiliar chemicals with no nutritional value. Some additives are quite harmless, but the safety of others is in question, despite testing that has been done on them. Frequently, additives are used to conceal the inferior quality of food, to heighten the appearance of damaged food, and to make the food more attractive to the consumer.

Chemical additives used in food processing must make the food more easily available, improve shelf-life, enhance nutritional value, increase quality or customer acceptability, or facilitate the food's manufacture or preparation.

The following summary describes the various types of food additives. (For more information on specific compounds, see *Recommended Books*, p. 304.)

PRESERVATIVES

About 100 chemicals called "antispoilants" are used to help prevent microbiological growth and chemical deterioration. They include antioxidants; "mold" inhibitors; fungicides; sequestering agents; and general purpose preservatives such as sulfur dioxide and propylgallate. Preservatives prevent changes affecting color, flavor, texture, or appearance. Traditional preservatives include salt, sugar, vinegar, spices, and wood smoke; however, wood smoke is no longer considered to be safe.

ACIDS, ALKALIES, BUFFERS, AND NEUTRALIZERS

To ensure product appearance and quality, the acidity or alkalinity of processed foods must be maintained. Acids and alkalies are added to foods for this reason. Acids provide tartness in candies, jams, gelatin desserts, sherbets, carbonated soft drinks, and fruit juices. Alkalies are used in confections, cookies and crackers, baking powder, creamed cottage cheese, ice cream, prepared pancake mixes, biscuit and muffin mixes, and bleached flours.

Buffers and neutralizing agents help to control acidity or alkalinity by absorbing or "neutralizing" excess acid or alkaline substances. Buffers are added to many processed foods, including breakfast cereals, baked goods, jellies and jams, and canned vegetables.

MOISTURE CONTENT CONTROLS

Substances that prevent loss of moisture are called humectants. Glycerine, propylene glycol, and sorbitol absorb moisture from the air and are frequently used as humectants. Calcium silicate and dextrose are added to prevent table salt from caking due to moisture absorption from the air.

COLORING AGENTS

Both natural and synthetic food colorings are used in processed foods to heighten acceptability and attractiveness. However, color can also be used to conceal damage or inferior quality.

Synthetic food colorings are preferred in the food industry over natural ones because of their better coloring power, uniformity and stability, and they are usually cheaper. Synthetic coloring agents, however, can cause problems for an allergic person. Those sensitive to petrochemical hydrocarbons will usually react to one or more of the certified food colorings.

Food colorings are added to thousands of foods, including baked goods, soft drinks, fruit juices, ice cream, gelatin desserts, maraschino cherries, oranges, sweet potatoes, sausages, prepared mixes, processed meats, cheeses, butter, cream, margarine, breakfast cereals, candies, jellies, and pet food.

FLAVORINGS

A wide variety of flavorings is used in processed foods, including spices, natural extracts, oleo resins, essential oils, and the numerous synthetic flavors produced by chemists. Flavoring agents are the most common food additives. There are over 2,000 flavoring agents in use, of which only 500 are natural.

Flavoring agents produce or modify the flavors of foods. Foods that lose their original flavor, as a result of processing, generally require flavoring agents to make them palatable. Flavorings are added to baked goods, beverages, candy, cottage cheese, fruit-flavored toppings, gelatin, ice cream, liquor, pickles, processed meats, puddings, shortening, and many other food items.

Flavorings—whether natural or synthetic—can pose a problem for the allergic person. Imitation (synthetic) flavorings contain very little, if any, natural materials. Unless a flavoring agent is made entirely from natural materials, it is considered to be an imitation.

Flavor enhancers are also added to foods, the most common being monosodium glutamate (MSG) and maltol. Flavor enhancers usually add no flavor of their own to foods, but heighten or modify existing flavor. Some researchers believe as many as 80 percent of our population will react to monosodium glutamate, with symptoms ranging from migraine headaches to a feeling of fatigue.

PHYSIOLOGIC ACTIVITY CONTROLS

Physiologic activity control chemicals serve as ripeners or antimetabolic agents for fresh foods. Ethylene gas is used to speed the ripening of bananas, and maleic hydrazide prevents potatoes from sprouting.

Some physiologic activity controllers are nontoxic enzymes of natural origin. Enzymes are used in fermentation and in the manufacture of bread, artificial honey, and frozen milk concentrates.

BLEACHING AND MATURING AGENTS

Bleaching agents are used to improve the appearance of food products, while maturing agents hasten their maturation. Both bleaching and maturing agents are added to flour. Fresh ground flour is pale yellow that slowly becomes white with storage. Processors add agents to the flour to accelerate its aging process, which improves its baking qualities and reduces storage costs, spoilage, and the possibility of insect infestation.

PROCESSING AIDS

Processing aids include sanitizing agents that remove bacteria and debris from products; clarifying agents that remove extraneous materials; emulsifiers and emulsion stabilizers that help to maintain a mixture and assure consistency; texturizers, stabilizers, or thickeners that are added to products to provide "body" and maintain a desired texture; and whipping agents or propellants in cans.

Sorbitan derivatives are a processing aid used to retard "bloom" on the surface of chocolate candy. Calcium chloride is added to canned tomatoes to prevent them from falling apart, and sodium nitrate and nitrite are used to develop and stabilize the pink color of meats.

Many people are allergic to these meat processing aids.

Since artificially sweetened beverages lack the "thickness" normally contributed by sugar, bodying agents or thickeners may be added to correct this problem. Some processors simply increase carbonation to make up for the lack of body.

NUTRITION SUPPLEMENTS

If natural nutrients have been removed and then replaced during processing, the food is labelled as enriched. Enrichment can also mean that yeast has been added. However, added nutrients always fail to make up for the number of nutrients removed in processing the food materials. A fortified food is one with nutrients added to make it more nutritious than it was before processing.

While not all artificial additives are harmful for everyone, not all natural additives are safe for everyone. The additives discussed in this summary are but a few of the many types used in the food industry, in packaging and processing, and in restaurants. It should now be obvious that eating fresh fruits, vegetables, and meats, together with cooking "from scratch," are vital for allergic persons!

Food Management

After food testing is completed, you may feel like saying: What am I going to eat? There is nothing left for me to eat. What am I going to do? I am going to starve! I don't have time to cook exotic foods. You have taken away all of my favorite foods.

Food management is necessary to help find your way through to health. Here are four approaches to controlling food allergies.

1. *Avoidance and retesting:* This allows the

best immune system repair, but nutrition may suffer if too many foods are avoided.

Foods that cause violent symptoms must be eliminated from the diet completely for a minimum of 30 days; depending on your health and the foods involved, this avoidance period may have to be extended. Study the food lists (pp. 81–106) to learn which food ingredients may be encountered in unsuspected places. Avoid all forms of the food, for even the smallest amount can cause reactions as severe as those caused by a regular serving.

Avoiding a food allergen allows our body to revert to a more normal state, which may initially be uncomfortable. Think of these feelings of discomfort as withdrawal symptoms. You may experience strong cravings for various foods. Whatever your withdrawal symptoms may be, they will last only a few days, and then you will begin to feel better.

At the end of the avoidance period you are ready to test your tolerance of the food. Re-introduce only one food at a time every four days, by eating a regular serving *once* for either lunch or dinner. If you experience no symptoms within 48 hours, then it is safe to try the food again in four days. If you still have no difficulty, you may add the food to your diet on a four-day rotation.

However, if you experience symptoms every time you eat the food, avoid it again for six months, and then try it with a 10-day interval between exposures. If you experience symptoms with each exposure to the food, it is possible that: 1) you have had inadvertent exposures when you thought you were avoiding the food, or 2) you have a fixed food sensitivity. With a fixed food sensitivity, you will react every time you eat the food, regardless of how long you have avoided it or how little of it you eat.

2. *Rotation diet and extracts:* This combination allows moderate immune system repair, and its nutritional support is better. Extracts protect the immune system, allowing it to rebuild. Rotation also prevents food reactions and allows enzyme function to repair. (Rotation diets are discussed in detail on p. 111.)

3. *Extracts only:* Extracts alone will lead to some immune system repair, but it will be slow since the body is constantly exposed to the same food. No enzyme repair occurs.

4. *Regular diet:* The same state of health is maintained. There is no chance for body repair, leading to increased debilitation and gradual loss of health.

If you continue to eat foods to which you are allergic, without rotation or extracts, you will experience reactions with every meal and snack. Continued masked reactions over a long period of time will weaken your immune system, which can ultimately lead to degenerative diseases and increased infections.

Children with untreated food allergies may suffer frequent earaches, eczema, bedwetting, asthma, hyperactivity, learning or discipline problems, and many other symptoms. Adults whose allergies are left untreated may have frequent headaches, "spaciness," spells of sleepiness, arthritic symptoms, depression, postnasal drip, sinus symptoms, hypoglycemic symptoms, frequent infections, and many other maladies. Both children and adults may experience outbursts of temper as a result of untreated food allergies.

Because your enzyme functions are unable to repair, your digestive processes will suffer, and will gradually degenerate. Improperly digested food is antigenic to your body and will cause an increase, over time, in the number of foods to which you are allergic. The situation quickly becomes a vicious circle.

THE ROTATION DIET

The rotary diversified diet, here referred to as the rotation diet, was developed by Dr. Herbert Rinkel. It is based on the fact that it usually takes four days for food components to "clear" our bodies. For some it may take seven to 10 days for the food to clear, but for most of us four days is sufficient. On the rotation diet, a food is eaten, and is then not repeated until it has cleared the body, preventing a cumulative effect from consuming offending foods.

Foods, both animal and vegetable, are divided into families according to their common biological and botanical properties. On a rotation diet these families are assigned and spread out over four days so that each day offers a selection of meats, vegetables, and fruits. Each day's selections are treated like a menu in a restaurant. You may chose only from what is on the menu for that day, omitting foods listed for another day.

For the more sensitive person, and for those who have a slower clearing time, the food families may have to be spread out over a seven-day or 10-day rotation. While this means less food to choose from each day, it prevents overlapping and allows these people to rotate foods safely.

A rotation diet also has other benefits. It prevents new food allergies from developing due to overexposure to a particular food; it preserves your tolerance for foods to which you are not sensitive; and it aids in identifying food sensitivities. Each time the cycle repeats, symptoms on a given rotation day signal an unidentified problem food. With only certain foods being consumed on a particular day, it is easier to identify the food allergen.

The strictness with which you follow a rotation diet depends on the severity of your food allergies and symptoms. Some people can eat only one food per meal, and cannot repeat the same food during a 24-hour period. Others are able to eat several foods in a meal and repeat foods if the meals are separated by a number of hours. The easiest way to do this is to begin your rotation day with supper and end it with lunch the following day. If you cook extra portions for supper, you will have "leftovers" for breakfast, lunch, or the freezer.

"Borrowing" Foods   There are many different versions of the rotation diet. If you have chosen a diet in which there are too many foods permitted on one day and not enough on another day, you can change the order of rotation. You may switch foods from one day to another, if you move the entire food family, and leave it on the day to which it was moved. If you are not careful to switch an entire food family at once, you will find you are no longer rotating.

For special occasions, you may temporarily "borrow" a food by using the following method: skip the food on the cycle just before the special occasion. Then eat the food for the special occasion. Skip the food on the next cycle, and add it back on the subsequent cycle. This method will allow you to cope with the diet on special occasions. However, beware of accommodating too many such occasions, or you will no longer be truly rotating.

Keep rotation meals very simple, and use only good-quality, additive- and preservative-free foods. Even though you may not have to eat single-food meals, try to limit the number of foods you consume at one sitting. Choose simple recipes and make any necessary substitutions. Remember, unless a food is permitted on a given rotation day, you should not eat it on that day.

If you are strictly rotating, grains may be consumed only on the day you eat foods from the grass family. For some whose sensitivities will permit, a grain may be eaten every other day, or gluten and nongluten grains may be alternated. Corn, rice, and millet are the nongluten grains; wheat, rye, barley, and oats all contain gluten in varying amounts. Buckwheat is not a grain, but it does contain some gluten. (For more information about gluten content in foods, see "Wheat," p. 81.) Now that amaranth, quinoa, spelt, and teff are available for baking, finding a bread substitute is not as difficult as it was several years ago. Bean flours are available and they make good pancakes and waffles. Potato flour can also be used to make bread substitutes.

In addition to wanting a bread for each rotation day, some people long for butter or margarine each day. Butter is allowable only on beef/milk days. Since most margarines contain whey combined with vegetable oil, they do not really fit in on any rotation day. An interesting margarine/butter substitute for vegetables is the oil-of-the-day in which spices for the day have been marinated.

Spices, teas, and oils must be rotated in the same way as all other foods. However, you may "float" spices or seasonings if you wish. For example, some people like onion and garlic, which are in the same family, for special dishes. They "save" the onion and garlic and use them only for these dishes, which they eat only once or twice a month. However, asparagus, chives, and leeks are also in this family. If you "float" onions and garlic, be careful that you have not eaten asparagus, chives, or leeks on another day of the same rotation cycle.

Keeping a notebook helps to make following a rotation diet easier. Keep your menu for one to two weeks (or for a length of time convenient for you) in the notebook. Your menu should include both meals and snacks, written out in detail. Also, you should note cooking plans; what to thaw, what to cook in advance, which will help when you are making your shopping list. You should also note any symptoms that occur on specific days either on your menu or on a record sheet in your notebook. This will enable you to identify additional problems.

Another helpful technique, particularly if you have children, is to "color-code" the rotation days. Snacks, freezer meals, shelves, or kitchen cabinets can be color-coded to correspond to rotation days. Children and family members can then easily find the food and snacks allowed on any given rotation day.

Even though all family members may not have allergies, it is easier on the person preparing the meals if the whole family rotates foods, so that only one menu need be cooked. A rotation diet is a healthy, balanced way to eat and includes meats, vegetables, and fruits from which to choose each day. The whole family can benefit from following a rotation diet; it will help identify allergies, prevent new allergies from forming, "protect" currently tolerated foods, and prevent any cumulative effects from eating a food or food group too often.

Easing into rotation gradually will probably make your family more cooperative—and perhaps even unaware that changes are being made. Start by rotating the protein portion of the meal (chicken, beef, fish, pork). After this has become commonplace in your menus, work on rotating vegetables, and then fruits. Leave grain rotation until last, because it is a bit more difficult. Alternative grains do not provide the same texture to baked goods as our old standby, wheat.

For more information on rotation diets, see *Recommended Books*, p. 304.

"But the Recipe Says …": Learning How to Substitute Foods

Following a rotation diet means that you will have the opportunity to create new recipes, something that most of us have never tried. In the beginning, God did *not* create recipes! That was left to those of us who need to provide for the well-being of our families.

Once you have learned about your family's food sensitivities, cooking will take on a new dimension. Rotating foods means that traditional recipes can seldom be used just as they are. This can be an overwhelming problem at first, but adapting recipes does become easier with time. The challenge and reward of creating satisfying, delicious meals for yourself or your family—plus the pleasure that comes from seeing them regain their health and positive outlook—make the time invested in the kitchen very worthwhile.

Fortunately, you are not the first person to attempt food rotation. Many good books are available, that are full of helpful hints and recipes. (Please see *Recommended Books*, p. 304.) Try to use as many of these as possible. At first, the foods, recipes, and menus may seem strange to you, but in time you will find that the unadulterated taste of high-quality food is wonderful. Your tastes, and those of your family, will become accustomed to new delights that you might not have otherwise tried.

The following are substitutions that you may use in recipes. You will find that substituting ingredients will cause variations in the texture and consistency of your recipes, but this is a part of the pleasure of expanding your cooking horizons.

Beverages

COFFEE

- Use one or two Tbsp. fig syrup to one cup hot water. Commercial coffee substitutes are also available.

SODA POP

- Make your own; mix carbonated spring water with fresh or concentrated fruit juices.
- Commercial "sodas" made from pure fruit juices and carbonated water are available.

SMOOTHIES

- Blend ice cubes and fruit juice until smooth. Add fruit for extra flavor and thickness.

Condiments

CATSUP

- Catsups sweetened with honey or rice syrup are available.

MAYONNAISE

- Several egg-free, cholesterol-free, honey sweetened mayonnaise products made with cold-pressed oils are available.
- For a tasty, no-fail, egg-free mayonnaise that may be substituted for oil, sweeteners, and spices, follow this recipe:

  In a blender, place three Tbsp. soy milk powder and ½ cup water. Blend well. Add one Tbsp. maple syrup or honey, one tsp. sea salt, and one green onion bulb, finely chopped. Mix. Slowly add one cup oil and continue blending on low until mixture is thick. Add ¼ cup lemon juice, blend, and refrigerate. This mayonnaise is not as thick as commercial products. Yields 1½ cups.

SALT

- Most brands contain dextrose (corn) and chemicals. Try using spices, sea kelp, or soy sauce (read labels). Non-iodized salt does not contain corn.

VINEGAR

- Vinegar contains yeast and should be avoided by those who have candidiasis or a yeast allergy. Substitute lemon or lime juice in an equal amount for vinegar.

Desserts and Chocolate

CHOCOLATE SYRUP

- Blend ½ cup roasted carob powder, ½ cup honey or maple syrup, ⅓ cup nut milk, and ⅓ cup water in a blender. Bring to a boil in a saucepan, stirring constantly. Boil for one minute. Remove from heat and beat in ⅓ cup tolerated margarine. Refrigerate syrup when cooled.
- Sweetened carob chips can also be used. Melt in a double boiler until smooth, and pour over ice cream or desserts.

COCOA (UNSWEETENED)

- Use equal amounts of carob powder in place of cocoa.

GELATIN

- Soften two Tbsp. agar-agar in one cup juice. Add the mixture to two cups hot liquid and boil for two minutes. Add sweetener if desired. When set, add fruit and nuts.

ICE CREAM

- If milk is a problem, soy-based brands are available.
- When soy and milk are a problem, try rice-based products and those sweetened with maple syrup.
- If chemicals and preservatives are a problem, try homemade ice cream. Combine one quart half-and-half cream with ½ jar of Knudsen flavored syrup and mix in an ice cream maker. "Clean" store brands of ice creams are also available.

ICINGS

- Blend mashed bananas with yogurt.
- Try unsweetened whipped cream with pure

concentrated juice or a touch of carob powder.
- Try cream cheese blended with maple syrup if milk products are not a problem.
- Use a regular icing recipe and substitute, as in the following adapted recipe:

The recipe calls for	Substitute
3 Tbsp. butter	3 Tbsp. oil
2 Tbsp. unsweetened cocoa	2 Tbsp. carob powder
1¼ cups instant powdered milk	½ cup puréed almonds
¼ cup water	same
⅓ cup mashed banana	same
¼ tsp. lemon juice	same
¼ tsp. vanilla	same

POPSICLES

- Freeze unsweetened fruit juice in paper cups or molds, or puree and freeze fresh or frozen fruits.
- To make creamsicles, add yogurt or milk to pureed fruits and freeze.
- Blend one cup plain yogurt, ¼ cup carob powder, and ¼ cup sweetener. Freeze and enjoy!

Eggs

AS BINDERS

In most recipes, substitutes can replace eggs without many changes. However, this depends on the recipe.

- Eggs can easily be replaced with three Tbsp. pureed fruit or vegetable for each egg required in the recipe.
- One Tbsp. flax seed mix may be substituted for each egg. Flax seed mix can be made by blending until smooth one cup ground flax seeds to three cups water. This mixture keeps well in a covered container in the refrigerator.
- Two parts arrowroot powder, one part tapioca

flour, and one part slippery elm powder makes an effective binding mixture. Use one Tbsp. of this mixture with two Tbsp. water to replace each egg.

- Many recipes work well when two Tbsp. oil beaten with one Tbsp. water is used to replace each egg.
- When needed for binding, one yolk equals two Tbsp. of the following mixture. Blend one part bean flour and two parts water, and heat in a double boiler for an hour. Use two Tbsp. of this mixture as a substitute for each cup of flour. Refrigerate in a covered container.

AS LEAVENING AGENTS

- For each egg to be substituted (not more than two), beat together two Tbsp. carbonated water with two tsp. baking powder.
- Or try substituting one Tbsp. bean flour and one Tbsp. oil for each egg.
- Another substitution is ¼ cup tapioca starch for each egg.
- When needed for leavening, one yolk = ½ tsp. baking powder and two Tbsp. bean flour.

Certain brands of egg replacer available at health food stores may also be substituted for eggs.

Grains

BISCUIT MIX:

- For each cup of biscuit mix, use one cup flour, 1½ tsp. baking powder, ½ tsp. sea salt, and one Tbsp. oil or shortening. Mix these ingredients well.

BREAD CRUMBS

- Crushed whole-grain cereals or whole-grain crackers work well.
- Crushed chips—rice, corn, potato, sweet potato, or taro—make a good substitute.
- Any dried 100 percent grain bread, or any ground nuts or seeds, may be used.

FLOUR

- Any type of flour may be substituted for white flour. When baking with alternative flours, the texture of the product will differ with each flour. Alternative flours should almost always be sifted before measuring, as this helps improve texture. Use amounts equal to those required of white flour in the recipe; the only difference will be in the amount of liquid needed to achieve the desired consistency. You may also have to adjust the temperature to prevent burning, particularly when baking cookies.

FLOUR IN GRAVY

Follow your usual recipe for gravy and substitute one of the following for each tablespoon of wheat flour:

- ½ Tbsp. arrowroot powder.
- ½ Tbsp. rice starch or flour.
- 1 Tbsp. buckwheat flakes or flour.
- Cooked, puréed, starch vegetable.
- Powdered brewer's yeast (very strong taste).
- 2 Tbsp. tapioca flour.
- ½ Tbsp. potato starch or flour.
- ½ Tbsp. cornstarch.
- 1 Tbsp. barley or rye flour.

NON-WHEAT BASED CRACKERS

- Norwegian flatbread.
- Rice cakes, or rice crackers.
- Some brands of Rye Krisp (read labels).
- Oat cakes.

Milk

All recipes work well with milk substitutes. In fact, interesting textures and tastes can be discovered with each substitute that is used.

Each item in the following list of milk substitutes is equal to one cup of milk:

- ½ cup plain yogurt plus ½ cup water.
- one cup goat's milk.
- one cup fruit juice.

- one cup soy milk, or infant formula.
- ½ cup nuts blended with water to make one cup.
- one cup water.
- water with ½ tsp. baking soda and lemon or lime juice or vinegar.
- one cup vegetable liquid.
- one cup tomato juice for casserole-type dishes.

ARTICHOKE MILK

- In a saucepan, combine two cups water and ½ cup artichoke flour. Mix together with an electric mixer. Bring the mixture to a boil and simmer for 20 minutes. Cool and sweeten if desired.

BUTTERMILK

- Substitute one cup plain yogurt, soy milk, or milk. To curdle, add 1 Tbsp. lemon or lime juice.

CHOCOLATE MILK

- To your choice of milk or milk substitute, add carob syrup to taste, or try the following non-dairy carob milk recipe.
- In a blender, blend 1½ cups nut milk, three Tbsp. roasted carob powder, five chopped dates, figs, or raisins, one Tbsp. nut butter, and a dash of pure vanilla (optional). Chill and serve. Makes two cups.

COCONUT MILK

- In two cups water, soak one cup unsweetened shredded coconut. Mix in a blender until very smooth and strain if desired. Milk drained from fresh coconut may also be used.

COTTAGE CHEESE

- Tofu pressed between paper towels and crumbled is a good substitute.

CREAM SAUCE

- Steam cauliflower until tender. Place it in a blender, and blend until smooth. Gradually add vegetable, meat, fish, or poultry broth until thick and creamy. Add ½ Tbsp. oil and spices if desired. This makes about one cup.
- A beautiful green sauce can be made using broccoli, peas, or spinach in the above recipe.
- Melt meat, fish, or poultry fat in a pan and add flour until the mixture becomes pasty. Slowly add broth and stir until desired consistency is obtained. Add spices if desired.

EVAPORATED MILK

- If milk is a problem, try using infant soy formula. Check the label for other allergens.
- If tolerated, try evaporated goat's milk.

NUT MILK

- Use one part water to ½ part nuts. Grind nuts or seeds in a blender. Add water and blend the mixture until smooth. If desired, add sweetener and vanilla. Commercial nut milk mixes are available at health food stores.

POTATO WATER

- Use water from cooked potatoes in place of milk. This is useful in baking and making sauces.

POWDERED MILK

- Try equal amounts of soy milk powder or powdered goat's milk, both available at health food stores.
- In some recipes, commercial nut milk powder can be substituted. It works well in icings.

SOY MILK

- Mix one cup soy flour, or any bean flour, with four cups water. Place the ingredients in the top of a double boiler and let them sit for two hours. Bring the mixture to a boil and simmer for 20 minutes. Cool and strain. Sweeten if desired, and keep the mixture in the refrigerator. Soy milk mixes are available at most health food stores, but be sure to read the label.

WHIPPED CREAM

- A whipped cream substitute can be made by adding a sliced banana to one egg white. Beat until stiff, and the banana will dissolve.

ZUCCHINI OR OTHER VEGETABLE MILK

• Blend one medium, peeled zucchini in a blender until smooth. Pour the liquid into a pan and heat on low. Add two Tbsp. sweetener and one beaten egg (the egg can be omitted) to the mixture, stirring constantly for about 10 minutes. If the mixture is overcooked, it will separate. Should this happen, pour the mixture into a blender and blend until smooth. Use as a milk substitute in recipes, or just chill and drink.

• Alternatively, peel and cut a zucchini into chunks, and then liquify in a blender. The pulp and seeds will constitute a thick liquid that can be frozen.

Sweeteners

CONFECTIONER'S SUGAR

This contains three percent cornstarch. Substitute:

• Non-instant dry milk powder.
• Goat's milk powder.
• Maple syrup granules, ground to powder in a blender.

MOLASSES

• Use equal portions of fig syrup or rice syrup.
• Try equal portions of all-fruit syrups.

SUGAR

• Honey, sorghum, maple syrup, and fruit syrups may be substituted for sugar, but use only half the amount called for in the recipe. Be sure other liquids are decreased (¼ cup for each cup of liquid sweetener).
• Date sugar and maple syrup granules are also good substitutes. Use ½ to ¾ cup date and maple sugars to one cup sugar.

Miscellaneous

BAKING POWDER

Most brands contain cornstarch. Corn-free powders are available at health food stores, or you can try making your own with the following recipes.

• Mix well ⅓ cup baking soda, ⅔ cup cream of tartar, and ⅔ cup arrowroot powder. Store in a covered container.
• Mix well ¾ cup cream of tartar, nine Tbsp. baking soda, and six Tbsp. potato, rice, or tapioca starch. Store in a covered container.
• Mix well ½ lb. rice or potato starch, ½ lb. cream of tartar, 5 oz. baking soda, and 1 oz. potash or tartaric acid (found at pharmacies). Sift these ingredients several times and store in a covered container.

BOUILLON CUBES

• Undiluted meat, fish, or poultry drippings may be frozen in ice cube trays and used in place of bouillon cubes.
• Another substitute is one Tbsp. soy sauce or one Tbsp. yeast in powder or flake form (caution: soy sauce frequently contains wheat).

CORNSTARCH

• Arrowroot may be substituted for cornstarch in recipes that will not be heated.
• Use 2½ Tbsp. potato starch or tapioca starch for 1 Tbsp. cornstarch.
• Flour works well in place of cornstarch for thickening sauces and gravies.

FLAVORED EXTRACTS

These contain sugar and alcohol.

• Extracts without sugar and alcohol are available.
• Vanilla flavor can be obtained by leaving a vanilla bean in honey. Use small amounts of the honey in a recipe that calls for both a sweet and vanilla taste.

SHORTENING

• All soy margarines or oils used in equal measurement work well as butter or shortening substitutes.
• Melted animal fat of any kind may be used. Poultry fat adds flavor, but goose and duck fat

are softer and more moist than butter. Pork and beef fat have about the same texture as butter, but lamb fat stays very firm at room temperature and has a stronger flavor.

Fast Foods

Fast foods are a nutritional and allergic disaster. Saturated fat, cholesterol, and sugar provide most of the high caloric content. Fast food meals always contain one or more major food allergens, as well as additives and preservatives, and yet the average North American seems willing to pay for convenience, spending more than $400 a year for fast foods. Two hundred customers order one or more hamburgers every second.

The smell of grease in most fast food restaurants tells us that fat is probably the biggest offender. The deep-fat fryer may contain highly saturated beef fat or hydrogenated vegetable oils. The constant heating and reheating of the frying oils converts the oil molecules to a form that is injurious to our body metabolism. Chicken and fish, which are coated with batter that absorbs large amounts of these frying fats and oils, may contain more fat than a hamburger. Still more fat is added by the use of condiments such as mayonnaise, sauces, and salad dressings.

Nearly all items on fast food menus contain large amounts of salt (sodium chloride). All foods contain some natural sodium, but 90 percent of our sodium comes from salt added to foods at the time of manufacture or consumption. Some fast food sandwiches contain ⅔ to ¾ tsp. of salt, more than half of the daily recommended sodium intake. Milkshakes may contain as much as 300 mg of sodium, 100 mg more than is in 10 potato chips. It is extremely difficult to determine by taste how much sodium foods contain. French fries, though they taste quite salty, frequently contain less sodium than do the burgers (salt is added to the outside of the French fries just before they are served, increasing the salty taste).

Sugar is also added to many poor-quality fast foods to improve appearance and taste. For example, molasses and corn syrup mixes are added to hamburger meat to reduce shrinkage and improve color, flavor, and juiciness. French fries may have a sugar coating that turns brown when it is immersed in hot grease. The batters on fried foods always contain some sugar, often sucrose, but more frequently they are corn sweeteners. Soft drinks, the common beverage at fast food restaurants, are the greatest single contributor of sugar to our diets. Excess sugar will disrupt blood sugar levels, cause pancreatic overload, disrupt function of neurotransmitters in the brain, and contribute to the likelihood of dental cavities.

The combination of salt and sugar in fast foods can cause problems for patients with high blood pressure. The hidden sugars are also a hazard for diabetics. Perhaps what is more dangerous for all of us is that fast food fans develop larger appetites for salt and sugar, and then crave and eat more salt and sugar on all of their foods.

Soft drinks sold at fast food restaurants usually contain caffeine. As a stimulant, too much caffeine can cause anxiety, irritability, muscle twitches, upset stomach, insomnia, rapid heart rate, and nervousness. Prolonged use or overuse of caffeine overstimulates adrenal function, which can lead to adrenal exhaustion. Caffeine also depletes B vitamins. Although a can of soda has only one-third of the caffeine that is found in one cup of coffee, its effect on a child's body is the same as the coffee would have on an adult. A child who drinks several sodas in a day may have trouble sleeping, as well as symptoms of hyperactivity, because of the caffeine.

Fruits, vegetables, and whole grains are necessary sources of fiber in our diets, and are not generally included on fast food menus unless there is a salad bar in the restaurant. These salad bars do provide small amounts of fiber, particularly if beans are offered. Beans are one of the best sources of soluble dietary fiber. A few fast food restaurants offer whole-grain or multi-grain buns. However, the percentage of whole grain in the buns is low and some contain brown food coloring rather than whole grains. A diet consisting largely of fast foods provides very little of the fiber needed for good digestion.

Fast foods are also low in nutrients, particularly vitamin A, biotin, folic acid, B_5, calcium, iron, copper, magnesium, B_6, and vitamin E. Salad bars can offer some foods with vitamin A, but the calcium-containing foods, such as cheese and milkshakes, are also high in fat. There is some iron in hamburger patties and in foods at the salad bar. Orange juice and potatoes contain vitamin C. However, a steady diet of fast foods and junk snack foods can lead to serious nutritional deficiencies.

Fast Food Allergens   The many common allergens found in fast foods create problems for the allergic person.

- *Beef:* Is in hamburgers, most Mexican food. The major meat served at all restaurants. May also be in frying oil.
- *Corn:* May be hidden in meats as a flavor additive; flour or starch may be added to the batter of deep-fat fried foods. The chief sweetener in soft drinks, corn, may also be added to dressings and sauces as grain vinegar.
- *Egg:* May be in the batter of deep-fat fried foods, or in salad dressings and sauces, breads,

doughnuts, pasta, or ice cream.
- *Milk:* Used in cheese on sandwiches, in garnishes, in milk shakes, ice cream, soups, doughnuts, and hot dogs. Milk solids, lactose, and whey are added to breads, desserts, salad dressings, and sauces.
- *Potatoes:* May be in salads, or served as baked potatoes or French fries.
- *Soy:* May be in hamburger patties. If the hamburger has a special name that does not include the word hamburger, soy and other extenders may be added. The most common oil used in all restaurants, soy is also used in cheeses.
- *Sugar:* Occurs in desserts, soft drinks, and batters on fried foods.
- *Tomatoes:* Used frequently in sandwiches, pizza, and spaghetti sauce, or served at salad bars.
- *Wheat:* Makes up the batter of deep-fat fried foods; used in sandwich bread and buns, pizza crust, and pasta.
- *Yeast:* Occurs in sandwich bread and buns, cheese, doughnuts, hot dogs, pizza crust, barbecue sauce, catsup, mayonnaise, and mustard.

In addition to common food allergens, fast foods also contain chemical additives. Artificial colorings are used to increase visual appeal. MSG (monosodium glutamate), a flavor enhancer, is frequently added to batters for breaded foods, salad dressings, gravy, soups, and croutons. At one time, sulfites were used extensively to preserve whiteness and freshness of fruits and vegetables. Because of fatal allergic reactions to sulfites in some people, restaurants may no longer add sulfites to their menu items. However, some foods may have sulfites added at the manufacturing level, particularly potatoes, stuffing, beer, wine, breaded shrimp, lime juice, and maraschino cherries. BHA and BHT are antioxidant chemicals that may be used in beverages, ice cream, baked goods, soup base, lard, shortening, and dry breakfast cereals. Aspartame, an artificial sweetener, is also found in some fast foods.

Recently many fast food chains have made an effort to reduce the fats in their foods. They have switched from saturated beef fat to vegetable oils for all products except French fries. Some companies are also seeking to eliminate dyes, particularly yellow dye #5.

Because ingredients may change daily in traditional restaurants, they are not required to label their food. However, fast food restaurants produce standard products that could easily be labelled on their wrappers or boxes. Because of allergy problems and nutritional concerns, such labels would be advantageous for the consumer. However, there are no government requirements for this, although government agencies do acknowledge that the restaurant industry has changed since 1938, when labelling rules were formulated. The restaurant industry is generally opposed to labelling, although some fast food restaurants have voluntarily disclosed the ingredients in their food.

For an allergic person, it would be best to avoid eating at fast food restaurants. If you are sensitive to the basic foods (corn, wheat, eggs, soy, yeast, milk, and sugar), it will be almost impossible for you to avoid these ingredients. One possibility, of course, is for you to take food extracts. If you can do so without symptoms, you might use a visit to a fast food restaurant as a treat, on only a very limited basis. Even with

the use of extracts, it is easy to overload. Fast food menus are definitely not part of rotation diets!

Surviving Fast Foods   If you do eat at a fast food restaurant, use the following guidelines to help make your meal as healthy as possible.

- Eat at restaurants where there is a salad bar. Eat only the fresh vegetables and the beans; use the dressings sparingly and avoid the pickled condiments.
- Order less than you want in order to conserve on calories. Avoid anything labelled big, deluxe, or whopper.
- Try to avoid fat by seeking out foods that are baked or broiled. Ask for the sauces, mayonnaise, cheese, and bacon to be omitted. If you order something deep-fried, peel off the batter or breading. Do not order "extra crispy."
- Ask that salt not be added to your meal. Avoid salted condiments, processed meats, and cheese.
- Reduce calories and sugar by avoiding soft drinks and desserts.
- If you suspect you will react to the restaurant water, bring your own from home.
- If the restaurant does not serve fruit you can eat as dessert, bring fresh fruit from home.
- Ask if the restaurant has an ingredients list for their foods. Read it carefully to avoid surprises!
- Instead of eating at the restaurant, take food home from the drive-in window or take-out counter and serve with healthy beverages, fruit, and vegetables.

CHAPTER 10

COMMON CHEMICAL SENSITIVITIES

What is Chemical Sensitivity?

Since the mid-19th century, developments in chemistry have radically changed our lives. Modern theories of chemistry have been developed, laboratory techniques and equipment have been refined, and thousands of new chemicals and compounds have been formulated. Chemical warfare agents were used toward the end of World War I, and after World War II, the chemical revolution began in earnest. While modern chemistry has given us wonderful products, it is not entirely a blessing. Over 500 billion chemicals are manufactured in North America each year, of which 500,000 are in common use. These chemicals have found their way into our homes, our food, our water, and our air, and, ultimately, into our bodies. Chemicals and their cumulative effects have a serious impact on our health.

Understanding of chemical sensitivity has developed slowly, primarily as a result of studying food allergy. Dr. Albert Rowe discovered in the 1930s that many of his patients had multiple fruit sensitivities. Rather than displaying an allergy to fruits in a particular family, these patients were allergic to all fruits. In the early 1950s, Dr. Theron Randolph found this was a problem with chemical contamination of the fruit rather than a true fruit allergy, since unsprayed fruits were tolerated by these patients.

Dr. Randolph is the father of chemical allergy. He first described chemical susceptibility in 1951, and in 1953 he outlined the effects of natural gas on sensitive people. In 1962 Dr. Randolph published *Human Ecology and Susceptibility to the Chemical Environment*, which identified the environmental chemicals—including indoor and outdoor air pollution, food additives and contaminants, cosmetics, toiletries, and drugs—responsible for a wide range of physical and mental illnesses. The concept of chemical allergy or susceptibility was born. Dr. Randolph used the term susceptibility to avoid debate over whether reactions to chemicals were allergies in the classical sense or hypersensitivity. Regardless of the mechanism, reactions to small doses of chemicals can cause severe symptoms.

Chemicals enter our body through the mouth and nose, and through direct skin contact. Chemically sensitive people acquire their susceptibility because of hereditary and genetic factors, lowered immunity, and inadequate or damaged body detoxification mechanisms. Chemical susceptibility usually develops as a result of repeated, low-level exposure to a number of chemicals over a period of time. However, it may also be triggered by a massive, overwhelming exposure to a chemical spill or fire, pesticide spray, or general anesthesia.

TYPES OF CHEMICAL EXPOSURES

Indoor Chemical Air Contaminants   Any chemical that pollutes the indoor environment is dangerous for the chemically susceptible person. Unfortunately, buildings themselves are frequently the largest contributors. Building materials, unless carefully selected, can be very toxic. Formaldehyde is found in large quantities in building materials and is dangerous to humans, even in low concentrations. Carpets contain large amounts of formaldehyde, while also trapping dirt, dust, and mold.

Combustion products from natural gas, fuel oil, coal, and heating systems fill the air. Gas stoves, hot water heaters, and dryers, as well as oil fumes (generated by running motors), contribute further to the problem. Fresh paint, cleaning supplies, deodorants, disinfectants, detergents, plastics, and insecticides all contribute to the toxic chemical pool. With the advent of more energy-efficient buildings, these indoor contaminants are trapped in our homes and workplaces. The workplace is becoming increasingly contaminated by the use of photocopiers, computers, correction fluid, carbon paper, and NCR (carbonless) paper.

Outdoor Chemical Air Contaminants   Outdoor air often is not safe to breathe. Traffic exhaust and smog raise outdoor pollution to unsafe levels in our cities. Despite government regulations and monitoring, some industries contribute to outdoor pollution. Oil refineries, wells, and storage tanks pollute the air for miles around them. Indiscriminate spraying of crops, forests, orchards, gardens, and lawns adds still more chemicals to the air. Paving and resurfacing roads and tarring roofs contaminate outdoor air. Woodstoves and fireplaces emit smoke from chimneys, fouling outdoor and indoor air.

Chemical Contaminants of Food and Water
Our food supply is contaminated with insecticide and fumigant residues, color and flavor additives, sweeteners, preservatives, sulfur agents, and many other chemicals used to make foods look, taste, and smell "right" to the consumer. Other chemicals find their way into our food from the containers in which they are packaged.

In some areas, chlorine and fluoride are added to drinking water that may already be contaminated by fertilizers and pesticides leeched from the soil. Inadequate or nonexistent sewage treatment may also contribute to water pollution.

Drugs and Medications   As pharmacology flourishes, reactions to drugs and medications become more abundant. Adverse reactions to all classes of medications have been reported. These reactions may be due to the substance itself, to the vehicle of the drug, or to the preservative. Many sensitive people are losing their "drug umbrellas." As their immune system dysfunction increases, they react to more and more drugs. Many are unable to tolerate any antibiotics or local anesthetics. There are no reserve medications under their umbrellas.

Clothing and Personal Care Products
With the advent of synthetic fabrics, reactions to clothing, bedding, and upholstery have become common. Natural fabrics can also cause reactions because of detergents, dry cleaning fumes, plasticizing starches or sizing, fabric dyes, or gas dryer residues. The rubber in elastic can also be a problem for some.

Most personal care products are no longer

natural or biological in origin. They are now formulated totally in laboratories, and most contain harsh chemicals that may sensitize a susceptible person.

Types of Chemical Reactions

According to Dr. Randolph, reactions to chemical allergens may be seen as part of a maladaptive process. When susceptible people are exposed to chemicals, their bodies adapt after the first exposures and no symptoms are obvious. As adaptation to our total load slows down, the maladaption spreads to related chemicals and even to foods. Chronic symptoms begin to develop, and the cumulative damage causes a gradual decline in health.

Some chemical reactions are IgE mediated; they involve an antigen-antibody response. Rashes, hives, and skin eruptions are symptoms common to this type of reaction. More research is needed to uncover the exact mechanism of most reactions. As with food reactions, chemical reactions can be immediate, so the offending substance can be identified.

Some chemically sensitive people experience reactions that differ from the acute, immediate response. These chemical reactions are delayed, making the connection to a particular chemical exposure unclear. Chemical reactions can also be occult, where damage is caused but no symptoms are obvious. Thermal reactions are those triggered by cold, heat, or light following a chemical exposure.

The toxicity of most chemicals is determined by animal studies. While these studies are helpful, they are not absolute. Animal physiology differs from human physiology, making the effects of a chemical different. Human drug doses that are simply extrapolated, based on weight, from animal doses, may not be accurate.

Perhaps the chemically sensitive people in our society can be likened to the canaries used in coal mines during the last century. Miners would take caged canaries into the mine shafts with them to act as sensors. If the canaries became sick or died, the shafts would immediately be evacuated. Death of the birds indicated the presence of methane gas.

Chemically sensitive people are the sensors of our polluted air, water, and food. They are the early warning signs that care must be taken to clean up our home and work environments. The chemically sensitive are those who have experienced overexposure or subtle, cumulative exposure to harmful chemicals that have damaged their detoxification pathways and immune system.

Symptoms of Chemical Sensitivity

The brain is the primary target organ in chemical reactions. Chemicals are deposited in fat cells, and the brain has a very high fat content. Smooth muscle is also a major responder in both food and chemical sensitivities. However, chronic symptoms and illness resulting from maladaption to various environmental elements can affect any system or organ of the body.

- *Cerebral*: Confusion, depression, anger, "brain fag," inability to concentrate, apathy, emotional instability, mental fatigue, light-headedness, and lethargy. Extreme reactions can result in psychosis, disorientation, regression, and sometimes hallucinations, delusions, and amnesia.
- *Respiratory*: Coughing, bronchitis, asthma, and "air hunger."
- *Gastrointestinal and urinary*: Excessive thirst, eating or drinking binges, diarrhea, constipation, urgency and frequency of uri-

nation, nausea and vomiting, gas, dry mouth, bad or metallic taste in the mouth, abdominal pain, difficulty swallowing, heartburn, and gallbladder symptoms.

- *Neurological*: Headaches, neck aches, nerve pain, muscle pain, arthritis, chest pain, fainting, restless legs, and numbness.
- *Ear, nose, and throat*: Ringing in ears, dizziness, cough, itching inside ears, hypersensitivity to noise, rhinitis, nasal obstruction, and stuffy nose.
- *Skin*: Hives, acne, blisters, eczema, itching, and burning.
- *Eye*: Vision disturbances, watery eyes, light sensitivity, eye pain, swelling around eyes, and drooping, itching, swollen, or red eyelids.
- *Musculoskeletal*: Fatigue, muscle pain, cramps, weakness, joint pain, stiffness, and lack of coordination.

Chemical reactions can also have cardiovascular effects. Dr. William Rea has shown in studies on nonatherosclerotic patients that angina symptoms can be triggered by exposures to various chemicals. Other cardiovascular symptoms include heart pounding, racing, palpitations and irregular beats; edema; fainting; flushing; pallor; phlebitis (vein inflammation); and purpura (hemorrhaging under the skin).

Chemically susceptible people can be masked to chemicals, just as others can be masked to food allergies. For example, sensitive persons can always identify a fresh paint smell as a problem, because it is not often encountered, but they may not recognize that the odor from a gas range is problematic because they are exposed to it daily and have become masked. If they avoid all natural gas exposures for four to seven days, symptoms will appear upon their return to the natural gas sources.

Chemically susceptible people may be addicted to chemicals just as food-sensitive people are addicted to allergenic foods. Those who are chemically addicted may say they love the smell of gasoline, nail polish, or fabric softener. One of our patients used to eat her father's lunch leftovers, which reeked of the oil refinery in which he worked. She eagerly awaited his return so she could eat this contaminated food, and she confessed it was the high point of her day. It is significant that her father felt so sick from his work exposures that he was unable to eat all of his lunch.

Chemically sensitive people have an extremely acute sense of smell and are more aware of odors and chemicals than those unaffected. However, they may not detect the very chemical or odor that is triggering a reaction. When exposed to chemicals, sensitive persons should always breathe through their mouths since chemical fumes entering the nose can directly affect the brain through interconnecting nerve pathways. Chemicals entering the body through the mouth must circulate through the bloodstream and pass through the blood-brain barrier before affecting the brain.

Those with chemical sensitivities are often misunderstood by friends, relatives, co-workers, and physicians who tend to label them as lazy, trouble-makers, or, worst of all, crazy. Many physicians immediately recommend psychiatric help or counselling after listening to their symptoms, and employers suspect psychological problems rather than symptoms from chronic chemical exposure. Chemically sensitive people can suffer a lifetime of impaired health unless they find proper diagnosis and treatment. They can become unable to work, and even existing comfortably can become difficult for them. However, there is hope. The following are ways chemically susceptible people can help themselves.

TREATMENT OF CHEMICAL SENSITIVITIES

You can avoid or reduce exposure to many chemicals by following these guidelines:

- Clean up your interior environment at home and at work. Complete information for accomplishing this can be found later in this chapter (p. 156).
- Eat a diet of "clean" foods, uncontaminated by pesticides, fertilizers, or processing.
- Drink only safe, uncontaminated water. (See p. 258.)
- Use an air cleaner both at home and in your car.
- Provide nutritional support for your immune system. (See *Nutrition and Allergies*, p. 227.)
- Seek out testing and immunotherapy with chemical extracts.

Implementing these measures requires some thought and effort, but it will help to create a "safe" haven and to reduce the overload on your immune system.

THE IMPORTANCE OF CLEAN AIR

Some chemically sensitive people must buy their air just as they buy safe water. There are many air cleaners on the market, in many price ranges. In general, the cheaper products remove particles such as dust, mold, bacteria, some viruses, cigarette smoke, and odors. These air cleaners don't contain enough activated charcoal to filter harmful chemicals.

You should purchase an air cleaner which:

- Contains enough activated charcoal to remove chemicals, including formaldehyde. Charcoal that has been impregnated with

potassium permanganate is available specifically for this purpose.
- Contains an odor-removing charcoal filter in addition to the formaldehyde filter.
- Contains a filter designed to remove dust, mold, bacteria, and viruses.
- Has the fan motor located so that the odors from the motor are filtered before the air leaves the cleaner.
- Has a stainless steel or baked enamel finish.

Some people may have difficulty tolerating the filter materials; they will have to investigate their tolerance to charcoal from various sources. The material used in the HEPA (High Efficiency Particulate Accumulator) filter in air cleaners may also cause a problem for some. A final filter, containing glass beads, may reduce these problems.

Extremely sensitive people should use a filter both in their homes and cars. Some air cleaners have electrical adaptors so they can be used in both places. House filtration systems can be purchased and fit into central heating and cooling units. There are also specialized air cleaners that fit over computers and printers to prevent their operating odors from filling the room.

It may be necessary to construct a box (with a glass front and vents to the outside) to hold your television set because chemicals released when the TV is in use can provoke symptoms. Reading boxes, vented to the outside, will eliminate problem fumes from paper and printers' inks.

Charcoal face masks, available in 100 percent cotton or 100 percent silk, have an activated charcoal filter. Using these masks makes trips outside possible for some very chemically sensitive people who otherwise could not tolerate the exposures.

ASSESSING UNAVOIDABLE CHEMICAL EXPOSURES

Even if all of the above guidelines are followed, you still face unavoidable chemical exposures at home, school, and work. You should be tested for the chemicals listed below if you experience any of the problems associated with them. Chemical neutralizing extracts can help control your symptoms.

Sources of Problem Chemicals	Chemical to Test For
Perfumes; solvents; artificial flavorings; tea; raspberries.	Benzyl Alcohol
Tap water for drinking, showers or baths, or dishwashing; water in swimming pools or hot tubs; laundry bleach; disinfectants.	Chlorine
Water for drinking, showers or baths, or dishwashing; hot water in tubs, swimming pools; toothpaste; dental fluoride treatment.	Fluoride
Clothing or fabric stores; carpets; mobile homes; new homes or additions; panelling; particle board; fresh paint; fresh concrete; glues and adhesives; air deodorizers; insecticides; hairsetting lotions; facial tissue; wood smoke.	Formaldehyde
Cosmetics; liquid and bar soaps; furniture polish; cough drops; toothpaste; hand lotion; vitamins (soft gelatin capsules).	Glycerine
Car exhaust; gas heat, stoves, or furnaces; oil heat or furnaces; airport fumes.	Petrochemicals (Gas or Diesel)
Car exhaust; gasoline; perfumes; liquors; gas heat, stoves, or furnaces; oil heat or furnaces; wood smoke; cleaning agents; airport fumes.	Ethanol
Perfumes; aftershaves; cosmetics; newspapers; canned foods; computers; aspirin or sulfa drugs; wood smoke; waterbeds; glues and adhesives.	Phenol

Each of these chemicals and possible sources of exposure are discussed in the following section.

Common Sources of Chemical Exposure

BENZYL ALCOHOL

Benzyl alcohol has a faint, sweet odor and a burning taste. It occurs naturally in tea, raspberries, jasmine, hyacinth, ylang-ylang oils, Peru and Tolu balsams, and storax.

Benzyl alcohol is used as a topical antiseptic, a local anesthetic, and a preservative in injectable medications. It is used frequently as the scent extractor in perfumes, as the flavor extractor in synthetic flavorings, and in many manufacturing processes.

Vomiting, diarrhea, and central nervous system depression are caused by ingesting large doses of benzyl alcohol. Stronger solutions are corrosive to skin and mucous membranes.

Sources of Benzyl Alcohol

Acne medications
Anesthetic (local)
Antiseptic (topical)
Artificial flavorings
Baked goods
Ballpoint pen inks
Beverages
Candy
Chewing gum
Cosmetics
Cough drops
Ear drops
Gelatin desserts
Heat-sealing polyethylene films
Ice cream
Ices
Nylon dyes
Ointments
Perfume
Photographic chemicals
Preservative in medications

Raspberries
Solvents
Synthetic flavorings and scents:
  Blueberry
  Cherry
  Floral
  Fruit
  Grape
  Honey
  Liquor
  Loganberry
  Muscatel
  Nut
  Orange
  Raspberry
  Root beer
  Rose
  Vanilla
  Violet
  Walnut
Tea

CHLORINE

In its elemental state, chlorine is a yellow-green gas with a suffocating odor. Because it is a very reactive element, it does not occur in a free state. It is found abundantly in compounds with other elements in the form of chlorides. Chlorides have properties and actions that are totally different from those of chlorine. Some chlorides, such as salt (sodium chloride), are not harmful and may even be beneficial.

Other compounds of chlorine release small amounts of chlorine gas when put in water, resulting in chlorine exposure. Reactions can occur to chlorine fumes rising from hot or cold running tap water. Symptoms include red eyes, sneezing, skin rashes, fatigue, abdominal pain, fainting, or dizziness. Taking a shower, washing dishes, or even washing your hands exposes you to chlorine.

Higher concentrations of chlorine can cause skin eruptions; heart swelling; severe respiratory tract irritation; swelling of the throat; delirium; coma; circulatory collapse; vomiting; erosion of the mucous membranes; and pain and inflammation in the mouth, throat, and stomach.

If you are chlorine-sensitive, set your drinking water out in an open glass bottle for 24 hours to let the chlorine dissipate. This should be done in a well-ventilated room or outside so that you are not exposed to the chlorine as it disperses. *Do not* store water in plastic containers, as it will absorb chemicals from the plastic. A water purifier may be used to remove the chlorine from your tap water, but it may be wise to supplement your diet with minerals since some filters also remove trace minerals.

Chlorine neutralizing extracts taken before a bath or shower—and before *and* after a swim or hot tub session—help to prevent chlorine reactions.

Sources of Chlorine Gas and/or Compounds

Aging and oxidizing agents
Anesthetics
Antiseptics
Bleaching of flour
Bleaching of textiles and wood pulp
Bleaching powder (Ajax, Comet)
Cleaning agents
De-tinning and de-zincing iron
Disinfectants
Fire extinguishers
Industrial preparations of various compounds
   (dyes, plastics, and synthetic rubber)
Laundry bleach
Metallurgy

Processing of meat, fish, vegetables, and fruit
Production of organic and inorganic
   chemicals
Refining of oil and sugar
Shrinkproofing of wool
Water sources:
   Bathtubs
   Hot tubs
   Municipal water systems
   Sewage systems
   Showers
   Spas
   Swimming pools

FLUORIDE

Fluoride is the name given to a class of fluorine compounds. In its elemental state, fluorine is a pale yellow gas. It is the most active of all elements, and so is found only in combination with other elements.

Dietary sources of fluorides include a wide range of foods, depending on regional fluoride content variations in the soil and water supplies.

Fluorides are plant-toxic pollutants because they accumulate in the leaves. These plants are then toxic to the animals and humans that eat their leaves. This type of plant contamination commonly occurs near ore smelters, refineries, and industrial plants which manufacture fertilizers, ceramics, aluminum, glass, and bricks.

Water is the greatest source of fluoride exposure for most people in North America. One part of fluoride per every million parts of water is added to aid in reducing dental caries, which has provoked an ongoing argument. Studies done in New Zealand, Japan, Canada, and Michigan have shown that fluoridated communities do not have lower levels of dental caries in the general population. The studies were done over a 10- to 15-year period, and results were compared to those from areas with unfluoridated water supplies. Some research demonstrates that fluoride actually damages teeth by interfering with the proper formation of proteins that make up the structural framework of growing teeth.

Excessive amounts of fluorides can be toxic to us, causing fatigue, weakness, mottling of the teeth, wrinkling of the skin, a prickly sensation in the muscles, kidney and bladder disorders, constipation, vomiting, itching after bathing, excessive thirst, headaches, arthritis, gum diseases, nervousness, diarrhea, hair loss, skin and stomach disorders, numbness, brittle nails, sinus problems, mouth ulcers, vision problems, eczema, bronchitis, and asthma. Too much fluoride can also reduce vitamin C levels, weaken the immune system, cause birth defects, and damage enzyme systems.

The following substances are, or contain fluorides, and can be a source of exposure:

Ammonium fluoride: Used as wood preservative.

Antimony fluoride: Catalyst for organic reactions.

Boron fluoride: Catalyst for organic reactions.

Calcium fluoride, hydrofluorosilicic acid, potassium fluoride, sodium fluoride, sodium silicofluoride: Used to fluoridate waters.

Chlorine trifluoride: Fluorinating agent.

Cobaltic fluoride: Fluorinating agent.

Cryolite: Solvent for aluminum oxide.

Fluoride lasers: Some, such as the Krypton fluoride (KrF) laser, contain fluoride as part of the medium.

Fluorite: Used as metallurgical flux.

Fluorspar: Used to prepare fluorides.

Freon: Refrigerant and propellant in spray cans.

Hydrofluoric acid: Used for etching glass, as a solvent, and as a catalyst in gasoline production.

Magnesium fluoride: Used in the optic industry to improve light transmission in glass.

Sodium fluoride: Insecticide and disinfectant.

Sodium silicofluoride: Used in water and toothpaste to prevent tooth decay (two parts/million).

Stannous fluoride, tin difluoride, fluoristan: Used in toothpaste and as a fluoride treatment to prevent tooth decay.

Sulfur hexafluoride: Gaseous electrical insulator.

Teflon: Non-stick compound.

Sources of Fluorides or Fluorocarbon Derivatives

Aluminum refining	Propellant in aerosols
Cutting steel	Refrigerants
Fire extinguishers	Rocket fuel
Insecticides	Rodenticides
Isotope separation	Soil-release agents
Lubricants	Solvents
Plastics	Textile treatments

FORMALDEHYDE

Formaldehyde is a potent chemical manufactured from methanol, natural gas, or lower petroleum hydrocarbons. At normal temperatures, it is a colorless, pungent gas, which irritates the eyes, nose, and respiratory tract. Other types of formaldehyde are trioxane, a crystalline solid form of formaldehyde; paraformaldehyde, a colorless, granular form of formaldehyde with the same irritating qualities; and formalin, an aqueous solution of formaldehyde. Formalin is the major form in which formaldehyde is marketed, containing 37–50 percent formaldehyde, stabilized by a water solution of methanol.

Annual formaldehyde production is measured in billions of pounds. The resinous compounds formed when formaldehyde is combined with other chemicals make it particularly important commercially. It has many industrial uses:

- To set dyes.
- To waterproof fabrics.
- As a germicide, disinfectant, and fungicide.
- In tanning and preserving hides.
- In printing and photography.
- In manufacturing building materials.
- In manufacturing artificial silks, cellulose esters, dyes, organic chemicals, glass mirrors, explosives, and resins.

Formaldehyde is a major, continuous indoor pollutant. Its odor can be sensed at levels as low as 0.05 parts per million (ppm). How much constitutes a safe level of formaldehyde is the subject of debate. Most people are unaware of formaldehyde if levels are maintained at 0.1 ppm, which is the safety standard. Health hazards are associated with this level and the standard should be reduced, since chemically sensitive people are affected by this and lower levels.

Average Concentrations of Formaldehyde

Source	ppm
Outside air	0.003
Textile manufacture	0.1–1.4
Clothing stores	0.13
Stores unpacking clothing	0.14–0.25
Treated paper	0.14–0.99
Fertilizer production	0.2–1.9
Fabric stores	0.60
Mobile homes	0.80
Plywood industry	1.0–2.5
Wet biology laboratories	1.70
Hospital autopsy rooms	2.2–7.9
Cigarette smoke	50.00

Indoor levels of formaldehyde can vary from day to day, and from hour to hour, according to fluctuations in temperature and humidity.

When relative humidity is between 50 and 60 percent, indoor formaldehyde levels peak, while on cold days they are usually lowest. Adequate ventilation in any building is important to reduce the indoor formaldehyde level.

Concentrations of formaldehyde also depend upon the type of building construction. Mobile homes have the highest concentrations—regardless of age, a mobile home contains formaldehyde. By the time a mobile home is two years old, its formaldehyde level will have dropped 20–30 percent; that level will be maintained for 10 or more years. Again, indoor ventilation is extremely important to lower formaldehyde levels.

There are many sources of formaldehyde exposure in our homes. To avoid these exposures, do not use items containing formaldehyde such as:

Air fresheners
Cosmetics and deodorants (some)
Glues
Insecticides
Leather
Mothballs
Paints
Soaps and shampoos (some)
Spray starch
Vinyl

Because new clothes, drapery and upholstery fabrics, and electronic equipment (televisions, computers, stereos) outgas (dissipate) a significant amount of formaldehyde, these items should be aired completely before use. Thoroughly wash new clothing before wearing it.

Carpeting is a significant, constant source of formaldehyde exposure that increases when carpets are wet. Formaldehyde is used to set the dye and in the backing to stiffen the jute. It takes at least three years for carpet to outgas the majority of its formaldehyde. Despite the age of the carpet, however, some formaldehyde will always outgas.

Composite panelling is another formaldehyde source. It takes about 18 months for panelling to outgas the major portion of formaldehyde; like carpeting, panelling will continue to emit the chemical.

Particle board (used in furniture, bookshelves, sub-flooring, home construction, and cabinet shelves) and plywood used in homes are also significant formaldehyde sources. Particle board outgases more formaldehyde than plywood. Formaldehyde release from these materials increases with moisture and heat.

Combustion also produces formaldehyde; gas stoves and heating systems, fireplaces, kerosene space heaters, and wood-burning stoves will cause problems for chemically sensitive people.

Because cigarette smoke contains extremely high concentrations of formaldehyde, chemically sensitive people should not smoke or allow smoking in their homes or cars.

Formaldehyde is also found in our food supply. Freshly caught fish may be washed with formaldehyde solution to prevent bacterial growth. Chicken may be dipped in a formaldehyde wash to whiten the skin. Formaldehyde may be used as a preservative in flour, and some maple syrup may contain formaldehyde from the pellets used on maple trees to keep taps open. Meat, from animals given feed containing formaldehyde, will be contaminated. At one time, formaldehyde was added to milk and eggs to increase shelf-life. This practice has been discontinued due to health problems caused by this chemical exposure.

Symptoms of Formaldehyde Exposure   Formaldehyde is extremely toxic. Exposures at concentrations from 0.1 to 5 ppm can cause asthma, contact dermatitis, nausea, chronic headache, diarrhea, memory lapse, fatigue, drowsiness, eye and respiratory tract irritation, nosebleeds, dry and sore throats, insomnia, and disorientation.

Higher exposures (10 to 20 ppm) may produce coughing, tightening in the chest, a sense of pressure in the head, and heart palpitations. Exposures at 50 to 100 ppm and above can cause serious injury or death.

Chronic or long-term health problems remain after formaldehyde exposure stops. It is a suspected carcinogen and it may be implicated in SIDS (sudden infant death syndrome) since most infant furniture is made of particle board. More research is needed to determine the role of low-dose formaldehyde exposure in chronic health problems and cancer.

Many people are sensitive to formaldehyde. There is strong evidence that it interferes with the functioning of the immune and detoxification systems, which causes sensitivities to an increasing number of substances. This is called the spreading phenomenon. An untreated formaldehyde sensitivity becomes worse with time so that one reacts to lower formaldehyde concentrations.

Formaldehyde exposures are a greater problem for those with candidiasis because the aldehyde detoxification pathway is already overloaded (see p. 196).

Sources of Formaldehyde

Acrylic, wool, and nylon fibers
Adhesives
Aerated waste
Aerosol insecticides
Agricultural seeds
Air and furnace filters
Air fresheners
Animal feed
Antihistamines
Antiperspirants
Antiseptics
Anti-slip agents
Anti-static agents
Automotive exhaust
Bactericides
Barber and beauty shop disinfectants
Binders and mineral wool insulation
Binders for sand foundry cases
Binding agents for machinery casting
Binding on paper bag seams
Biology laboratories

Brake drums
Butcher paper
Buttons
Car exhaust
Carpeting
Catalytic heaters
Chalk
Chemistry laboratories
Chewing gum
Chickens (may be washed with formaldehyde to whiten the skin)
Chip board
Cigarettes and cigarette smoke
Clothing
Clothing stores
Coated papers used for cartons and labels
Coatings for appliances
Concrete or plaster
Cosmetics
Cotton fabric (some)
Cut flower arrangements (some)

Dental fillings
Deodorants
Detergents (some)
Dialysis units
Disinfectants
Disposable sanitary products
Drapery fabrics
Dry cleaning (disinfectant in cleaning solutions)
Dust sterilizing solutions
Dyes (some)
Eggs (formaldehyde sometimes used to increase shelf-life)
Electric shavers and mixers (in housing)
Electrical insulation parts
Electronic equipment
Embalming fluid
Enamels
Explosives
Fabric stores
Fabrics (used to improve color stability, wrinkle and shrink resistance, water repellency, moth proofing, and flame retardation in both synthetic and natural fabrics)
Facial tissues
Fertilizers (nitrogen)
Fiberboard
Fish (used as a preservative rinse on fresh or frozen)
Flame retardants
Flock adhesives
Floor coverings
Flour (preservative)
Foam insulation
Formica
Foundries
Fuels
Fungicides
Fur
Furniture adhesives

Gas stoves
Glass manufacturing
Glues
Gum (chewing)
Hair setting lotions
Hair waving preparations
Hardeners
Hardware or hardware store
Hospital bed sheets
Incinerators
Insecticides
Instant coffee
Insulation (urea-formaldehyde foam; fiberglass, and wool)
Kerosene stoves
Lacquers
Laminates
Latex paint
Lawn and garden equipment
Leathers
Lubricants (synthetic)
Maple syrup (some)
Mascara
Meat smokehouses
Medicines (some)
Melamine tableware
Mildew prevention
Milk
Mimeographed paper
Mineral wool production
Mobile homes
Molding compounds
Mothballs
Mouthwash
Mushroom farms
Nail hardener
Nail polish and undercoatings
Napkins
Napping agents
Newsprint
Non-woven binders

Nylon fabric
Oil-based paints
Orthopedic casts and bandages
Panelling
Paper products
Particle board
Pesticides
Phenolic thermosetting resins
Photochemical smog
Photographic developing solutions
Plaster
Plastics
Plumbing fixtures
Plywood
Polishes
Preservatives
Razor blades
Reclaimed paper products
Refrigerator hardware
Resins
Rubber hose production
Sanforized cottons
Shampoo

Soap
Soap dispensers
Softeners
Solvents
Sporting goods
Spray starch
Sterilizing solutions in barber and beauty
   shops
Tires
Toilet seats
Toothpaste
Upholstery fabrics
Urethane coatings and resins
Utensil handles
Vaccine preparation
Vinyl resins
Water filters
Water softening chemicals
Waxed paper
Waxes
Wood-burning stoves
Wood finishes

GLYCERINE

Glycerine—also called glycerol—is a clear, thick liquid about half as sweet as cane sugar. As the base of fat and oil molecules, it is a familiar chemical to our body, which uses glycerine as a source of energy or as a starting material for making more complex molecules. Many foods naturally contain glycerine. Any foods from which oil can be extracted, such as corn, peanuts, safflower, coconut, and animal fat, contain natural glycerine. It can also be processed from hydrocarbons.

Glycerine is used extensively in the food industry. Because it is a humectant (absorbs water from the air), manufacturers add it to foods to maintain a specific moisture content and to prevent foods from drying out and becoming hard. Glycerine is used as a humectant in tobacco, marshmallows, pastilles, and jelly-like candies. Glycerine is a solvent for oily chemicals, especially flavorings, which are not water-soluble. Glycerine serves as a bodying agent in combination with gelatins and edible gums and as a plasticizer in edible meat and cheese coatings. Beverages, liqueurs, confectionery, baked goods, chewing gum, gelatin desserts, meat products, and fudge toppings all contain glycerine.

Glycerine is also used in the manufacture of

nitroglycerine (dynamite); cosmetics; liquid soaps; blackening, printing, and copying inks; lubricants; elastic glues; and lead oxide. It helps to keep fabrics pliable, preserve printing on cotton, and to keep windshields frostfree. Glycerine is also found in automobile antifreeze, gas meters, hydraulic jacks, and shock-absorber fluid, and is used as a fermentation nutrient in antibiotic production.

In the cosmetics industry, glycerine is used in many products—read the labels! Mixed with water or some other suitable liquid, glycerine acts as a moisturizing agent when applied to skin. However, rather than acting as a humectant, glycerine first draws whatever moisture it can from the underlying tissues of the skin. Because it absorbs water from the tissues, glycerine keeps our body in a state of dependence. As long as glycerine is applied, the external skin surface will have some semblance of elasticity and softness, but when the applications cease, the skin takes on a dry, raspy feel. Any preparation containing glycerine can be damaging to delicate skin tissues. Glycerine is absorbed through the skin.

Sources of Glycerine

Adhesives
Animal fat:
  Beef
  Chicken
  Lamb
  Pork
Antifreezes
Astringents
Capsules (soft gelatin)
Coconut
Cosmetics (especially cake or compact form)
Cough drops
Disinfectants
Dry cleaning agents
Emollients
Eye drops
Fabric softeners
Face masks
Fire retardant for textiles
Flavorings
Food additives
Freckle removal lotions
Glues, cements
Hand lotion

Inks:
  Ballpoint pen
  Copy machine
  Felt-tipped pen
  Permanent marking
  Printers'
  Rubber stamp
  Stamp pad
  Water-soluble
Latex paints
Leather
Margarines
Modelling clay
Mouthwashes
Oven cleaners
Paper
Perfume
Pharmaceuticals
Plastics
Polishes:
  Floor
  Furniture
  Nail
  Shoe

Polyurethane foam (auto dashboards, carpets,
   flooring, furniture, mattresses, pads, seat
   cushions)
Regenerated cellulose
Shaving creams and lotions
Shortenings
Soaps

Solvents
Styptic pencils
Suntan preparations
Textile finishes
Tobacco
Toothpastes
Window cleaners

PETROCHEMICALS

Petrochemicals are compounds produced by distilling crude oil. They may be solids, liquids, or gases.

Exposure to petrochemicals usually occurs through inhalation, skin contact, or ingestion of foods that contain them. Exposure can occur both in and away from the home. Odors from nearby gas stations, garages, storage tanks, refineries, and producing wells can affect sensitive people both indoors and outdoors. Driving a car or filling the gas tank is a petrochemical exposure that should be minimized if possible.

Within your home, you should also eliminate all possible exposures to petrochemicals. Thoroughly air new plastics and paints for several weeks or longer before trying to live around them. Although some petrochemical products may continue to outgas for two to three years, the older the product (car, plastic shower curtains, painted walls, carpets, furniture) the less toxic it will be. However, an extremely sensitive person may never be able to tolerate some products that contain petrochemicals.

Forms of Petrochemicals	
Solid	Plastics; Synthetic fibers Wax coatings on fruits and vegetables
Liquid	Diesel oil; Gasoline; Other oil products
Gas	Natural and bottled gas Fumes from solids such as plastics Fumes from liquids such as gasoline Odors from soaps, perfumes, scented stationery, cleaning compounds, polishes, paints, and insecticides Oil evaporating from electric motors in household appliances Exhaust from automobiles and buses Fumes from chemicals used in copying or duplicating machines, inks, newspapers, typewriters, cosmetics, fabric softener sheets, medications, hair products, lipsticks

Some personal care products contain petrochemicals; use toiletries that are prepared without these chemicals.

Latex paint slowly releases petrochemical gases. To speed up this dispersion process, add baking soda to the paint before applying it. Some paints will become gluey when soda is added, so experiment with a small amount of paint first (one tablespoon baking soda to one cup of paint). Then paint a small board with this mixture, letting it dry outdoors for several days before bringing it inside to determine whether you will experience symptoms.

Mix the baking soda into the paint as follows:

One gallon of paint: Add one cup baking soda.

One quart of paint: Add ¼ cup baking soda.

One pint of paint: Add ⅛ cup baking soda.

Mix the paint outdoors while wearing a mask (and if possible, paint during the summer months for good ventilation). Stir the baking soda mixture thoroughly. It will bubble and cause rapid dispersion of the petrochemicals.

ETHANOL (ALCOHOL)

In many petrochemical environmental exposures, ethanol is a common denominator. It is a clear, colorless liquid that has a pleasant odor and a burning taste. Industrial ethanol is synthetic, while "organic" ethanol, also called ethyl alcohol or grain alcohol, is made by fermenting such natural substances as grains (corn, barley, rice, rye), sugars (molasses, cane sugar, any sweet fruit juice), and potatoes. Ethanol makes up the alcohol content in liquors.

Whether organic or synthetic, ethanol can cause central nervous system depression, anesthesia, feelings of exhilaration and talkativeness, impaired motor coordination, dizziness, flushing, nausea, vomiting, drowsiness, headache, wheezing, vision problems, impaired perception, disorientation, stupor, coma, and death. Alcohol is rapidly absorbed through the gastric and intestinal mucosa, and it can magnify an allergic reaction four times. Ethanol forms naturally in the intestinal tract from the fermentation of sugar, alcohol, and simple carbohydrates. It is formed in excess in the lower bowel by the action of *Candida albicans*.

Sources of Petrochemicals and/or Ethanol

Because of their widespread use, it is impossible to provide a brand-name listing of all products containing petrochemicals. Although reading labels helps, an ingredients label is not required on most of these products. When in doubt, consider a product to be of petrochemical origin until you can obtain more information from the manufacturer.

Ethanol neutralizing extracts are helpful both in preventing and alleviating symptoms caused by a petrochemical or ethanol exposure.

The following items are sources of one or the other of these chemicals.

Air fresheners
Alcoholic beverages
Anesthetics
Baked goods
Bath oils
Beverages
Bubble bath
Butane

Candy
Catalytic heaters
Chapstick
Cigarette smoke
Cleaning agents containing naphtha
Coal heat
Colognes
Copy machines
Cosmetics
Deodorants
Detergents
Diesel oil
Dried fruits
Dyes derived from coal tar
Exhaust fumes
Explosives
Face creams
Facial tissue
Fireplaces
Flavoring agents
Frozen pizza crust
Fruits (all sprayed, even if scrubbed and
    peeled)
Fumes from:
    Any engine that burns petrochemicals
    Any motor lubricated with machine oil
(electric mixers, sewing machines)
    Buses
    Cars
    Lawnmowers
    Outboard motors
    Trucks
Garage fumes
Gas appliances (propane and natural gas
    stoves, ranges, water heaters, refrigerators,
    dryers, oil or gas furnaces and space
    heaters, and the pilot light for any gas
    appliance)
Gasoline
Gelatin desserts
Glycerol

Hair care products
Hair pomades
Hand lotions
Ice cream
Ink
Insecticides
Kerosene
Lighter fluid
Lipstick
Liquors
Lotions
Machine oil
Meat (stored in the animal's fat cells)
Metal polish
Mineral oil
Mineral spirits
Motor oil
Nail polish and polish remover
Newsprint
Oil heat (furnaces)
Oil in electric appliances
Paints and stains
Paraffin
Perfume
Petroleum jelly
Photographic film
Pine scent
Plastics
Polyester
Preparation of:
    Essences
    Tinctures
    Extracts
Printers' ink (newsprint)
Propane gas
Rubber
Rubbing alcohol
Sauces
Soaps
Space heaters
Spray propellants

Stationery
Sterilization of medical instruments
Synthetic fibers
Tires
Toilet tissue
Varnish
Vaseline

Vegetables (all sprayed, especially the
  cabbage family)
Wax-coated fruits and vegetables
Wax-coated paper cups
Waxes
Wood burning byproducts

GASOLINE EXHAUST

Emissions from automobiles (gasoline exhaust) have long been considered a prime source of pollutants involved in smog formation and ozone production. A large percentage of these emissions is composed of hydrocarbons (compounds of hydrogen and carbon).

These hydrocarbon emissions can be divided into three classes, each class containing several compounds: Paraffins; olefins; and aromatics.

The amount of hydrocarbons in the air is measured in relation to the amount of nitrogen oxides and is the determining factor in the production rate of photochemical smog. As this ratio increases, the immediate potential for ozone production decreases. Nitrogen dioxide is also produced.

Automobiles also emit some unburned fuel hydrocarbons, carbon, a small amount of sulfur (an impurity in gasoline), and tars (heavy, poor-burning components of gasoline and oils). The carbon combines with oxygen to form carbon monoxide. Similarly, the sulfur combines with oxygen to form sulfur dioxide. Some of this is emitted from automobiles as an air pollutant, but a larger percentage is released by fossil-fuel burning plants.

Tiny specks of lead also float out of exhaust systems along with lead bromide, which escapes as a gas. Lead can cause anemia, kidney disease, mental retardation, blindness, and death. Although enough lead is not emitted to kill anyone, it is a health hazard for urban children who put into their mouths things that have touched the street.

Ammonia, organic acids, and solids, including zinc and metallic oxides, are also found in gasoline exhaust. Gasolines also contain antioxidants, metal deactivators, anti-rust and anti-icing compounds, detergents, and lubricants. Fragments of these compounds are also found in exhaust.

Sensitivity to gasoline exhaust can cause sleepiness; mental confusion and loss of reasoning ability; loss of memory; headache; nausea; dizziness; paranoia; anger; irritation of eyes, nose, and throat; and wheezing and coughing. Many of the components of exhaust are fat-soluble and have a special affinity for the nervous system. The most important route into the body for the chemical composition of exhaust is through the nasal passages. The smell receptors of the brain are located directly behind the uppermost cavities in the nose.

Diesel Exhaust

Diesel exhaust odors and irritants are generall considered to be nuisance pollutants. However, diesel exhaust is a potent allergen for many people. Symptoms caused by diesel exhaust exposure include nausea; headache; cough; disturbances of sleep, digestion, and appetite; irritation of eyes, nose, and throat; and mental confusion.

Diesel oil is composed chiefly of aliphatic hydrocarbons, but amylnitrate is added to raise octane and improve fuel ignition. Operating conditions affect chemical emissions; for example, as a diesel engine goes from idle to high speed, full load emissions are reduced. There are two sources of odors in diesel engines: unburned fuel and its thermal breakdown products (hydrocarbons and some nitrogen compounds); and products of incomplete combustion.

Nitrogen dioxide, sulfuric acid, formaldehyde, acrolein, and phenol are also present in diesel exhaust and are known to act as irritants. Other aldehydes in addition to formaldehyde are also present. The total aldehyde level in diesel exhaust is frequently higher than levels known to produce irritation.

Auto hydrocarbon, ethanol, formaldehyde, and phenol extracts are available from some physicians and are effective in controlling symptoms to vehicular exhaust. The extracts should be used daily, and extra doses should be taken when one is exposed to heavy traffic conditions.

Phenol

Phenol or carbolic acid is a colorless, crystalline solid that absorbs water from the air to become a liquid. It is poisonous and caustic, with a sharp burning taste. In weak solution, it has a mild, sweet taste and is a component of coal tar and wood odor.

Several phenols occur naturally. Natural phenol is part of the toxic agent in poison ivy and poison oak. It may also be present in spring water as a result of humus or natural coal around the spring.

Phenol is rapidly absorbed through the skin; it can cause skin eruptions, peeling, swelling, hives, burning, numbness, nausea, vomiting, cold sweats, headache, irritability, and wheezing. More serious effects of phenol exposure include gangrene, circulatory collapse, respiratory failure, paralysis, convulsions, coma, and death. It is also a suspected carcinogen.

Half of the total production of phenol is used in the manufacture of plastics. One-quarter goes toward manufacturing medications of coal tar origin, such as aspirin and sulfa drugs. Phenol is often used as a preservative in many injectable medications, including some allergy extracts. It is also used in producing nylon. Thyme oil, a compound chemically similar to phenol, is used in producing menthol.

Any product that has been manufactured with phenol will later outgas the chemical, which means that phenol is a major environmental exposure in our air, food, medications, and surroundings at home and work. Common phenol exposures include phenol emissions from computers, televisions, plastics, waterbeds, cleaning products, and newsprint.

Those who are allergic to phenol should also avoid phenol derivatives and chemically similar compounds. If you (or any member of your family) are phenol-sensitive, it is very important that no member of the family wear perfume, aftershave, or cologne. Avoid phenol exposures away from home as much as possible.

A phenol neutralizing extract can provide relief from symptoms resulting from unavoidable phenol or phenol-derivative exposures.

Sources of Phenol

Usage is so widespread that it is impossible to list all brand-name products containing phenol, phenol derivatives, or chemically similar compounds. Read labels! If you are not certain whether a product is phenol-free, do not use it.

In some cases, you may need to write to the manufacturer for confirmation.

The following are some sources of these compounds. Do *not* use products containing these compounds if you are sensitive to phenol.

Phenol Derivatives

Coal tar
Creosote
Cresols (ortho, meta, and para)
Hexachlorophene
Hexylresorcinol

Juniper tar
Parachlorophenol
Pine tar
Resorcinol
Trinitrophenol (picric acid)

Chemically Similar Compounds

Benzene
Benzoic acid (widely used in foods and
    beverages)
Benzoin
Camphor
Menthol (Bengay, Mentholatum, menthol
    cigarettes, Vick's Vaporub)
Parabens:

Butyl
Ethyl
Methyl
Propyl
p-Dichlorobenzene (mothballs, moth crystals)
Toluene
Xylene (Xylol)

Phenol

Aftershave
Allergy extracts (some)
Aluminum foil (the plastic on the dull side
    outgases phenol when heated; put shiny
    side against foods)
Antiseptics
Aspirin and other medications
Bakelite (molded articles, such as

    telephones, toys)
Bronchial mists
Calamine lotion
Canned foods (the golden liner in the can
    contains phenol)
Carbolated vaseline
Chloraseptic (lozenges, mouthwash, spray)
Cleaning products

Cosmetics (especially Revlon products):
- Cream blushes
- Liquid eyeliner
- Mascara

Deodorants, scented

Detergents

Dyes

Epoxy

Equal (sugar substitute—has a phenol ring in its chemical structure)

Explosives

Gasoline additives

Hair products:
- Dyes
- Hairsprays
- Setting lotions
- Shampoos

Hand lotion

Herbicides and pesticides

Laminated boards

Lysol, Lysol spray

Nasal sprays (Afrin, Neo-Synephrine)

Newsprint

NutraSweet (has a phenol ring in its chemical structure)

Nylon

Ointments (first aid cream, etc.)

Over-the-counter drugs:
- Antihistamines

Aspirin

Cold capsules

Cough syrups

Decongestants

Eye drops

Perfumes (all):
- Aftershave
- Deodorants
- Hand lotion
- Powder

Pesticides

Phenolic resins (hard plastics that outgas phenol vapors when warmed—TV sets, computers, radios)

Photography solutions

Pine Sol

Plastic coatings on electric wires

Plastic dishes and wraps (when heated in microwave)

Polyurethane

Preservatives in medications

Refrigerator storage dishes

Scotch tape

Sunscreens and suntan lotions

Thermal insulation panels

Vaccines

Wallpaper (vinyl-coated)

Waterbeds

Jewelry and Metal Allergy

A metal allergy is a special type of chemical allergy that usually manifests as contact dermatititis. The metal itself may not be toxic, but hypersensitivity to the metal may cause the problem. Metals that can cause reactions include chromium, cobalt, copper, iron, nickel, and mercury. Mercury is, of course, an extremely toxic metal.

Nickel is the most common metal cause of contact dermatitis. As our perspiration dissolves the metal, it attaches to our cells. Bonded to the cells, this nickel prompts symptoms long after the offending object has been removed.

One out of 10 women are nickel-sensitive, usually because they have had their ears pierced. Women with allergic tendencies should wear high-quality gold or stainless steel posts and wires. Stainless steel does contain nickel, but it is tightly bound and perspiration cannot cause its release. Some women can wear sterling silver, but silver also tends to corrode in the presence of perspiration. There have been cases reported of women who developed dermatitis from the internal use of metal containing a minute amount of nickel (for example, stainless surgical steel sutures and copper-7 IUDs).

On some people, metal jewelry tends to turn dark or leave black marks on the skin. This is not an allergic reaction to the metal, but rather an indication that the person's pH (acid/base) levels are too acidic.

The following items are common causes of contact dermatititis:

Bra clips
Bracelets
Buckles
Buttons
Clips
Costume jewelry
Earrings
Frames for metal glasses
Garter clips
Necklaces
Rings
Snaps
Scissors
Thimbles
Watch bands
Watches
Zippers

Cosmetics and Toiletries

Cosmetics and toiletries have been used in some form throughout history. Early cosmetics and toiletries included simple unguents, and lotions made from flowers, fruits, vegetables, and herbs. Some unlucky people even tried arsenic and lead, leading to their deaths.

Today's cosmetics and toiletries are formulated in chemical laboratories and contain harmful ingredients. Yet, despite their harsh contents, they are widely used. They are glamorized, advertised, made irresistible and the consumer ignores warnings that they may be unsafe. It was not until 1976 that the Food and Drug Administration (FDA) required the contents of cosmetics to be labeled. Even now, fragrances and trade secrets are exempt from this requirement. Illnesses, injuries, and allergies have been caused by the use of cosmetics.

Many chemically sensitive people have problems with cosmetics and toiletries. Some must avoid them totally; others are able to use some carefully selected products. Cosmetics worn by others can also affect the chemically sensitive. Ethanol, phenol, benzyl alcohol, and orris root extracts provide prevention of and relief from allergic reactions to cosmetics and toiletries.

Hypoallergenic products are supposedly free of irritants and allergens, but they still contain potentially harmful chemicals. The FDA admits that there are no official standards for hypoallergenic products, other than that they must be less likely to cause adverse reactions than other similar products. While manufacturers of natural cosmetics genuinely try to make health and beauty products that are superior, due to individual sensitivities, these products can still cause problems. There is no such thing as a nonallergenic cosmetic. Reading labels is as critical with cosmetics as with other products.

PERFUMES

One reaction-causing substance, alone or as part of other products, is perfume. Perfumery is considered an art, and much secrecy surrounds the industry. There are three basic types of perfumes:

- Essences or extracts, which are referred to as perfume, usually contain 10 to 20 percent perfume oil dissolved in alcohol.
- Colognes contain 3 to 5 percent perfume oil dissolved in 80 to 90 percent alcohol, the balance being water.
- Toilet waters are 2 percent perfume oil in 60 to 80 percent alcohol with water as the balance.

Perfume oils or essential oils, used as the scents in perfumes, are obtained by a variety of processes from leaves, needles, roots, peels, whole flowers, petals, gums, and resins of plants. Essential oils usually carry the taste and smell of the original plant, and most of them are easily vaporized. A large number have antiseptic, germicidal, and preservative properties, but are used primarily for their scent. Orris root (a highly allergenic substance) is the oldest, most widely used, and most expensive ingredient used in perfumes. It is obtained from the root of the iris plant.

Animal exudates, formerly used in perfumes, were obtained by slow evaporation of substances such as castor from the beaver, musk from the male musk deer, ambergris from the sperm whale, and civet from the civet cat. Synthetic chemicals that simulate natural aromas are now used in perfumes, and petrochemicals and coal tar are the source of raw materials for still other chemicals added to them.

Most perfumes are blends of flower oils, animal substances, synthetics, alcohol, and water. Alcohol is added to animal or plant substances and heated; water is used for dilution. Alcohols used include benzyl alcohol, methanol, and ethanol. Some perfumes have as many as 200 ingredients blended to create that "special" scent.

The substances found in a perfume relate to its usage. The expensive perfumes contain rare flower oils, whereas inexpensive perfumes and perfumes in soap come from artificial materials. Perfume aromas usually last longer than toilet waters and colognes, but there is no standard to dictate how much perfume oil must be used for a product to qualify as a perfume.

Perfumes are frequent allergens and are deleted from hypoallergenic products. Allergic symptoms from perfume include headaches, dizziness, rash, hyperpigmentation, violent coughing, vomiting, skin irritation, and asthma.

LIPSTICKS

Lipsticks are a mixture of oil and wax in stick form with staining dyes, pigments, flavorings, and perfumes dispensed in oil. Typical lipstick formulas contain:

65 percent castor oil
15 percent beeswax
10 percent carnauba wax
5 percent lanolin
Soluble dyes
Insoluble pigments
Perfume

Frosted lipsticks also include a pearlizing agent. Sheer lipsticks contain transparent coloring and no indelible dyes to create a more natural look. Medicated lipsticks, which treat or prevent chapping, usually contain petrolatum, mineral wax, and oils. Color-changing lipsticks contain iodine.

Many women suffer lip peeling caused by lipstick allergies. Sensitizing lipstick ingredients cause lips to react to the sun, become irritated, then crack and bleed. Even hypoallergenic lipsticks can cause these problems. Lipstick reactions reported to the FDA include burns, cracks, excessive dryness, lacerations, numbness, rash, and swollen gums.

Lip balms and gloss, when made from beeswax and vegetable or nut oils, will prevent chapped lips and help chapped lips heal. Vitamin A and D ointment is also soothing and healing for chapped, peeling, or cracked lips.

FOUNDATION MAKEUP

Foundation makeup is used to cover blemishes, to control skin oiliness, to protect skin from wind and cold, and to give a healthy appearance to skin.

Pigmented foundation creams, which tint and cover the skin, are 50 percent water and contain:

Mineral oil
Stearic acid
Lanolin
Cetyl alcohol
Propylene glycol
Triethanolamine
Borax
Insoluble pigments

Foundation may also contain emulsifiers, detergents, humectants, lanolin derivatives, perfumes, preservatives, thickeners, and waxes.

Allergic symptoms caused by foundation makeup include rashes or itching on the face, arms, and chest; swollen eyes; inflammation; and skin swelling and eruptions.

ROUGE

Rouge is one of the earliest types of makeup and is intended to give the wearer a rosy, healthy look. It usually contains ferric oxide.

Cake rouge may contain:
Talc
Kaolin
Brilliant red pigment
Zinc oxide
Zinc stearate
Liquid petrolatum
Tragacanth (plant gum)
Mucilage
Perfume

Cream rouge contains:
Erythrosine for coloring
Stearic acid
Cetyl alcohol
Potassium hydroxide
Glycerine
Water
Sorbitol
Lanolin
Mineral oil
Color pigment
Perfume
Carnauba wax
Ozokerite (hydrocarbon mixture)
Isopropyl palmitate
Titanium dioxide
Talc
Petrolatum

Although consumer complaints about rouge are not common, eye irritation and fungal contamination have been reported.

POWDERS

Face powder is applied at the end of the make-up process to remove shine. It may be loose or compacted. Talc is the principal ingredient, but face powders also contain:
Clay
Kaolin
Calcium carbonate

Zinc oxide
Zinc stearate
Magnesium carbonate
Pigments
Barium sulfate
Boric acid
Cetyl alcohol
Titanium dioxide
Rice starch or cornstarch
Perfume
Pigments used include:
Yellow ocher
Sienna
Red ochers
Calcium pigment
Umbers
Burnt sienna
Ultramarine blue and violet
D & C red #7
D & C orange #4

Dusting powders, used after a bath or shower for absorbing moisture, contain talc, perfumes, and zinc stearate. Toxicity of powders includes mechanical blocking of pores, causing irritation, and breathing difficulties from prolonged inhalation.

Eye Shadow

Eye shadow is used to color the lid and area under the eyebrow. Eyeshadows may contain:
Titanium dioxide
Petrolatum
Lanolin
Beeswax
Aluminum
Ceresin
Calcium carbonate
Mineral oil
Sorbitan oleate
Talc
Eye irritation is a common complaint arising from eyeshadow use. Eye shadows are easily contaminated by bacteria both in the factory and by the user.

Mascara

Mascara is used for coloring eyelashes, and it contains insoluble pigments, carnauba wax, triethanolamine stearate, paraffin, and lanolin. Pigments include carbon black, iron oxides, chromium oxide, ultra-marine, or carmine.
Other ingredients include:
Beeswax
Cetyl alcohol
Mineral oil
Glyceryl monostearate
Gums
Perfume
Vegetable oils
Preservatives
Isopropyl myristate
The newer lash extenders contain tiny fibers of rayon or nylon that make lashes appear longer and thicker.

Mascara may cause allergic reactions and is easily contaminated by bacteria, which may result in eye infections.

Hair Spray

Hair spray is used by both men and women to hold hair in place. In the past, hair spray contained insect shellac, alcohol, perfume, triethanolamine, and water. These sprays caused the hair to shine, but made it brittle.

Today's hair sprays contain polyvinylpyrrolidone (PVP) dissolved in glycerine with perfume, polyethylene glycol, cetyl alcohol, and lanolin. Pressurized hair sprays contain:
PVP
Alcohol
Sorbitol

Water
Lanolin
Perfume
Shellac
Silicone
Sodium alginate
Gums
Freon

Hair sprays can cause headaches, dizziness, tinnitus, hair loss, rash, change in hair color, eye and lung damage, and throat irritation.

SHAMPOO

Coconut, castille, and glycerine soaps were originally used to wash hair. Shampoos are relatively new, and today there are many different types.

Liquid shampoo, the most popular, usually contains:

Triethanolamine dodecylbenzene sulfonate
Ethanolamide of lauric acid
Perfume
Water

Cream shampoo contains the same ingredients as liquid shampoo, but has added lanolin. Sequestering agents, finishing and conditioning agents, antiseptics and preservatives may also be added to shampoos.

Problems with shampoos include eye irritation; scalp irritation and itching; loss of hair; hardened hair; split and fuzzy hair; shortness of breath; and swelling of the hands, face, and arms.

A safe shampoo can be made by simply dissolving baking soda in water.

HAND CREAMS AND LOTIONS

Hand creams and lotions are emollients which soften the skin. They must apply easily without being sticky, and have a pleasant odor. Most of them have a pH of 5 to 8.

Hand creams contain:
2 percent cetyl alcohol
2 percent mineral oil
1 percent lanolin
13 percent stearic acid
12 percent glycerine
0.15 percent methylparaben
1 percent potassium hydroxide
68 percent water
Perfume

Hand lotions contain:
0.5 percent cetyl alcohol
1 percent lanolin
3 percent stearic acid
2 percent glycerine
0.1 percent methylparaben
0.75 percent triethanolamine
85 percent water
Perfume

Rashes, blisters, peeling skin, and swollen hands and feet have resulted from use of hand creams and lotions.

NAIL POLISH AND REMOVERS

Nail polishes contain:
Cellulose nitrate
Butyl acetate
Ethyl acetate
Toluene
Dilbutyl phthalate
Alkyl esters
Dyes
Glycol derivatives
Gums
Hydrocarbons
Ketones
Pigments
Phosphoric acid
D & C red #19 or #31 are commonly used for coloring.

Skin rashes of the eyelids and neck are common allergic symptoms to nail polish. Complaints to the FDA include reports of nail area irritation, discolored nails, nails permanently stained black, splitting and peeling of nails, cracking of the cuticle with subsequent infections, headaches, dizziness, and nausea.

Nail polish remover is highly volatile and is even more damaging. It contains:

Acetone
Toluene
Alcohol
Amyl acetate
Butyl acetate
Benzene
Ethyl acetate

Other ingredients include:

Castor oil
Lanolin
Cetyl alcohol
Olive oil
Perfume
Synthetic oil

Many of these components are extremely toxic and can cause central nervous system depression.

DEODORANTS AND ANTIPERSPIRANTS

The action of bacteria and chemicals on human sweat create the sometimes unpleasant smell of body odor. Deodorants control perspiration odors by inhibiting the growth of microorganisms. Antiperspirants retard the flow of perspiration. Deodorants may contain:

Hexachlorophene
Bithionol
Ammonium compounds
Aluminum chloride
Urea
Propylene glycol

Water
Sodium stearate
Sorbitol
Alcohol

Deodorant/antiperspirants may contain:

Aluminum chloride
Propylene chloride
Aluminum chlorhydroxide
Sorbitan monostearate
Poloxamers
Stearic acid
Boric acid
Urea
Water
Petrolatum
Perfume
Propylene glycol
Cetyl alcohol

There have been many side effects related to using deodorants: stinging, burning, itching, fatty cysts, enlarged sweat and lymph glands, pimples under the arms, and lung and throat irritation. Lung tumors, vision problems, and death have been linked to inhalation of deodorant sprays.

AFTER-SHAVES, PRESHAVES, AND SHAVING CREAMS

After-shave lotions soothe skin irritated by shaving. Early after-shave preparations, such as bay rum and witch hazel, were merely substitutes for water. Today, after-shaves fall into two categories: alcoholic and nonalcoholic. Alcoholic after-shaves contain alcohol, glycerine, water, certified color, and perfume. Menthol antiseptics and alum may also be added. Nonalcoholic after-shaves resemble hand lotions and may contain:

Stearic acid
Triethanolamine
Cetyl alcohol
Glycerine
Distilled water
Small amounts of lanolin
Preservatives

Other fats, waxes, perfumes, coloring, and emulsifying agents may also be added. All of the ingredients in both alcoholic and nonalcoholic after-shaves are potential allergens.

Problems reported to the FDA include face irritation, burned or peeling skin, and eye irritation.

Because dry hair is difficult to cut with a razor, shaving creams are used to make beards softer and easier to shave. Some shaving creams are soaps which, when applied with a brush, form lather. The brushless preparations are emulsions of oil and water, and are creams rather than soaps. Washing and rinsing the face with hot water a few minutes before shaving softens the beard as well as any type of shaving cream.

Men who use electric razors frequently use preshave to temporarily tighten the skin before cutting the beard. These products may contain:

Aluminum phenolsulfonate
Menthol
Camphor
Water
Perfume
Alcohol

Oily types of preshave may contain:

75 percent alcohol
Isopropyl myristate or isopropyl palmitate
Water

Preshaves made for regular razors contain:

Coconut oil
Triethanolamine

Alkyl arylpolyethylene glycol ether
Fatty acids
Water
Perfume

Insects and Pest Control

Insects are the most plentiful life form on earth. The number of insect species is conservatively estimated at about 1.5 million. Insects like to inhabit our homes and eat our food, yet most of us are unwilling to share, and so we look for ways to get rid of these pests.

There are many chemical insecticides (pesticides) that are advertised as the answer to any insect problems. When these compounds are sprayed on insects, the tiny animals supposedly die. However, many insects are unaffected, while others reproduce so quickly that insecticides have little effect on the overall population of that particular species. Insects often become resistant to insecticides so that more potent and different chemicals are required to kill them.

Insecticides are more dangerous to us than to the insects—many contain neurotoxins that can cause permanent damage. Once used, insecticides can linger for many years. For example, Chlordane has a half-life of 30 years. (Half-life is the length of time it takes half of the material to decompose. It takes another half-life for the "half of the half" to decompose, and so on.) Chlordane can cause cancer, nerve damage, and immune system damage. There is no safe level for this pesticide. Although the use of Chlordane was banned in 1988, residues may still linger in the foundations of older homes.

In many areas of the continent, building codes require soil preparation with an insecticide before a foundation is laid. Many patios, sun rooms, and solar heat collection areas are floored with brick or flagstone on a bed of sand. The ground under these areas is often sprayed with insecticide before the sand is spread. Any immunocompromised person should ask in detail about prior use of insecticides in any dwelling where they intend to reside.

Pesticide exposure is not limited to attempts to control insects in the home. Pesticides used to control crop pests can get into the food chain. Unused pesticides are poured down drains and sewers, and eventually enter our water supply. Pesticides from gardens also find their way into the water supply.

People can suffer severe health problems and permanent damage from exposure to numerous pesticides in food, water, and air, even though the exposure level for each is below the federally defined safe tolerance level. Pesticides are absorbed through the lungs, skin, and gut. Most insecticides are fat-soluble, being deposited in the fat cells of exposed persons and animals. Those who have had numerous exposures to insecticides carry a large toxic load in their fat cells, unless they go through detoxification. (See *Detoxification,* p. 250.) Symptoms and damage will continue unless their bodies are cleansed of the insecticide. As a result, these people may not respond well to immunotherapy, nutrient therapy, and exercise programs.

Controlling Household Insects

Insects in the home must be controlled in the most nontoxic way possible, but this takes hard work and the understanding that there are no magic solutions. Careful home maintenance is the most important factor in pest control. You will not get instant results or 100 percent suc-

cess, but you can have a home with very few insects.

The first step in insect control is keeping your home in good repair. Most insects need only a fraction of an inch to crawl through and enter a house. Cracks in walls, openings around plumbing pipes, broken window screens and sills, loose flashing around grills and vents, and rusted-out floor drains all provide doorways for insects to enter your home. Sliding glass doors allow garden crawlers to get in the house.

Be sure your yard is not attracting insects, by paying attention to the landscaping around your home. Plants should not hug outside walls. A clear strip of concrete or sand against your house's foundation will act as a barrier for crawling insects.

Try to prevent dampness next to the foundation of the house. Moisture both outside and inside the house draws insects; they feed on the mold that may grow in hollow wall construction or in moist areas on slab foundations. Lush foliage and damp crawlspaces also draw moisture-loving insects.

Cleanliness is the most important factor in insect control. Adult insects, larvae, and eggs can be removed by vacuuming, which also eliminates food crumbs that might serve as their food. Spring cleaning disturbs and rids the home of insects, while clutter attracts both insects and rodents. Rotate your wool clothes so that all garments are worn, brushed, and cleaned regularly. Move your furniture from time to time and remember to clean under it.

Proper food storage is also extremely important. Food should be stored in glass and metal containers to keep insects out. Separate older food from new food so that any infestation will not be spread, and avoid storing food for long periods of time.

Cockroaches

Cockroaches are a common household pest. They are immune to insecticides, and while they prefer carbohydrates, they will eat almost anything. Cockroaches will nest anywhere, including in refrigerator insulation. While they prefer the kitchen and bathroom, they will spread to all parts of the house.

Roaches are known carriers of boils, dysentery, plague, polio, hepatitis, salmonella, typhus, and toxoplasmosis (a disease affecting the central nervous system).

The following procedures will help fight cockroaches:

- Store food in glass or metal containers.
- Do not leave dishes unwashed.
- Cover pet food and water overnight.
- Sweep up crumbs and spills promptly.
- Wipe off containers before returning them to cupboards.
- Put your garbage out every night.
- Do not save grocery sacks or cardboard boxes.
- Do not buy any packaged foods or drinks with spilled beverages or food on them.
- Use commercial or technical-grade boric acid to kill roaches. It penetrates the insects' outer covering, and can be picked up on their feet and swallowed while the roaches preen themselves. Sprinkle boric acid (with a small amount of sugar added) on surfaces where roaches are likely to crawl, such as behind appliances and under the sink. The sugar attracts the insects so they will walk across the boric acid. Wear a mask and gloves while distributing the boric acid, and do not sprinkle the mixture where you store food. Keep the mixture out of reach of children and pets.
- Use roach traps. Wrap the outside of a jar with masking tape, and fill the jar half-full with beer or a few boiled raisins. Smear a band of petroleum jelly one or two inches below the rim inside the jar so the roaches cannot crawl out. Drown the victims of these traps in hot, sudsy water. Be sure to wash your hands thoroughly.
- Put "food" out for the cockroaches. Mix equal parts of oatmeal with plaster of Paris. Spread on the floor of infested areas. Or, sift and mix together one oz. trisodium phosphate (TSP), six oz. borax, and four oz. flour. Spread where needed. Another fatal roach food is a mixture of two tablespoons flour, one tablespoon cocoa, and four tablespoons borax. Spread in roach traffic areas. Repeat these treatments in four days and again in two weeks in order to kill newly hatched cockroaches.
- Heat kills roaches—temperatures of 130°F will kill any insects in heating system ducts. Roaches will also die when temperatures dip below 23°F. Open the window on a freezing day and wipe out cockroaches, silverfish, and clothes moths.

Kitchen Pests

There are four categories of kitchen pests, which get into stored food.

- **Beetles:** Eat flours, dried soups, herbs and spices, cereals, cake, cookie and pancake mixes, and cured meats.
- **Weevils:** Eat grains and dried beans of all kinds.
- **Moths:** Adults do not feed on anything, but larvae eat cornmeal, grains, dried fruit, and nuts.
- **Mites:** Eat previous items plus barley, caramel, cheese, rotting potatoes, sugar, and wine.

The following will help eradicate these insects:

- Do not buy damaged packages at the grocery store.
- Keep your kitchen cool and dry.
- Rotate your food stocks; eat older foods first.
- Store foods properly and discard any food with holes in the containers.
- Heat or freeze foods suspected of infestation.
- Keep your kitchen and pantry scrupulously clean.
- Put a bay leaf in flour and cereal boxes or containers.

HOUSEFLIES

Flies have caused more human and animal deaths than any other insect. They are carriers of bacterial, parasitic, and viral disease. Flies eat and lay their eggs in filth, and when they get into our houses, they bring larvae, bacteria, and excreta. Flies very rapidly become immune to chemicals. The following will aid in controlling houseflies:

- Sanitation is vital, since flies have a keen sense of smell. Keep all dishes clean, and rinse containers before putting them in the trash. Keep your garbage covered and dispose of it at the end of each day.
- Garbage should be kept in covered cans. Dispose of diapers hygienically.
- Use proper lawn-care methods, such as spreading manure thinly so that maggots and eggs will die. Do not leave lawn clippings to decompose on the lawn. Pick up animal droppings and dispose of them properly.
- Make a fly trap; put a paper cone into a baited jar.
- Use fly swatters to kill flies in the house. Since flies are drawn to light, darken a room and open a screened door or window. The flies will alight on the screen. At night, cover all windows, but leave an open slit at one of them. Flies will collect there overnight.

- Be sure that all screens on your house fit well.
- Some herbs will repel flies—clove, tansy, and pine oil are helpful. Camphor trees close to the kitchen door repel flies.

MOSQUITOES

Mosquitoes also cause many human diseases. They are carriers of malaria, yellow fever, dengue fever, and encephalitis. There is no effective treatment for the latter two illnesses.

Mosquitoes are able to develop immunity to almost all pesticides. The life cycle of the mosquito has four stages: egg, larvae, pupa, and adult. The males never bite, but females require a blood meal in order to lay fertile eggs. All eggs are laid on still water. If the water dries up before the eggs hatch, the larvae will hatch the next time water accumulates, even if the interim is as long as five or six years. Water management is the most important aspect of mosquito control.

The following measures will help in mosquito control:

- Eliminate all objects around your house that will hold water.
- Fill any holes, cavities, or pools that can hold water.
- Be sure flat roofs drain well.
- Be certain you have no leaky faucets.
- Help your community control all breeding sources for mosquitoes.
- Be certain your screens fit well and have no holes.
- Use natural mosquito repellants: oil of citronella; garlic; pennyroyal mint; tansy; and basil.
- Use minnows in ponds for mosquito control.
- If you are particularly prone to mosquito bites, wear long sleeves and keep your pant legs tucked in. Try taking B_1 (thiamine) before going outdoors. This works for about half

of those people affected by mosquito bites.

- Bug control lights are effective if they are hung about 100 feet from the house or outdoor living area.
- If you live in an area that supports blue martins or swallows, erect a habitat that will attract these birds. They will devour a large number of mosquitoes.

SILVERFISH

Silverfish eat paper, textiles of vegetable origin (linen, rayon, and cotton), and cereals. They enter the house on secondhand books and cardboard boxes. Damaged papers and books signal their presence.

The following measures will help with silverfish control:

- Fill in holes around pipes entering the house and repair any plumbing leaks.
- Vacuum your bookshelves and books frequently.
- Check your books periodically by opening and shaking them.
- Carefully inspect any secondhand books and old papers before bringing them into the house.
- Check lined draperies for silverfish between the drapery and the lining.
- Make a trap for silverfish, by covering a jar with masking tape to provide a good foothold for the insects and baiting the jar with flour.
- Sprinkle boric acid, flour, and sugar on a piece of paper and place it in a corner or on a window ledge.

TICKS

Ticks do not normally pose a problem for city dwellers, unless your home is close to a forest or a wilderness area. Some species of ticks are dangerous, carrying Rocky Mountain spotted fever, tularemia (a disease caused by bacteria), relapsing fever, and Lyme's disease. The species of tick that carries Lyme's disease is a smaller variety.

The following will aid in controlling ticks:

- Prevention is the best cure; check your dogs and cats regularly and remove any ticks. Make your home rodent-proof to keep out tick-carrying animals.
- Remove ticks with tweezers. Be careful that you do not crush the body, and be certain not to leave the insect's head in the wound. Place the ends of the tweezers as close as possible to the skin before pulling out the tick.

FLEAS

Fleas are unusual insects, capable of pulling 400 times their weight and lifting objects 150 times their mass. They have incredible jumping ability and many hiding places. Although not as dangerous as mosquitoes, fleas can spread plague (bubonic, pneumonic, and septicemic) typhus, tularemia, and tapeworm. Flea bites can also provoke allergic reactions.

Fleas are very difficult to eradicate. They are able to survive for long periods without food and can move from one host to another. Four species are important to humans: the human flea, the dog flea, the cat flea, and the rat flea, which is the plague carrier. Flea eggs cannot hatch if the temperature is lower than 40°F. or the humidity less than 40 percent. Wet winter and spring seasons increase flea populations.

Fleas may live in upholstery, carpets, cracks in wooden floors, attics, basements, and walls, as well as in the yard. Even if you do not have pets, it is possible to have a flea infestation.

Anti-flea sprays, flea powders, and flea collars are toxic to both humans and animals. Many people are allergic to these chemicals, while it is doubtful whether flea insecticides bother fleas.

The following will help to control fleas:

- Prevention is most important; keep dogs outside and do not let them roam around the neighborhood. Cats that go outdoors will have flea problems, so comb your pet daily for fleas.
- Take precautions outdoors. Destroy all rodent nests, making sure the outside of your house is in good repair. Overwater or dry out the yard to kill fleas. Get rid of stray animals.
- Vacuum your house frequently and empty the dust from the vacuum, being careful to bag and burn it, or bake it in the sun.
- Have your upholstery and carpets steam-cleaned.
- Wash pet beds every two days (eggs take two days to hatch).
- Use repellants—brewer's yeast in pet food seems to help protect some animals. Some herbs that help repel fleas are citronella, eucalyptus, pennyroyal mint, and rosemary. Use these in your animal's collars.
- Washing your pet's fur with lemon infusions helps to keep dogs free of fleas. To make the treatment, cut four lemons into eighths. Cover with water and bring to a boil, then simmer for 45 minutes. Cool, strain, and store in a glass container. Brush the infusion into the fur; allow to dry and brush again.
- Frequent bathing of animals can control fleas, since they drown easily.
- Light and water traps may be helpful. Make one by filling a shallow dish with water and detergent. For one month, place a lamp over the dish and leave the light on all night.

ANTS

Ants are found everywhere on earth, in all types of climates. They live in structured societies and eat everything that humans eat. Ants are beneficial to us because they prey on other insects, including cockroaches, mealy bugs, conenose bugs, larvae of filth flies, termite queens, and scale insects. They also enrich the soil and eat mosquito eggs.

Ants are most likely to invade a home after their nests have been flooded. It is easier to keep ants out than to try to get rid of them once they are established inside your house.

The following help to control ants:

- To prevent their entry, cut plants away from the house. Do not overwater the garden.
- Wipe up spilled foods and rinse dishes before putting them in the dishwasher. Store foods and leftovers properly, and sweep the kitchen floor daily.
- Seal entry holes with petrolatum, putty, or caulking.
- Use mint or tansy to temporarily repel ants. Honey and boric acid on small pieces of paper placed in the path of ants will help control them.
- Destroy ant nests outdoors by pouring boiling water or hot paraffin into the nests.

CLOTHES MOTHS

Moths are notorious for destroying clothes of animal origin, particularly wool. These moths are found mainly in warmer areas, and signal their presence by making holes in your clothes and upholstery. The larvae, which cause the damage, will eat straw, rayon, cotton, paper, fur, tobacco, hemp, and felt. The adults of one species will even eat mothproofed fabric.

To prevent clothes moth infestation:

- Seal all small openings into the house and attic. Clean closets and stored clothes regularly. Vacuum in all the cracks, backs of furniture, and under the furniture. Sun, air, and brush your clothing regularly.
- Freezing clothing, pressing with a steam iron, dry-cleaning, and heating your clothes in an

oven at 140°F will kill all stages of insect life.

- Store clothing carefully, sealing it in plastic bags or clean cardboard boxes.
- Mint, tansy, bay leaves, rosemary, lavender, cloves, spearmint, and cedar will repel moths.

TERMITES

Termites are divided into two groups: those that live in the earth and those that live above it. Subterranean termites live in colonies under the ground but feed above it. Drywood termites nest in the wood they eat and do not need ground contact. Those that live in the earth cause more damage. The termite problem is getting worse in North America—the only region free of termites is Alaska.

All houses, including brick houses, are vulnerable to termite infestation. Homes over 35 years old are likely to have termites. Signs include shelter tubes or fecal pellets, and wood flooring with dark or blistered areas.

Although most insects can be handled by nontoxic methods, eradicating termites almost always requires chemicals. Drywood termites are treated using a "drill and treat" method if the infestation is local; chemicals are injected into drilled holes. Electroguns are a more recent and effective method, sending a current of electricity through the galleries in the wood and killing the termites.

Subterranean termite infestations were treated primarily with Chlordane until 1988, when its use was banned. Dursban, which is more immediately toxic to humans, is still in use. It is an organophosphate and many people, including exterminators, react to it. Many companies now use either Tribute or Dragnet, which are pyrethrin compounds. Pyrethrin is a compound (found naturally in some flowers, such as chrysanthemums) that has insecticidal properties. It appears to be effective in both killing and controlling termites. While it is considerably less toxic than Dursban and Chlordane, the pyrethrin compound can cause allergic reactions and symptoms in some individuals exposed to it. Its chronic exposure effects are not yet known.

To prevent subterranean termites:

- Keep your home as dry as possible. Be sure the lot drains adequately away from the house. Check that doors and windows are adequately flashed. Attics and crawlspaces should be adequately ventilated, and walls should be fitted with vapor barriers.
- Be sure all wood debris is cleared away from the house, particularly from the fill dirt under porches and steps.

To prevent drywood termites:

- Silica aerogel dust in wall spaces will kill insects that crawl over it.
- Arrange an annual termite inspection of your home.

To keep houses termite-free:

- Keep plumbing in good repair.
- Make sure there is a foundation of concrete or concrete-filled block under all wood portions of your house.
- Avoid wetting stucco and wood siding.
- Fill all cracks in and around the house. Keep gutters and downspouts in good repair.

Ants pose the greatest threat to the termite. If you see them around your house's foundation, let them be—they will help protect your home from termites.

FINDING AN EXTERMINATOR

Should you need the help of a professional termite exterminator, be certain you find a competent pest control company.

- Contact at least three companies for information.

- Find out how much of the company's business comes from termite control.
- Find out how well the employees are trained and whether they receive continuing education. Will they be supervised when they apply the pesticide?
- Find out what kind of insurance the company carries. Coverage against errors and omissions is important.
- Find out what types of chemicals they use and whether they are familiar with new, non-chemical controls, such as the Electrogun.
- Ask for information on the toxicity of any of the chemicals to be used. Double-check this information at a library.
- If fumigation is necessary for a drywood infestation, find out: How will foods, plants, photographic equipment, artwork, leather, and rubber items be affected and protected? How will weather affect the fumigation? How will your home be secured to prevent burglary? How long will the fumigant last? How will it be determined when the house is safe to reoccupy?
- If you are chemically sensitive, ask your physician for information about the chemical ingredients of the materials to be used.
- Beware of a company that tries to pressure you into doing something quickly. Check the reputation of the company you choose with a consumer protection agency.
- When the company employees arrive at your home, check whether the workers, their clothing, and their truck are clean.

Insect Stings and Bites

While there are useful, helpful insects, like the ladybug and the praying mantis, we focus on those that are a problem for us. Insects are disease vectors (they carry disease-causing organisms). Their bites can cause swelling, itching, and systemic reactions. (See "Bee or Insect Stings," p. 264.) Insects can kill either through their toxic venom or through causing severe allergic reactions to venom and other substances injected through a sting or bite. Insects cause more deaths each year than poisonous snakes.

After an insect sting, consult a physician if any of the following systemic reaction symptoms occur.

- Wheezing or difficulty breathing.
- Constriction in the throat and chest.
- Drop in blood pressure.
- Thickened speech.
- Difficulty swallowing.
- Dry, hacking cough.
- Numerous hives.
- Nausea, vomiting, and abdominal pain.
- Dizziness.
- Severe itching.

Whether or not one is sensitive, a physician should be consulted immediately if the insect sting is in the throat, face, nose, or eye area. Those who are acutely sensitive and who have life-threatening reactions to insect venom and bites should be carefully desensitized with extracts. In addition, they should carry insect bite kits containing adrenalin.

Keeping a Chemically Clean Home Environment

If you are chemically sensitive you need to "clean up" chemical exposures in your home as much as possible. When you are not constantly reacting to chemical exposures at home, you will be more able to tolerate unavoidable exposures away from home. To clean up your home, follow these guidelines as closely as possible. It would be overwhelming to accomplish all of these suggestions at once. Try to incorporate a few improvements at a time until your house is safe.

- Run an air purifier continuously and change the filters frequently.
- If possible, use a water filter in the shower and in the kitchen. For the extremely sensitive, whole-house filters are better since all water sources will be filtered.
- If you do not have a filter, let your drinking water stand in an uncovered glass jar for 24 hours to allow the chlorine to evaporate. The jar should be kept in a well-ventilated area to help prevent chlorine exposure.
- Do not use gas appliances, as they are among the primary sources of chemical exposure in the home. Unless you are electromagnetically sensitive, electric ranges, furnaces, hot water heaters, and clothes dryers are recommended. If it is too costly to replace or move the furnace or hot water heater to an outbuilding, you should weatherstrip (with felt stripping) the access doors to reduce exposure to combustion products.
- Use appliances with the least amount of interior plastic. Avoid aluminum and Teflon coatings on all appliances. The following are "safe" appliances:

Blender: Use only glass or stainless steel container.

Broiler: Use only stainless steel or porcelain.

Crock pot: Use only those with removable, stoneware interiors.

Dishwasher: Porcelain or stainless steel interior is best.

Electric oven: Porcelain-lined bake/broil section; ceramic top burners. *Never* use a continuous cleaning oven. (Self cleaning is dangerous. Leave the house until cycle is finished and oven is cooled.)

Iron: Stainless steel soleplate. Use distilled water only.

Juicer: All stainless interior.

Refrigerator/freezer: Porcelain interior and exterior.

Vacuum cleaner: Water-trap vacuum, double-filter vacuum, or built-in central vacuum system. Use disposable dust bags and wash outer bag frequently.

Washer/dryer: Porcelain and stainless steel interiors are best. Locate appliances in a room that can be closed off and vent your dryer outside.

- Cook in glass, china, or stainless steel. Some people are able to tolerate cooking with cast iron. However, food particles from previously cooked meals will be released from the porous iron surface. Do not use aluminum, copper, or Teflon cookware, and do not coat cookware with "non-stick" cooking sprays.
- Store food in cellophane, in aluminum foil with the shiny side next to the food (the dull side is coated with plastic), or in glassware. Do not use plastic wrapping or soft plastic containers.
- Clean the house with *safe* cleaning products only. (See "Lemon for Household Cleaning and Deodorizing," p. 160, *Recommended Books*, p. 304, and *Recommended Sources and Organizations*, p. 299.) Stop using and remove all "non-safe" cleaning products, such as furniture polish, ammonia, and dishwashing detergents, from all areas of the home— including the kitchen, laundry room, and bathroom. Even if the lids are on these containers, these items are chemical exposures; offending items *must* be removed.
- Do not use *any* aerosol sprays such as room or

rug deodorants or spray starch. Discard any existing aerosol products.

- Do not use any insecticides, pesticides, or fungicides. Remove any existing containers from the home.
- Do not allow any tobacco smoking in your home.
- Do not use a wood-burning stove or fireplace. Do not burn candles or incense.
- Remove all glues, adhesives, lighter fluids, shoe polish, mothballs and crystals, and canned or spray paints.
- If any member of the household has a hobby involving the use of glues, adhesives, paints, or chemicals of any kind, be sure that hobby is never performed inside the house.
- Remove as many rubber and plastic items as possible.
- If a garage is attached to your house, use weather stripping to make sure any adjoining doors seal tightly. Do not idle vehicle engines in the garage. Some very sensitive people may not be able to park their cars in their garages.

Personal care products, unless selected carefully, can be a constant source of chemical exposure. The scents as well as the skin contact pose problems for the chemically sensitive person. Because there are many chemical exposures over which you have no control, it is important that you limit or eliminate all possible exposures.

- Stop using and remove all standard commercial scented products from the house. Even when sealed in plastic bags, the following items are sources of chemical exposure:

  Aftershaves
  Bar soaps
  Body lotions
  Body powder
  Colognes
  Cosmetics
  Deodorants
  Hair conditioners, oils, sprays, and tonics
  Hand creams and lotions
  Makeup
  Mousse
  Nail polish and removers
  Perfumes
  Setting gels
  Shampoos
  Shaving cream

- Stop using bleach, scented laundry soap, and fabric softener (substitute ½ to 1 cup baking soda in the rinse water). Remove these items from the house.
- Stop using standard commercial toothpaste and mouthwash.
- Do not use aerosol spray hair-care products or standard deodorants.
- Baking soda can be used both as a toothpaste and an underarm deodorant.
- Do not wear dry-cleaned clothes or leather garments. Wear natural fiber clothing as much as possible.

Making a Bedroom Oasis

The extremely sensitive person will need a virtually allergen-free place to allow his or her immune system to rest and repair. Dr. William Rea suggests creating an environmentally safe "oasis." Since we spend the majority of our time at home in the bedroom, it is best to make this the oasis—free of chemical, inhalant, and food exposures. To prepare a bedroom oasis, follow these guidelines carefully.

- Always keep the bedroom door closed. If the door does not seal tightly enough, put felt weather stripping around it.
- Block the air vents from forced-air heaters with aluminum foil. Portable electric heaters may be used in cold rooms. (Electrically sen-

sitive people may have problems with this heat source.)

- Clean the room with *safe* cleaning products only.
- Use an air purifier; run it continuously and change the filters regularly.
- Prohibit tobacco smoking in this room!
- Do not eat or bring food into this room.
- Remove all plants from the room.
- Do not use any insecticides, pesticides, or fungicides.
- Do not allow pets in the room.
- Remove all synthetic materials (carpeting, drapery, bedding). Use only natural fabrics, such as linen, cotton, silk, or wool (if tolerated).
- Pillows may be either cotton, kapok, or feathers (if tolerated). You can make a pillow by folding cotton batting, a cotton blanket, or cotton diapers and covering them with a pillow case. Do not use sponge or foam rubber pillows.
- Do not use electric blankets, as the heated wires give off chemical fumes. The current in the wires can also cause electromagnetic problems. Even when unplugged, these blankets are not safe because of the wire configuration.
- Hardwood floors with a urethane finish are acceptable; however, allow sufficient time for the finish to outgas before using the room for a sleeping area. Use sanded wood for flooring, but do not use pine, cedar, or spruce wood as they have a high terpene (hydrocarbon) content. If floors cannot be replaced, use a foil barrier and cover it with cotton carpeting.
- Remove particle-board furniture. Unless you are electrically sensitive, use metal dressers. Older, solid wood furniture is fine unless it has been treated with insecticide.
- Remove *all* scented cosmetic items—per-

fumes, colognes, hand and body lotions, powders, deodorants, hair sprays, hair products, nail polish and remover, aftershave lotions or astringents.

- Do not keep freshly polished shoes in the room until all of their odor has dissipated. Remove any leather clothing, which is processed with tannin, a potent allergen.
- Clean out closets. Remove any possible contaminants (such as mothballs, old books, shoes, boots, clothes with scents on them). If there is an access door to a crawlspace in the bottom of the closet, seal it with weather stripping in order to prevent mold exposure from the soil.
- Do not wash clothes in scented products or use fabric softeners or static control products, and do not store any clothing in the room on which these products have been used.
- Wash new clothing before storing in the closet, drawers, or shelves.
- Dry-cleaned clothes should not be stored in the room.
- Remove books, magazines, and printed materials from the room. The ink and paper are phenol and formaldehyde exposures.
- Remove candles from the room.
- Do not use clock radios, TVs, hairdryers, computers, or any other electric appliances in the room. You may use a transistor or wind-up clock.
- See also the sections on "Dust" (p. 174) and "Molds" (p. 167) for information about inhalant allergens.
- Because of the electromagnetic polarity of the earth, it is important to position the head of the bed facing north. (See "How to Reduce Electromagnetic Effects," p. 57.)
- Determine where the main electric current enters the house and do not use this room as a bedroom.

- Do not use a waterbed; the plastic covering is a phenol exposure and the electric components are a problem for electrically sensitive people.

Lemon for Household Cleaning and Deodorizing

Freshly cut lemon, lemon peel, or lemon juice may be substituted for commercial household cleaning and polishing products. This is important for chemically sensitive people who cannot tolerate the usual chemically loaded products.

However, as with any substance, some people will react to lemon; the only way to know whether you can tolerate this use of lemon is to try it. Anyone who is already aware of a lemon sensitivity should not try these cleaning procedures.

Always wear gloves while cleaning with any product to prevent absorption of the substance through your hands. Extremely sensitive people may also need to wear masks.

Commercially bottled lemon juice can be substituted for fresh lemon, but it will not clean as well as the fresh fruit.

- *Appliances:* You can remove soap film from the interiors of ovens and refrigerators by adding fresh lemon juice to the rinse water after cleaning.
- *Baby bottles:* Add lemon juice to the water when boiling bottles to remove mineral deposits.
- *Brass and copper:* Rub with lemon juice or a slice of lemon sprinkled with baking soda. Rinse with clear water and dry with a soft cloth. For heavy corrosion, rub with a paste made of lemon juice and salt. Rinse with clear water and dry with a soft cloth.

You can also use a paste made of lemon juice and cream of tartar. Rub the paste on gently and leave it for five minutes. Rinse in warm water and dry with a soft cloth.

- *Chinaware:* To restore the original shine, scour chinaware with lemon juice and salt. To clean inside a china decanter, use one part salt and two parts lemon juice.
- *Chrome:* Rub with lemon peel and rinse with clear water. Polish with a soft cloth.
- *Faucets (kitchen and bath):* To remove spots and shine faucets, rub them with lemon peel and wash with a soft cloth. Then polish with a dry, soft cloth.
- *Furniture polish:* Use a solution of one part lemon juice and two parts of any vegetable oil.
- *Garbage disposal:* Put used lemons in the garbage disposal to help keep it clean and deodorized.
- *Glass:* Soak glass in lemon juice and water or rub it with cut lemon to clean and remove spots. Dry with a lint-free cloth.

   Shake a small piece of freshly cut lemon and a small amount of water inside glass decanters to renew their sparkle.
- *Glass surfaces:* Clean glass surfaces as above with lemon juice or cut lemon to remove dirt and spots. To remove dried paint, apply hot lemon juice with a soft cloth and leave it on until it is almost dry. then wipe it off with a soft cloth.
- *Insect bites and bee stings:* A drop of lemon juice rubbed on insect bites and bee stings instantly relieves the irritation.
- *Ivory (piano keys):* Rub ivory with half a lemon or a paste made of lemon juice and salt. Wipe with a clean, wet cloth to rinse. Dry with a clean, dry cloth.
- *Leather: (picture frames, book bindings, furniture):* Apply a mixture of equal amounts

lemon juice and warm water. Wipe clean with a dry cloth.

- *Lipstick stains on fabric:* For white, washable fabrics, use full-strength lemon juice to remove lipstick stains. Use diluted lemon juice for colored, washable fabrics.
- *Mildew stain on fabrics:* Rub salt and then lemon juice on the mildew stain. Place the fabric in the sun to dry.
- *Paint brushes (hardened):* Dip hardened paint brushes into boiling lemon juice and immediately lower heat. Leave brushes in the juice for 15 minutes before washing in soapy water.
- *Pastry boards and rolling pins:* Rub occasionally with a freshly cut lemon half to bleach out stains.
- *Refrigerators:* Place a freshly cut lemon half on the refrigerator shelf to absorb odors.
- *Rust spots on fabrics:* Cover the spot with a paste of lemon juice and salt. Let it dry in the sun or hold the fabric over steam until the spot is gone.
- *Silverware:* Rub with lemon juice or a slice of lemon. Rinse with hot water and polish dry. For heavy oxidation, soak the silverware in lemon juice for five minutes before rinsing and polishing.
- *Tile:* Rub tile with a cloth soaked in lemon juice. Polish tile with a dry, soft cloth or chamois.
- *Tubs and sinks:* Rub with half a lemon dipped in borax. Rinse with clear water and dry with a soft cloth.
- *White marble:* To clean, rub with half a lemon or a paste made of lemon juice and salt. Wipe with a wet cloth and dry with a soft, dry cloth.
- *Wine stains on fabrics:* For washable fabrics only, spread a paste of lemon juice and salt on the wine stain. Rinse. Wash in soapy water.
- *Wooden furniture (scratches):* Mix equal amounts of lemon juice and any vegetable oil. Apply this mixture to the scratches on wooden furniture and rub gently with a soft cloth until they are no longer visible.
- *Woodwork:* Will keep its gloss if the juice of one lemon is added to one quart of water for the last rinse after cleaning. This also works for any painted, enamelled, or linoleum surface.

THE ALLERGENS WE INHALE

What is Inhalant Allergy?

We breathe in more than two tablespoons of solid particles every day. Inhalants (substances that are inhaled when breathing) include: pollens from trees, grasses, and weeds; mold; animal danders (dog, cat, horse, rabbit); mold; dust and dust mite; fibers (cotton linters, kapok, jute); feathers and down; orris root; tobacco; and other substances. Sensitive people can develop allergic responses to inhalants.

Inhalant allergy symptoms include sneezing; hoarseness; increased mucus production; scratchy throat; runny nose; hay fever; itchy, red, watery eyes; and sinus symptoms of headache, pressure behind the eyeballs, pain in the frontal area, tenderness over the cheekbones, and aching teeth. Those affected have allergic shiners (dark circles under the eyes), and many, particularly children, will show signs of the "allergic salute." The allergic salute produces a horizontal crease across the nose from wiping a runny nose upwards with the palm of the hand. However, both allergic shiners and the allergic salute crease can also be from sensitivity to foods and chemicals.

Allergic responses to inhalants can also appear as multiple systemic symptoms such as eczema, cold and flu-like symptoms, insomnia, asthma, fatigue, depression, cramps and diarrhea, headaches, hives, swollen lymph glands,

flushing, skipped heart beats, panic attacks, and many others. Some women may experience irregular periods, toxemia of pregnancy, or uterine hemorrhaging during pollen season, particularly when ragweed is pollinating. The same processes that cause symptoms in response to pollen can affect any organ of the body.

Most inhalant reactions of our bodies are IgE mediated and many people with severe inhalant allergies will have high IgE antibody levels in their blood. IgE molecules attach to various tissues, including lung tissue and tissues in the nasal passages. When the allergen attaches to two adjacent IgE molecules on a mast cell or a basophil, chemicals are released, which cause the symptoms of an inhalant allergy. These released substances include histamine, heparin, kinins, enzymes, and leukotrienes.

Some people have low IgE levels in their blood, but experience significant inhalant symptoms. Their reactions may possibly be IgG mediated. These people must be tested by a method different than the high IgE people in order for them to receive relief with allergy extracts.

Unfortunately, most inhalants cannot be totally avoided (especially pollens, mold, dust, dust mite, and tobacco), and lessening sensitivities to these substances depends on making environmental changes as well as treatment. Using antihistamines or oral steroids to treat allergic symptoms is only palliative, as these substances treat only the symptoms and do not decrease sensitivity to the allergen. In fact, sensitivity to allergens may actually increase, even though symptoms are being lessened with antihistamine or oral steroid medications. These medications can be hazardous, as they both can produce serious side-effects in some people.

Most antihistamines cause drowsiness, thus someone who is already fatigued from allergic reactions becomes more tired. Two new antihistamines, Seldane and Hismanal, cause drowsiness in only 10 percent of those taking them but, as with other such medications, afford only symptom relief. Orally administered steroids (cortisone) can lead to cataracts, high blood pressure, ulcers, diabetes, edema, and suppression of adrenal gland function.

Steroid nasal sprays and Nasalcrom (cromolyn sodium) are two relatively new types of medications that may be helpful, and that do not cause the side-effects seen with antihistamines and oral steroids. Nasalcrom is thought to stabilize mast cell membranes, thus inhibiting the allergic response. Inhaled steroids decrease both inflammation and the late phase of the allergic reaction.

Allergy testing for inhalant allergies and treatment with extracts affords safe relief of symptoms while decreasing sensitivity to the substance over a period of time. Supportive treatments for the immune system are also helpful.

Common Inhalant Allergens

POLLEN

All seed-bearing plants produce pollen (analogous to human sperm) as part of their reproductive cycle. Pollen can cause problems for humans; however, not all pollen-producing plants cause allergic symptoms. There are about 100 plant species which produce pollen that can be significant in human sensitivities.

Plants that cause pollen problems in humans must:
- Be abundant and widely distributed.
- Produce pollen in large quantities.
- Produce pollen that is windborne.
- Produce pollen light enough to be carried some distance.
- Produce pollen containing specific antigens for hypersensitivity.

Generally, plants that display brightly colored, perfumed flowers do not affect the allergic person. (There are exceptions, such as goldenrod.) These plants have heavy pollen that is spread by insects and birds, and if the pollen does fall it will stay on the ground because of its weight and will not become airborne.

Trees, grasses, and weeds are the wind-pollinated plants that cause allergy problems. These plants have small, unattractive flowers that lack odor or nectar and they produce pollen grains that are "dry," containing no fats, pigments, or waxes. They also have a mechanism to arrest pollen release so that it occurs only as a result of the shaking motion of the wind.

To be airborne, pollen must be between 15 and 50 microns in diameter. When inhaled, these small grains enter the nose and pass into the small ducts of the bronchi, causing mild to severe problems, depending on the nature of the pollen and the person's sensitivity. Some pollens contain as many as 15 allergenic compounds, while others contain only one or two.

Plants producing windborne pollen fill the air with literally tons of pollen, most of which is protein in nature. For example, one acre of ragweed can produce 60 pounds of pollen in one season. This large production ensures that the pollen will be spread by rather sporadic breezes. In addition to being lightweight, different types of pollen grains frequently have efficient structures that aid in their dispersal so the wind can carry them for many miles. Fortunately, most pollen travels only a few feet from the parent plant.

There are several factors affecting the amount of pollen in the air. Heavy rains prevent distribution and help destroy the pollen more quickly. Since most pollen is released between 6:00 a.m. and 9:00 a.m., afternoon rains do not help. However, high humidity weighs down the pollen and slows its movement. On dry, sunny days the slightest breeze can send it far and wide. Even after a frost, which stops plants from pollinating, existing pollens can still be spread by wind for a short period of time.

Recognizing Pollen Allergies   You should suspect a pollen problem if you experience symptoms, or if the symptoms are worst:
- In the early spring when trees pollinate.
- In the late spring and early summer when grasses and weeds pollinate.
- In the autumn when weeds are a continuing factor.

When symptoms occur from spring to first frost with a peak in the fall, mold often is the prime offender. If you experience symptoms during the winter, suspect allergy to housedust, dust mites, and/or the gas furnace (combustion products and airborne allergens are circulated by the forced air).

Symptoms of a pollen sensitivity are:
- Itching of eyes or nose with thin, watery nasal discharge.
- Worse outdoors from 8:00 a.m. to 12:00 noon.

- Worse on clear, windy days.
- Improved on rainy days.
- Improved indoors with the house closed and air conditioning and filtration on.
- Worse when going from an air-conditioned room to open air when the pollen count is high.
- Worse at peaks of specific pollen seasons.
- Improved after the first light frost.

If the whole eye itches, pollen allergy is likely to blame. However, if the inner canthus (inside corner of the eye) is itchy, this suggests a food allergy, even though it may be pollen season.

If you experience any of the above symptoms you should suspect a pollen allergy. Because pollens are difficult to avoid, you should consider some form of testing and treatment for pollen sensitivity. Air cleaners help to create a pollen-free environment in the home and are a must for the extremely sensitive person. Filters in air cleaners should be changed or cleaned as needed. Wearing a mask when outdoors will also filter out pollens.

Pollen Activity Dates   Pollination dates vary from year to year, depending on weather conditions. The timing of the first and last freeze will affect the dates. However, pollination dates usually fall within a given time span, making it possible to predict, within limits, when a particular plant will pollinate. Amount of rainfall and temperature will also affect the amount of pollen produced.

The following Regional Zone Maps show the different pollinating zones within the continental United States and Canada. Spring flowering plants bloom and pollinate from south to north, and fall flowering plants bloom and pollinate from north to south. In most areas, trees pollinate from late winter until spring, grasses pollinate from spring until early summer, and weeds pollinate from summer until early fall.

Below are listed the general pollinating times for each zone. These are broad time frames; pollination times within a particular zone will vary between states or provinces, and within the states or provinces themselves. The variation depends on the size of the area, the type of terrain, and the plant species in each state or province. Varying altitudes and proximity to seacoasts also affect the length of the pollen season. More detailed information should be available from your environmental medicine physician, county agent, or appropriate government agency.

United States

Zone 1
Trees	February–July
Grasses	February–September
Weeds	April–October

Zone 2
Trees	December–October
Grasses	January–October
Weeds	April–October

Zone 3
Trees	December–July
Grasses	February–September
Weeds	April–October

Zone 4
Trees	February–July
Grasses	February–October
Weeds	April–October

Zone 5
Trees	January–October
Grasses	January–October
Weeds	April–October

Zone 6
Trees	January–October
Grasses	January–October
Weeds	March–October

Zone 7
Trees	February–July
Grasses	March–September
Weeds	April–September

Zone 8
Trees	February–September
Grasses	February–August
Weeds	March–November

Zone 9
Trees	Year-round (some trees pollinate every month)
Grasses	January–October
Weeds	March–November

Alaska
Trees	March–July
Grasses	April–August
Weeds	May–September

Hawaii

The pollen season in Hawaii is less easily defined than it is in the continental United States. At lower elevations, Hawaii's growing season is essentially continuous with a few peak periods for grasses and weeds.

Canada

Zone 1
Trees	February–June
Grasses	April–September
Weeds	May–September

Zone 2
Trees	March–May
Grasses	April–August
Weeds	May–October

Zone 3
Trees	April–June
Grasses	April–September
Weeds	April–October

Zone 4
Trees	February–April
Grasses	May–September
Weeds	May–October

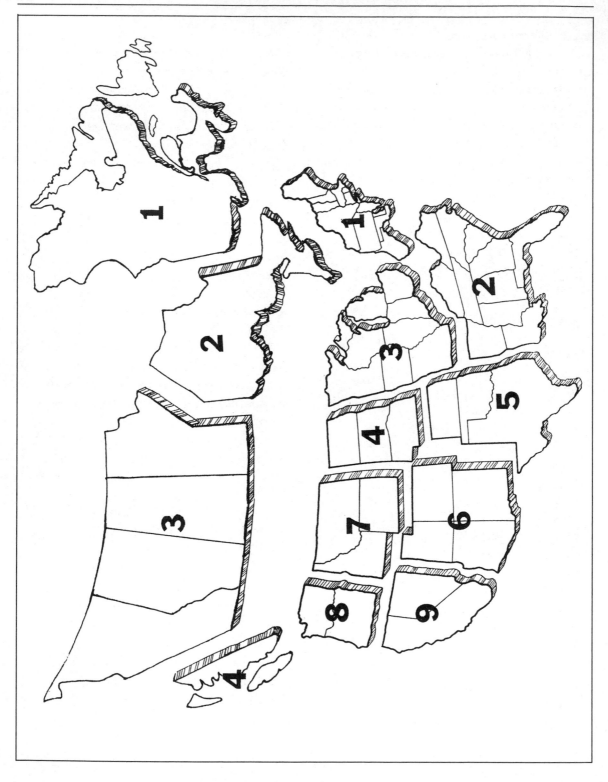

TERPENES

Terpenes are types of unsaturated hydrocarbons occurring in both animals and plants. They are most widely distributed in plants, particularly in the essential oils and resins, and are responsible for the plant's odor and taste. There are many classes of terpenes, depending on their chemical structures. Turpentine, rubber latex, and vitamin A are examples of plant terpenes. Cholesterol is an animal triterpene.

Terpenes are found in all parts of the plant—the pollen, stems, leaves, and flowers—but terpene concentration is highest in the stems, leaves, and flowers. Terpene production increases before flowering and then decreases rapidly. Terpenes are responsible for some of the blue haze seen over the mountains, for the smell of freshly cut grass, for the pine scent of all conifers, and for the sweet smell of lilacs. The unique taste of meat broiled over mesquite wood charcoal comes from the mesquite terpene.

Many sensitive people experience adverse reactions to both terpene and pollen of plants. This is evident in those who develop pollen symptoms long before pollen appears. These symptoms coincide with the rise in terpenes that occurs just before trees, grasses, and weeds flower. Some of these people will receive symptom relief or control using only pollen extracts, while others require testing and treatment with allergy extracts for both terpenes and pollens.

MOLDS

Fungi make up a portion of the plant world that does not contain chlorophyll and therefore cannot synthesize food from water and carbon dioxide. Many of these fungi are familiar to us: mushrooms, toadstools, puffballs, and various yeast and molds. There are over 100,000 fungi,

which fall into the classes listed below:

- *Lichens:* Grey-green patches on rock.
- *Phycomycetes:* Water molds.
- *Basidiomycetes:* Mushrooms, toadstools, puffballs.
- *Ascomycetes:* Industrial yeasts.
- *Fungi imperfecti:* Pathogenic yeasts (Candida species) and molds.

Molds are part of *Fungi imperfecti*. They are widespread, found in great numbers in soil and in the air. Molds do not have a season, but are present all year, except when there is snow on the ground. Molds require abundant moisture for growth and spore dispersion. They also need a supply of organic matter and oxygen. Molds are hardy, thriving at 70° to 90°F, but some can endure subfreezing temperatures; they will remain dormant until thawed and then will grow again. In general, molds grow best at room temperature, since intense heat and excessive dryness are detrimental to them.

Mold growth can take place in any part of the continent. Molds send their spores into the air when it rains and when snow thaws. Peak spore production months for these molds are from midsummer until fall. After the first hard freeze, spore production becomes minimal.

Molds grow well in an environment containing sugar, as well as under acidic conditions in which bacteria cannot grow. These properties enable mold to develop on the surfaces of foods such as jellies, jam, and pickles.

Molds can be found in homes, schools, factories, hospitals, farms, and outdoors. There is no environment devoid of molds. They can grow on food, plants, soil, paint, wallpaper paste, wood, leather, hay, animal waste, paper, and many other fibers. Mold can contaminate food, such as bread, or it can be an essential added ingredient, as in the production of cheese. Roquefort, Blue, Havarti, and Camembert are examples of mold-ripened cheese. One of the best-known mold products is the antibiotic penicillin, which is produced by *Penicillium notatum*.

Molds can be highly destructive agents. They are one of the chief causes of disease in cultivated plants, causing considerable loss of stored seeds. Molds cause deterioration of many products, such as wood, leather goods, rubber articles, paper, fabrics, and even glass lenses.

Household Mold   When mold spores are plentiful outside, they dominate the indoors also. Molds originating indoors are more obvious when buildings are closed; a musty smell signals the presence of mold. Indoor mold levels are proportional to the relative humidity. Ventilation is extremely important in controlling household mold.

In the home, mold is frequently found in the basement, since this area is usually a little damp. Basement mold can send spores throughout the house. Mold production is also high in bathrooms and kitchens. In the bathroom, mold grows on the caulking between the tub and the tile, on the shower curtain, and on the floor behind the toilet. In the kitchen, mold frequently develops at the sink-wall junction and around the bottom of the cold-water pipe. The surplus water tray on self-defrosting refrigerators is a particularly notable mold source. Sunrooms, atriums, or other areas of the house that contain houseplants are major sources of mold from the soil. Hot tubs that are not properly maintained or that have small leaks may also be a mold source. The rugs and flooring beneath water beds are also a prime spot for mold growth.

Walls in adobe houses that have been placed directly on soil rather than on concrete foundations frequently have a great deal of mold from upward seepage from the ground. Flat-roofed houses also have mold problems because of leakage into ceilings and walls. Insulation and wallboard can be moldy before it is possible to detect any mold on the painted surface.

Outdoors, mowing the grass and raking leaves constitutes a mold exposure. In farming areas where there are grain crops, harvesting the grains is an enormous exposure, not only for the harvesters but for the surrounding communities. Mold spores can be spread by winds, insects, and humans. Because they are microscopically small, spores can be carried by the wind for 15 to 20 miles.

Symptoms of Mold Allergy   Molds can be significant in many clinical disorders. When they are inhaled, mold spores can be an important cause of nasal symptoms. Respiratory complaints, such as hypersensitivity pneumonitis, can result from contact with airborne spores or mycelial fragments. Dermatitis can be caused by inhalation of fungal material, as well as by absorption from skin colonization or by invasion of other tissues. Urticaria (raised, itchy skin patches), secretory otitis (fluid behind the ear drum), gastrointestinal distress, cerebral symptoms, depression, and other complaints can be caused by mold sensitivity.

Many people with chronic sinus problems have mold colonizing their nasal passages and sinuses. The possibility of mold growing in the lungs should be examined in those with asthma and bronchitis-type symptoms.

Treatment of mold infections is determined by their location in the body. If you have an infection in the lungs, a systemic antifungal, such as Nizoral or Diflucan, will be necessary. For an infection in the nose and sinuses, sodium thiosulfate nosedrops are very effective. Treatment with an allergy extract containing the appropriate molds is imperative, regardless of the location of the infection, as sufferers are always acutely mold-sensitive.

For a typical mold-sensitive person, symptoms will be:

- Worse outside between 5:00 to 9:00 p.m., in the cool evening air.
- Worse in damp places (woods, or particular rooms in a house, especially the basement and bathroom).
- Worse when mowing or playing on grass, or when raking leaves.
- Worse when exposed to hay (fields, haystacks, barns).
- Distinctly worse from August until heavy frost.
- Ongoing after the ragweed season.
- Improved inside a closed house when the air conditioning or furnace is on.
- Improved when temperature drops below freezing and snow covers the ground. Snow covers outdoor sources of mold: decayed vegetation, dry leaves, and grass.
- Worse when eating foods made by fermentation: beer, wine, sharp cheese, sauerkraut, tofu, pickles, and vinegar.
- Worse following ingestion of mushrooms, other fungi, and seaweed.
- Worse after exposure to a number of days of damp weather in succession.

With mold allergies there is no itching of the eyes and nose; those symptoms strictly relate to pollens or foods. With pollens, the entire eye becomes itchy. With foods, only the inner canthus (inside corner) itches. Allergy extracts are very useful in controlling a mold allergy.

Molds can cause other problems for us in addition to allergic responses. Mycotoxins are poisons produced by molds when they grow on particular food substances. Only certain species of mold produce these poisons, and only under certain environmental conditions and on certain foods, such as rye, peanuts or wheat. These toxins can cause mild to severe symptoms in animals and humans. These symptoms include destruction of blood vessel and liver tissues, overgrowth of fibrous tissue, convulsions, hematomas, vertigo, rashes, swelling of the heart, destruction of brain cells, hemorrhage, and even death.

More investigation of these toxic substances is necessary, but it is quite likely that more diseases will be found to be directly attributable to these toxins.

Controlling Mold Allergies

GENERAL

- Avoid eating mold-laden foods: cheeses, fermented beverages, cider, vinegar, pickles, mayonnaise, sauerkraut, dried and candied fruits, tofu, mushrooms, sour cream, buttermilk, smoked meats, and spices (which may become moldy during processing and drying).
- Avoid old dust (which is full of mold) found in attics and unoccupied buildings.
- Avoid anything that smells musty (mold produces this odor).
- Avoid using mildewed items. Mildew is caused by mold.

INDOORS

Avoiding mold is the best strategy for those who are sensitive to it. Controlling dampness and increasing air circulation are helpful in preventing mold growth.

It is important to determine the mold population of your home, particularly in rooms in which you spend long periods of time, or which are notorious for the presence of mold. The bedroom and bathroom are important for these reasons, as is the den or family room. Mold counts can be determined by using mold diagnostic plates from Mold Survey Services (See *Recommended Sources and Organizations*, p. 299.) The results can help you determine which parts of your house require more attention for mold control.

BASEMENT

- Clean and check regularly for mold. Take care with items that support mold growth. These items should not be stored in damp places, particularly the basement.
- If the basement humidity exceeds 50 percent, use a dehumidifier. Clean and check it regularly for mold.
- Correct and clean up after any flooding or seepage problems.

BATHROOM

- All bathrooms should be well ventilated to decrease dampness. Dry off the shower walls, floor, and fixtures with a towel to decrease the amount of standing water.
- Pick up bath mats and dry after use. Carpeting should not be used in bathrooms.
- Never put damp clothing or towels into a hamper or closet. Allow these items to dry thoroughly before putting them away.
- Shower curtains frequently grow mold and should be discarded if they cannot be cleaned thoroughly.
- Wallpaper should be checked frequently for mildew.
- Check for dampness accumulating from condensation at the base of the toilet.

KITCHEN/LAUNDRY ROOM

- Clean the drip pan of self-defrosting refrigerators regularly. Check for mildew on refrigerator seals.

- Do not allow molded fruits, vegetables, or leftovers to remain in the refrigerator.
- Vent your clothes dryer to the outside.
- In damp climates, soiled clothes in hampers or baskets sometimes produce mold, as do clothes washed and not yet dried. Do not leave wet clothes in the washing machine. Keep the lid of the washing machine open when not in use in order to provide air circulation and prevent mold growth.
- Garbage cans should be cleaned regularly to prevent mold growth.
- Dirty dishes will grow mold if allowed to sit; wash after each meal.

BEDROOMS

- If you have items that have molded, you must discard them. These may include old newspapers, books, or magazines, old furniture, bedding, carpet, clothing, and pillows.
- Furniture and bedding made of latex rubber or urethane will harbor mold. These need to be covered with barrier cloth.
- Stringent dust control procedures also help prevent mold growth.
- Carpeting with foam-rubber backing or padding can foster mold growth and should not be used.
- Check for leaks under waterbeds.

MISCELLANEOUS

- Houseplants may harbor mold, both on the plant and in the soil. Watering plants causes them to release mold spores into the air. In cases of severe mold allergies, these plants must be removed from the house.
- Dried flowers may sometimes be moldy. If so, they should be discarded.
- Do not use a humidifier unless absolutely necessary. Humidifiers frequently grow mold

and then dispense spores into the air. If you do use them, they should be cleaned frequently. Most manufacturers include a compound to prevent mold growth, but a chemically sensitive person may not be able to tolerate these chemicals.

- Air conditioners, particularly "swamp coolers," may be sites of mold growth because of their dampness. Change the pads frequently.
- Car air conditioners can also be a potent source of mold, sending spores throughout the car each time they are turned on.
- Mold grows on tree bark. Do not keep fireplace logs in the house.
- Air sleeping bags thoroughly after each use.
- Before using them, air out cabins or houses that have been closed for the winter season.
- Avoid storing mattresses, pillows, upholstered couches, and bedding in unheated cabins.

Mold is frequently brought into the house on work clothing, shoes, and boots. If a family member works where there are large numbers of mold spores, work clothes should be changed and left outside the house. This includes the following occupations, businesses, or activities: sawmills; dusty factories; mattress or furniture factories; breweries; cheese factories; floral shops/nurseries; farmers; botanists; lumberjacks; hikers; or gardeners.

OUTDOORS

An acutely mold-sensitive person should:
- Avoid raking, burning, or jumping in leaves.
- Avoid walking through weedy fields or vacant lots.
- Avoid hay, straw, peat moss, compost, or sawdust.
- Avoid playing under shrubbery or climbing trees.
- Avoid stacking or playing on fireplace logs.
- Avoid deep woods and caves.
- Avoid clean-up chores in the yard, as well as mowing grass.
- Avoid combing, shovelling, or storing grains.
- Avoid live Christmas trees and evergreen decorations.
- Avoid sweeping porches, basements, and garages (approximately one-third of cement dust is mold).
- Avoid greenhouses.
- Keep the exterior of the home free of leaves and debris.
- Remove vines on outside walls of house.
- Remove shrubs resting against the walls of the house.
- Eliminate areas of standing water, and remove obstacles that cause constant shade.
- Clean leaves and debris from gutters on and around the house.

Mold Clean-up and Control
- Use soap and water and wash thoroughly, scrubbing with a brush if possible.
- Bleach will kill mold, but those sensitive to chlorine/chemicals should not use it.
- Zephiran (17 percent aqueous solution) diluted 1 oz/gal in distilled water will kill mold. It has no odor when diluted, and it is available at drugstores.
- Adding Impregnon, a fungal retardant, or Taheebo tea to houseplant water will retard mold in the potting soil. Both are available at health stores.
- To kill mold in the dirt under the house (pillar and post foundation), spread copper sulfate or borax crystals.
- Borax sprinkled in moldy places will retard mold growth. Mix borax and water in a spray bottle and wash the walls of your shower or

bathroom. Let it dry on the walls to prevent mold growth.

- Keep all areas dry and well lit. Allow space for air circulation behind furniture to keep the walls dry.
- Heat will kill mold, drying it into a powder that can be brushed off. You can use a hair dryer or a portable electric heater to heat, dry, and kill the mold. However, the spores remain viable unless the temperature is extremely high.
- Air cleaners will remove mold spores from the air. Be sure to change or clean the filters as needed.
- Ozone generators can be used to kill mold. These can be rented from some physicians, cleaning companies, or fire departments. They produce an ozone gas, which penetrates all parts of the room in which the generator is operating. People, animals, and plants must leave the room while the generator is producing ozone; exercise caution and follow directions carefully when using an ozone generator.
- A mold-sensitive person should avoid cleaning chores associated with mold clean-up. If this is not possible, wear a mask and gloves during the clean-up, keep the area well ventilated, wash clothing immediately, and take a shower (including hair-washing) when you are finished.

Common Airborne Molds

ALTERNARIA   This mold grows on organic debris in the soil; on the leaves, stems, flowers, and fruits of many vegetables; on cereal grains; and on ornamental plants (such as tomatoes, beans, chrysanthemums, and cabbage). Its spores easily become airborne and are very common from late spring until fall, especially between noon and 3:00 p.m. In September,

symptoms caused by *Alternaria* are frequently mistaken for ragweed symptoms. *Alternaria* is one of the two major widespread molds that produce allergic symptoms, and it is probably the most clinically reactive airborne fungus allergen.

ASPERGILLUS   A common soil fungus, *Aspergillus* also grows on stored food products under damp conditions. One species is common on wet surfaces in bathrooms and in drip pans of refrigerators and other appliances. *Aspergillus* also grows on damp hay, grain, fruits, and sausage. Indoor and occupational exposures are common.

AUREOBASIDIUM (PULLULARIA)   The spores of this mold are most plentiful in the air during the afternoon (1:00–5:00 p.m.). When they germinate, fungus colonies have a slimy, yeast-like appearance, due to the numerous spores that bud off from the fungus growth. *Aureobasidium* is found in soil, but also grows on decaying vegetation and plants. It frequently occurs in large numbers.

CLADOSPORIUM (HORMODENDRUM)   These spores are very plentiful in the air, sometimes making up half of the total spore count. These spores are released in large numbers after rains and damp weather. The highest levels occur from mid-summer until December, and spore counts peak between 11:00 a.m. and 3:00 p.m. This mold grows on decomposing plants, leather, rubber, cloth, paper, and wood products; it may also be a parasite on the living leaves of some plants. *Cladosporium* and *Alternaria* are the primary widespread molds that produce allergic symptoms.

FUSARIUM   The spores of this mold are often produced in a slimy mass, and the mold colonies are usually prominently colored. They need water-splashing to be dispersed, and so may be especially common in the air after a rain. Many *Fusarium* species are parasitic on vegetable and field crops, such as peas, beans, tomatoes, corn, sweet potatoes, rice, and cotton. *Fusarium* is also found on decaying plants. Its spores may be released from infected grasses and cereals, and from stored fruits and vegetables such as cucumbers, tomatoes, and potatoes.

HELMINTHOSPORIUM Found on cereal grain plants, such as corn, wheat, oats, and rye, *Helminthosporium* spores are fairly common in the air, and are also dispersed by grain-threshing operations. The daily peak of *Helminthosporium* production is at about 2:00 p.m.

MUCOR A soil inhabitant, *Mucor* is found around barns and barnyards growing on animal waste. It also grows on food residue and leaf litter. While this mold is plentiful in the soil, its level in the air is usually low. Because of ground water seepage and dirt tracked into the house, *Mucor* can flourish indoors and contribute to inhalant allergies.

PENICILLIUM Normally a soil inhabitant, *Penicillium* can grow on breads, cheese, citrus fruits, jams, apples, other foods, leather, and organic materials. Colonies of this fungus are often blue or green. Its spores are plentiful inside houses during the winter, and peak at about 2:00 p.m. (Mutant strains are used to produce the antibiotic penicillin.)

PHOMA This mold grows on paper products, such as books and magazines, and also on some paints and plants. *Phoma* spores arise in flask-shaped organs and are extruded in mucinous masses of slime spores. These spores are dispersed by dew and raindrop washout. *Phoma* reactivity is common and is similar to *Alternaria* allergy.

RHIZOPUS This mold grows on bread; cured meats; harvested root vegetables; and sugary, stored food products (bakery goods, fruit, and sweet potatoes). It also grows on a variety of plants and is widespread in nature.

ANIMAL DANDERS

All animals, including humans, shed dander into the air. Dander is composed of skin scales and scurf (dandruff). It is light, airy, and floats about freely, and it may remain in an area for days after the animal has been removed. People may be allergic to both animal and human dander, as well as to animal serum and saliva. Reactions to animal dander or saliva can include hives, difficulty breathing (asthma), headaches, loss of voice, itching or watering eyes, and sneezing.

Cat dander and saliva are extremely potent allergens; the saliva is more allergenic. The dander is very lightweight and difficult to remove from an area. Many people develop symptoms after being licked by a cat, and saliva can cause a reaction even when it has dried on the cat's fur. Cat-sensitive people can be affected by more than just housecats, and should avoid leopard coats, tiger rugs, and lion and other feline cages at the zoo. Although not common, cat fur can also be found in toys, gloves, slippers, imitation fur, upholstered furniture, bathrobes, and caps. Dry-cleaning these items can reduce the potency of the dander or saliva, but avoiding them is best.

Dogs are the second most common source of animal dander, hair, or saliva allergies. All species of dogs, short- or long-haired, can cause sensitivities. Many sensitive people also react to licks from dogs. All dogs share common allergens, as well as having special, breed-specific antigens. Because of this, some people may tolerate one breed better than another. Also, some dog breeds shed very little, and if these are kept clean and trimmed, they are less of a problem. Dog hair is sometimes used to make fur coats, rugs, and robes.

Horse dander can also be a potent allergen, but it is less of a problem now than in the early part of this century because there are few horses in our cities. Horse hair is no longer used as often in upholstered furniture, mattresses, mattings, padding, and felt. However, exposures are likely in rural areas and certain for those who ride for recreation. Horse hair is also found in manure, posing a problem for those who use it to fertilize gardens and lawns. Because horse dander is antigenically similar to horse serum, people allergic to horse dander should be careful about receiving horse antisera shots, such as snake venom antiserum, antivenom for black widow spider bites, and tetanus antitoxin. Rugs, upholstered furniture, carpet padding, blankets, pillow stuffing, mattress stuffing, clothing, drapery, and some toys may still contain horsehair.

Rabbit dander and fur may also cause allergic reactions. Fur coats and hats, fur trimmings, fur pillows, toy animals, fabrics, linings of gloves and slippers, angora yarn, the sounding hammers of pianos, and some felts constitute exposure to rabbit fur or dander.

Sensitivities to cattle, pig, and goat hair and dander, sheep wool, sheep dander, and lanolin are also possible. The hair and wool from these animals are found in cushions, clothing, cloth, bedding, carpets, and wigs.

You should suspect an animal dander sensitivity if your symptoms occur or worsen when:

- You are exposed to animals, such as cats, dogs, or horses.
- You are exposed to animal hair (rabbit, mohair, wool) in blended form (sweaters, gloves, liners, blankets), rug padding, or furniture stuffing.
- You are licked by an animal.

The degree of animal sensitivity varies from person to person. For some people, animals must be removed from the home environment. For others, reducing contact (by keeping animals outside) may be sufficient. Regardless of the intensity of your sensitivity, animals should never be allowed in the bedroom or on the bed.

Animal dander can be spread throughout the house by a forced heating or cooling system. Even after an animal has been removed from your house, it may take years to completely remove all traces of hair and dander from carpeting and furniture. Cat dander has been found in homes that have never housed cats, and in houses under construction. Air cleaners aid in removing animal dander and hair from the air.

Regular bathing of cats and dogs helps decrease their allergenicity. However, to comfortably bathe cats, you must begin regular baths when they are very young kittens. Animals should never be groomed in the house, and certainly never by the person who is allergic to animal danders. For the very sensitive person, animal hairs or dander on the clothing of another person can trigger symptoms. Animals in the classroom can pose a problem for the sensitive child. Allergy extracts for animal danders can afford relief and protection.

DUST

Outside dirt is basically inorganic. Housedust, on the other hand, is considered organic dirt, because it is so laden with organic matter. Housedust is a very complex mixture, composed of the breakdown products of the following items:

Plant
Cellulose:
  Cotton
  Jute

Kapok
Linen
Wood
Food remnants
Mold spores
Pollen

Animal
Camel hair
Felt
Fragments:
  Ants
  Beetles
  Cockroaches
  Cocoons
  Feathers
  Fleas
  Flies
  Mosquitoes
  Moths
  Silverfish
  Spiders
  Webs
Furs
Hair
Horsehair
Housedust mites
Human dander
Insect feces
Mohair
Pet dander
Rabbit fur
Silk
Wool

Inorganic
Acrilan
Cigarette smoke
Dacron
Fiberglass
Fireplace soot

Lycra
Nylon
Orlon
Paint
Paper
Plastic
Rayon
Rubber
Spandex

Housedust contains mold spores, and is a bigger problem in damp climates than it is in drier areas. When molds release their spores, they are sent throughout the house and into the air we breathe.

Another major component of housedust is the housedust mite. This is a microscopic insect (arthropod) which, in damp climates, is found in abundance in the dust of homes. (See the following section on "Dust Mite.")

No matter how well we clean our houses, we will be surrounded by some dust and we breathe it continually. An average six-room house accumulates 40 pounds of dust in a year. Dust is formed when materials that make up household articles, furniture, and clothing age and deteriorate. It also collects in stored articles and furniture. Housedust could be considered an occupational hazard for the homemaker, as housecleaning stirs up enormous quantities of dust.

Housedust can produce year-round symptoms, but they occur principally during the months when the house is closed and the furnace is operating. The harder the furnace works—and the drier the house—the greater the problem of housedust allergy.

The following are possible indicators of a dust and dust mite sensitivity. Symptoms occur or worsen:
• Indoors, and improve outdoors.

- When the heating season starts (symptoms improve in the spring).
- When the house is swept or dusted.
- When the bed is being made.
- When sitting on upholstered furniture.
- In a library.
- In the bedroom.
- When you arise in the morning, improving during the day.
- When you have been in bed for 30 to 60 minutes.

While all of us could probably benefit from some dust-control measures in our homes, the acutely sensitive person may have to take extreme measures. These procedures should be used all over the house; however, the bedroom should receive the most attention. Cleaning should be done while the extremely sensitive person is out of the house (if a sensitive person does any housecleaning, a mask must be worn). Consider investing in a double-filtered or water-filtered vacuum cleaner in order to reduce recirculating dust particles.

To prepare a dust-free bedroom:

- Empty the room of furniture and clean thoroughly to eliminate all traces of dust. Wash the walls, and scrub the woodwork, baseboards, and floors. Clean the closets; empty and clean them thoroughly before returning appropriate items.
- Take the bed outside the room and clean thoroughly. Vacuum, then wipe with a damp cloth.
- For extreme sensitivity problems, cover the mattress and pillows with barrier cloth.
- Eliminate under-the-bed storage.
- Use only freshly laundered linens. Blankets and spreads should be washed once a month; avoid blankets that have not been washed. Avoid fuzzy blankets and chenille bedspreads, and do not use any bedding or pillows that cannot be washed.

- Clean each item of furniture thoroughly before returning it to the bedroom. Upholstered furniture is taboo!
- *Never* allow pets in the bedroom.
- Eliminate carpeting and padding. Remove books and bookshelves unless the shelves are covered.
- Keep all clothes in the closet with the doors shut at all times. Use closets only for storing laundered clothes. If you're extremely sensitive, you may have to store clothes outside the bedroom.
- Empty and clean drawers with a damp cloth. Use drawers only for storing laundered clothes.
- Eliminate drapes and blinds; use washable curtains.
- Dust the bedroom once a day with a damp cloth, and vacuum frequently.
- Remove dust-catchers, such as pennants, pictures, trophies, books, models, and dried or silk flower arrangements.
- Use an air cleaner with a dust filter and change the filters or clean them as needed.
- Open the windows to blow away the dust you raise, particularly when vacuuming. (In winter, wear a coat if you have to.) Close the windows after you have finished cleaning, and keep them closed.

For other parts of the house:

- Vacuum upholstered furniture and rugs daily for acute cases, and one to two times per week for mild cases.
- Do not sit on upholstered furniture or feather pillows. Be sure anything that has been stored is thoroughly cleaned and aired before using.
- Avoid knick-knacks. Do not use brooms or dusters.
- Do not allow birds, animals, or reptiles in the house.

- Dust with rags dampened with water or a safe cleaning product. Do not use commercial dusting oils or other scented preparations.
- Replace furnace air filters at least twice a year.
- Spend most of your time in the cleanest, barest rooms—the bedroom and the kitchen.
- Dust-sensitive children should not play with stuffed toys. They should play in their clean rooms with clean toys.

Dust-sensitive people should avoid attics, closets, basements, or storerooms. They should not rummage in drawers, handle dusty items, or handle items that have been stored for a long period of time. Avoid clothing made from linty materials. New sweaters, fleece-lined fabric, and chenille garments should be washed several times before wearing, as should new bath and kitchen towels.

Live Christmas trees are a source of dust and molds and should not be used in the homes of dust-sensitive people. Exercise care when using Christmas and other decorations also, as these items are usually stored in dusty attics or storerooms. Clean and seal all decorations in plastic bags before placing them in storage boxes. When unpacking the decorations for the next season, open the storage boxes outside and bring only the clean decorations into your house.

The severity of your dust sensitivity will determine how you will use these measures. Dust extracts are also beneficial. Anything you can do to minimize your allergic load contributes positively to your health.

Dust Mite

Dust mites, which are related to ticks and spiders, make up a microscopic insect component of housedust. There are 15 species living around the world. They eat the 50 million skin scales people shed every day. They cannot survive on living skin. Mites are harmful only to people who are allergic to them. Mites and their excrement induce bronchial inflammation and hyperreactivity, leading to asthma and other forms of breathing difficulty. Other symptoms caused by dust mites include rhinitis, sneezing, congestion, and itchy, watery eyes. Allergy extracts for dust mites are helpful in controlling these symptoms.

Live mites are not inhaled, as they have sticky feet that cling to surfaces. It is the feces and mite carcasses that are inhaled. In damp climates, mites are found in abundance in dust, and their carcasses and excrement float about, entering our lungs. The average dust mite produces about 20 highly allergenic fecal pellets per day, enough to equal its own weight in just a few days. The pellets are so light that they stay in the air for 10 minutes after being disturbed. They are covered by a membrane so strong that soaking for 16 hours does not affect it.

Signs of dust mite allergy include:
- Persistently stuffy nose or ears.
- Repeated sneezing on awakening.
- Worsening of symptoms when beds are made.
- Improving symptoms outside the house.

Dust mites colonize in mattresses, carpets, and upholstered furniture; they also live in stuffed toys. It is difficult to rid a house of dust mites—vacuuming removes only dead ones. Heat and low moisture appear to be the best ways of prevention, although hot washing will destroy mites in bedding. Chemical measures have not been practical; they are hazardous to people and the mites are resistant to most chemicals. However, there are now two chemicals available to aid in mite control. Tannic acid destroys dust mite allergen, and benzyl benzoate powder kills mites. It is not clear which product is best for repeated use in the home. Chemically sensitive individuals may not be able to tolerate these products. Even if they are tolerated, they should be applied by other people.

Controlling humidity is the single most important factor in curbing dust mites. They thrive in 70 percent humidity and tend to hit their population peak in late summer. When home heating systems come on, the numbers of mite colonies drop off, hitting their lowest point in January. Their numbers increase again in the spring when the heat goes off and the humidity rises.

Other measures of dust mite control include washing drapes regularly, vacuuming carpets and upholstery once a week, and disposing of the vacuum cleaner bag immediately. Shampooing carpets has only a temporary effect. Remove area rugs for the summer, which is the peak mite season. Beat them to remove the residues in which mites hide, and return them to the floor in the fall.

FEATHERS AND FIBERS

Feathers Many people are sensitive to chicken, goose, and duck feathers. The feathers of canaries, parakeets, parrots, pigeons, turkeys, and sparrows rarely produce reactions. Pillows, comforters, quilts, jackets, sleeping bags, and beds are common sources of feather exposure. Because feather allergens are usually products of decomposition, most feather-sensitive people are able to eat the meat and eggs of the fowls without problems. They also do not usually experience allergic reactions from egg-containing vaccines.

You should suspect a feather allergy if your symptoms occur or worsen when:

- You are exposed to feathers (in pillows, down sleeping bags, comforters, and jackets).
- You are exposed to chicken, geese, or ducks.
- You are exposed to someone working with fowl.

Down pillows, comforters, and sleeping bags should not be stored in a sensitive person's bedroom nor used by them, and they should not keep any type of bird for a pet. Feather extracts help to prevent and control allergy symptoms from feathers.

Rubella vaccine cultured on duck embryo tissue can produce an allergic response in those sensitive to feathers. Skin testing with measles, mumps, rubella (MMR) vaccine can be done prior to immunization if the person is extremely feather- or egg-sensitive.

Cotton Linters Cotton linters are not the same fibers used in cotton cloth, which are usually safe for people with health problems. Linters are the short fibers that cling to the seed after longer fibers have been removed, and they contain fragments of the seeds. The short fibers, when inhaled, can cause local irritation in the nasal passages.

Cotton linters are used to make cotton wadding or batting in pads, cushions, comforters, some mattresses, and upholstery. Linters may also be found in stuffed toys, some carpets, and rope. Contact with some types of varnish should be avoided because it may contain ingredients made from cotton linters. Examples of this type of varnish are those used to coat metals and artificial leather, and those used in waterproofing.

Jute In this age of synthetic fibers, allergies to natural fibers are frequently overlooked. Jute is a natural, tropical fiber that may trigger asthma in some people. Jute is found in burlap, carpet padding, grass place mats, hula skirts, and hemp braided rugs.

Kapok Kapok is another natural fiber that can be a potent allergen. Its silky fiber, obtained from the Indonesian silk-cotton tree, is used as stuffing for cushions, mattresses, pillows, life jackets, and toys. Exposure to kapok can cause asthma, sneezing, itching of the skin, and itchy, watery eyes.

ORRIS ROOT

Orris root comes from the iris plant. The roots are washed, dried, and then stored for three years, during which time they acquire their fragrance. The fragrance is faintly violet with a fruity undertone. After drying, the roots are pulverized and distilled to extract their yellow, semi-solid oil. The majority of orris root production takes place in Italy, with the distillation process done mostly in France. It is one of the oldest, most expensive, and most widely used perfume ingredients.

Orris root is also used in cosmetic powders and toiletries because its oil and fine starch granules hold perfumes. Many manufacturers have stopped using orris root powder in cosmetics because of its high allergenicity. However, even if orris root powder is not listed on the label, a cosmetic may contain tincture of orris root. Reactions can include infantile eczema, hay fever, stuffy nose, red eyes, headaches, nausea, and asthma. Orris root extracts help to control these symptoms.

Orris root may be found in bakery goods, dusting powder, face powder and creams, gin factories, hair tonic, lipstick, lotions, perfumes, rouges, sachets, scented soaps or shampoos, shaving creams, sunburn lotions, teething rings, and toothpaste or tooth powder.

TOBACCO

Tobacco smoke is a major contributor to indoor pollution. About one-third of the adult North American population smokes tobacco, and everyone is exposed to tobacco smoke in varying degrees. A major irritant for both smokers and nonsmokers, tobacco smoke causes burning eyes, nasal congestion and drainage (rhinitis), sore throat, cough, headache, and nausea. Even those who enjoy smoking find the irritating "sidestream" smoke from smoldering tobacco to be unpleasant. Smoking one cigarette releases three mg of carbon monoxide and 70 mg of dry particulate matter. Cigar and pipe smoke is even more irritating to the eyes, nose, throat, and breathing passages.

There are two types of smoke: mainstream smoke, which is the smoke drawn through the tobacco during inhalation (active smoking), and sidestream smoke, which arises from burning tobacco (passive smoking). Ninety-six percent of the gases and particulates (small solid particles) produced when cigarettes burn become sidestream smoke. They are found in higher concentrations in the sidestream smoke inhaled by the nonsmoker than in the mainstream smoke inhaled by the smoker.

Results from studies show that compared to mainstream smoke, sidestream smoke contains:

- Twice as much tar and nicotine.
- Three times as much 3,4 Benzo(a)pyrene (a suspected carcinogen).
- Five times as much carbon monoxide.
- Five times as much ammonia.

Gases and Vapors Present in Sidestream Smoke

ACETALDEHYDE Acetaldehyde damages the cilia, which line the upper respiratory tract. This damage lessens our body's ability to protect itself against infection, because the capacity to remove particulates from the respiratory tract is impaired. Coughing and wheezing result. Acetaldehyde can also depress and disrupt the central nervous system.

AMMONIA   Ammonia vapors are present in sidestream smoke, irritating the eyes and mucous membranes.

CARBON MONOXIDE   The National Ambient Air Quality Standard for carbon monoxide is nine ppm (parts per million); the allowable concentration in industry is 50 ppm. In rooms and vehicles where cigarettes are being smoked, carbon monoxide concentrations may range from 12 to 90 ppm. One study shows that if seven cigarettes are smoked in one hour, even in an average-sized ventilated room, the carbon monoxide level goes up to 20 ppm. In the seat next to the smoker this level will be 90 ppm, almost twice the maximum allowable level set for industry.

Carbon monoxide, even in small amounts, can cause:
- Diminished ability to distinguish relative brightness.
- Diminished ability to judge time intervals.
- Diminished attention to sounds.
- Difficulty with hand-eye coordination.
- Headaches, dizziness, fatigue, and nausea.

Ventilation helps lower the carbon monoxide level, but not right next to the smoker. A carbon monoxide "hangover" lasts for three to four hours after leaving a smoky area.

FORMALDEHYDE   Formaldehyde is found in sidestream smoke, as are other aldehyde compounds resulting from chemicals sprayed on the tobacco. Formaldehyde causes coughing; eye, nose, and throat irritations; fatigue; headaches; nausea; skin reactions; wheezing; and other symptoms.

HYDROGEN CYANIDE   Hydrogen cyanide is a poisonous gas that attacks respiratory enzymes. Levels above 10 ppm are considered dangerous; the concentration of hydrogen cyanide in ciga-rette smoke is 1,600 ppm.

NITROGEN DIOXIDE   Nitrogen dioxide concentrations in sidestream cigarette smoke are 250 ppm; five parts per million is considered a dangerous level. Nitrogen dioxide causes irritation, inflammation, and fluid retention in the air passages in the lungs, triggering "tightness" in the chest, coughing, and wheezing. It destroys cellular and sub-cellular structures in the lungs and induces emphysema in laboratory animals.

Particulates Present in Sidestream Smoke

NICOTINE   Nicotine is a toxic alkaloid that constricts blood vessels, increases blood pressure, increases pulse rate, and aggravates respiratory disease. It acts both as a stimulant and as a depressant on the nervous system and can cause mental confusion.

BENZO(A)PYRENE AND DIMETHYLNITROSAMINE   These substances are carcinogens that are measurable in small amounts in sidestream smoke. Cigar and pipe smoke contains even more of these compounds than cigarette smoke.

PHENOLS   Phenols interfere with the function of respiratory tract cilia. This leads to coughing and wheezing because our body's ability to remove particulates from the respiratory tract and to protect itself against infection are destroyed.

CADMIUM   Cadmium is toxic to humans and is measurable in sidestream smoke. In high concentrations, cadmium is a poisonous metal. Only minute amounts are inhaled in smoke, but the metal builds up in the body in direct proportion to the amount of smoke inhaled. Cadmium accumulates in the liver, kidneys, and lungs, where it stays permanently. There is more cadmium in sidestream smoke than in inhaled mainstream smoke.

Radioactive lead and polonium can also occur in sidestream smoke.

Other Components of Sidestream Smoke

2-napthylamine	Fluorides
4-aminobiphenyl	Furfural
Acetone	Hydrocyanic acid
Acetonitrile	Hydrogen sulfide
Acetylene	Hydroquinone
Acrolein	Isoprene
Acrylonitrile	Lead
Ammonia	Metals
Arsenic	Methacrolein
Benz(a)anthracene	Methane
Benzene	Methanol
Butadione	Methyl alcohol
Butylamine	Methyl chloride
Carbon dioxide	Methyl nitrite
Creosol	Methylamine
Crotonamitrile	Methylethylketone
DDT	N-nitrosamine
Dimethylamine	Nickel compounds
Endrin	Nitric oxide
Ethane	Propane
Ethylamine	Pyridine
Ethylene	Tar

About 4,000 known compounds are generated by burning cigarettes. The composition of tobacco smoke varies with the type of tobacco, the soil in which it was grown, the method of curing the leaves, and the temperature of combustion during smoking. Unlike other manufacturers, cigarette companies are not required to label the contents of their products. This is a problem because:

• There are pesticide and fertilizer residues on the tobacco.
• Tobacco is flue-cured with wood, so smoke residues are left on the leaves.

• The quality of cigarette paper varies from brand to brand.
• Sugar is mixed with the tobacco in some brands of cigarettes.

Tobacco Smoke and Disease Out of 16 waking hours in a day, a two-pack-a-day smoker spends from three to four hours with a cigarette in his or her mouth, hand, or ashtray, and takes about 400 puffs, inhaling up to 600 milligrams of tar. The average employee who smokes wastes six percent of working hours with the smoking ritual, takes 50 percent more sick leave, uses the health care system 50 percent more, and causes the employer to spend more money to meet building code air standards.

Inhalation of tobacco smoke during active cigarette smoking is the largest single preventable cause of death and disability in North America. Over 350,000 people die prematurely each year of diseases linked to smoking. Cigarette smoking is a major cause of cancer. The risk of developing lung cancer is 10 times greater for smokers than nonsmokers, and smokers account for 83 percent of all cases of lung cancer. Lung cancer is the primary cancer killer of American women.

Cigarette smoking is most strongly implicated in cancers of the lung, pharynx, larynx, and respiratory tract, but it also causes cancer of the pancreas, bladder, esophagus, and mouth; chronic obstructive lung disease (emphysema); and cardiovascular diseases, including aortic aneurysms, coronary heart disease, and atherosclerotic peripheral vascular disease (deposits in the arteries).

Cigarette smoke penetrates deep into the lungs and reaches small airways and alveoli (air sacs). The portion of the smoke deposited in the lungs is high because most smokers do some breath-holding following inhalation, resulting in increased lung burdens of toxic smoke.

Lung cancer is very difficult to detect in its early stages. Only 13 percent of lung cancer patients live five or more years after diagnosis. In lung cancer, the hair-like cilia that filter the air disappear from the lining of the bronchi. Extra mucus is then secreted to substitute for cilia function and to trap pollutants. This mucus remains in the lung until forced out by a smoker's cough. If one quits smoking before cancerous lesions form, the bronchial lining will return to normal.

Emphysema destroys lung elasticity, and this affected tissue can never be repaired or replaced. Emphysema victims become respiratory cripples, struggling to obtain oxygen and expel carbon dioxide. Some of the air sacs in their lungs burst and collapse, creating tiny craters, while others balloon and become permanently enlarged.

Pregnant women who smoke have a higher rate of premature births, miscarriages, stillbirths, and complications during pregnancy. A fetus is more sensitive to passive smoking than is an unhealthy adult. The risk of infant mortality is significantly higher in smoking mothers, and babies born to them are significantly smaller than babies born to nonsmokers. The risk of sudden infant death syndrome is increased for infants whose mothers or fathers smoke. A study from Denmark shows cigarette smoking may reduce a woman's ability to breastfeed; women who smoke stop breastfeeding their infants at an earlier age because of decreased milk production. There is also an increased risk of leukemia in children of mothers who smoked during their pregnancies.

Involuntary smoking (exposure to sidestream smoke) also causes disease, including lung cancer. Second-hand smoke causes more lung cancers than all other air pollutants in the environment. Spouses of smokers suffer an increased incidence of lung cancer over those of nonsmokers. Medical researchers believe that each year about 120,000 people will die of lung cancer caused by smoke they breathe at work from cigarettes of coworkers.

The children of parents who smoke, compared with those of nonsmoking parents, have 50 percent more respiratory infections, increased respiratory symptoms (bronchitis, asthma, trachea inflammation, and laryngitis), and a lower rate of increase in lung function as they grow older. These children are more likely to be hospitalized for bronchitis and pneumonia during their first year of life. This may increase their susceptibility to developing lung disease as adults. Cigarette smoke in the home can aggravate symptoms in some children with asthma, and can even trigger asthmatic episodes. Children of smokers also have more frequent chronic coughs and excessive amounts of mucus. Middle-ear effusions (fluid behind the eardrum) and ear infections are also more common in these young children.

Separating smokers and nonsmokers in the same airspace reduces but does not eliminate exposure to tobacco smoke and its damaging effects. Environmental tobacco smoke is made up of extremely small particles that are distributed rapidly throughout the room by air streams and convective currents. Everyone in the room is forced to breathe the smoke-filled air. Smoke odors cling to walls, carpeting, furnishings, draperies, clothing, hair, and other materials. These odors are released slowly, over days, weeks, and even months. Allergic people frequently react to these smoke residues. A tobacco extract will help to prevent symptoms from tobacco exposures.

Rooms in which tobacco is smoked generally require four to seven times more ventilation, and even where there is effective ventilation, smoke odors may persist. Because energy conservation has become important, air is frequently recirculated instead of being exchanged for outdoor (fresh) air, causing a higher concentration of and greater exposure to tobacco smoke.

The tobacco industry spends over $2 million each year for advertising. It also has other programs to encourage smoking, such as:

- Budget brands (25-cigarette packs for the price of a 20-cigarette pack).
- Rebate coupons.
- Distribution of free samples on city streets, at state fairs, at amusement parks, at rock concerts, and at other youth-oriented events.

Tobacco industry giants Phillip Morris and R.J. Reynolds now own General Foods and Nabisco, which are the top suppliers of North American supermarkets. This gives the tobacco industry an influence over supermarket chains, and cigarette ads are appearing on the food pages of newspapers.

Protecting Yourself from Tobacco Smoke

To protect yourself from the harmful effects of tobacco smoke, consider the following:

- If you are a smoker, stop smoking *immediately*. The risk of lung cancer mortality is reduced when smoking is stopped. Former smokers who quit 15 or more years ago have lung cancer mortality rates only slightly above those for nonsmokers.
- Your smoking also endangers the health of those nonsmokers around you, including your spouse, children, relatives, friends, and others. The sidestream smoke from your tobacco can cause many health problems and even death for these people.
- Smokers who have quit are less likely to backslide if surrounded by spouses and friends who do not smoke.
- For most people, quitting smoking "cold turkey" seems to work better than gradually tapering off.
- Smokers of low-tar and low-nicotine cigarettes find it easier to quit than do smokers of high-tar and high-nicotine cigarettes.
- Only one-third of smokers who quit gain weight. One-third lose weight when combining a general fitness program with their efforts to stop smoking.

If you continue to smoke, in consideration to nonsmokers:

- Smoke only in designated areas.
- Smoke only in well-ventilated areas.
- Put out your cigarettes quickly and completely. Do not let them smolder in ashtrays.
- Use smokeless ashtrays.
- Do not smoke in the presence of children or nonsmokers.
- For the sake of your health and that of your family, try to quit smoking.

If you are a nonsmoker, you should:

- Never allow smoking in your home or car.
- Dine only in restaurants with a nonsmoking section.
- Stay only in motels or hotels with nonsmoking rooms or floors.
- Insist on high air quality at your workplace.
- In social situations, politely insist that no one smoke in your presence.

Do Your Own House Survey

The following form is a modified version of the one used by our staff when determining the allergenic safety of a person's home. By applying the material in *Common Chemical Sensitivities* (p. 121) and *The Allergens* *We Inhale* (p. 162), along with the information on this questionnaire, you can do your own house call and determine what should be changed to make your home an environmentally safer place to live.

General Information

- Age of house_____ How long have you lived here?_____
- Did you have allergies before moving into this house?_____
  Did your allergies begin after moving into this house?_____
- In which part of the house do you feel best?_____ worst? _____
- In which part of the house do you spend the most time? _____
- Do you feel better: Inside?_____ Outside?_____
- In which season do you feel the best?_____ worst? _____
- House heated with: Electricity_____ Gas_____ Solar power_____
  Wood-burning stove/furnace_____ Forced hot air_____ Water-circulated_____
  Furnace location(s): _____
- Water heated with: Electricity_____ Gas_____ Solar power_____
  Heater location(s): _____
- Insulation in house: Batting_____ Foam_____ Spray-in_____ Other_____
  If solar, materials used: _____
- Storm windows made of: Glass_____ Plastic_____ None_____
- Garage: Attached_____ Detached_____ None_____
  Location:_____
- Construction of house: Slab_____ Pillar and post_____
  Outside walls: Stucco____ Wood____ Masonite____ Aluminum____ Brick____ Adobe____
  Roof: Flat_____ Pitched_____ Attic_____

- Greenhouse: Attached_____ Detached_____ None_____
  Location: _____
- Humidifier: Built-in_____ Portable_____ Hot_____ Cold_____ None_____
- Termite-proofing: Yes_____ No_____ Date: _____
  Part of house treated: _____
  Ground pretreated before construction of house?_____ Material used: _____
- Sprays with which your yard is treated: _____
  How often? _____
- Renovations to your house since you moved in (include dates of renovations):
  Additions _____
  Paint _____
  Insulation _____
  Stain _____
  Appliances _____
  Floor coverings _____
  Carpeting _____
  Panelling _____
  Wallpaper _____
  Outside: Stucco_____ Siding_____ Paint_____ Stain_____
- Gas meter_____ Propane tank_____ Location _____

Specific Information

- How often and where do you use these items?
  Insect strips _____
  Room deodorizers _____
  Furniture oils _____
  Spray or other waxes _____
  Floor cleaner _____
  Oven cleaner _____
  Cleansers _____
  Glass cleaner _____
  Ammonia _____
  Rug shampoo _____
  Disinfectants _____

Scratch remover _____

Lye _____

Plastic glasses/plates _____

Plastic tablecloth _____

Air cleaners (type, location) _____

Space heaters _____

Plants (check for molds) _____

Mothballs _____

Sachets (hangers, etc.) _____

Shoe polish _____

Cedar closet _____

Nail polish/remover _____

Scented soaps _____

Scented deodorant _____

Scented makeup/after-shave _____

Electric rollers _____

Curling brush/iron _____

Perfume _____

Hair spray _____

Clothing fabrics _____

Dry-cleaning _____

Leather clothing/accessories _____

New clothes/shoes _____

Pets in house _____

Pets sleep with anyone? _____

In bedroom? _____

Kitty/pet litter (location) _____

Dog bed (material, location) _____

Kerosene _____

Gasoline _____

Solvents _____

Pesticides _____

Weedkillers _____

Fertilizers _____

Oil (used, new) _____

Paint (stored) _____

• Changes needed: _____

_____

_____

_____

_____

Electrical Information

• Note where the main electrical current enters the house: _____

• Distance

to nearest building_____ to nearest power line_____

to nearest ponds/water_____ to nearest transformer_____

to nearest antennae_____ to nearest wire fence _____

to nearest electric meter/pole_____

Living Room

• Note type and age of:

Floor covering_____

Furniture_____

Curtains _____

Wall covering _____

• Fireplace used: Never_____ Sometimes (how often?) _____

Location:_____ Heatilator?_____ Gas igniter?_____

• Wood-burning stove used: Never_____ Sometimes (how often?)) _____

Location:_____

Airtight?_____ Fuel burned _____

• Ceiling fan: Yes_____ No_____ Location: _____

• Wood stored for fireplace use_____ Type of wood_____ Location: _____

• List other living room items not covered above (include age of item): _____

_____

_____

• Closets: _____

Unusual contents _____

_____

• Changes needed: _____

_____

_____

_____

Kitchen

• Appliances (note if gas or electric):

Stove_____ Fan_____ Refrigerator_____ Dishwasher_____

Exhaust fan_____ Ceiling fan_____ Garbage disposal_____

Microwave_____ Microwave plastic dishes_____

• Floor covering (include age): _____

• Wall covering (include age): _____

• Food storage containers and wraps:

Soft plastic_____ Foil_____ Glass_____ Plastic wrap_____ Wax paper_____

• Mold (check under sink, dishwasher, refrigerator): _____

• List other kitchen items not covered above (plants, deodorizers, insect strips, cleaning agents):

_____

_____

• Closets and cupboards

Unusual contents _____

_____

• Changes needed: _____

_____

_____

_____

Laundry Room

• Dryer: Gas_____ Electric_____ Vented to outside_____

• Type and use of:

Detergent _____

Fabric softener_____

Bleaches _____

Spot remover _____

Rinses _____

Sprays _____

Other _____

- Ironing board cover: _____
- Molds, spills: _____
- Location of laundry room in house: _____
- Closets_____
  Unusual contents _____

  _____

  _____

- List other laundry room items not covered above: _____

  _____

- Changes needed: _____

  _____

  _____

  _____

Bathroom

- For each bathroom, note type and age of:
  Floor covering_____
  Wall covering _____
  Shower/tub walls_____
  Shower door/curtain _____
- Note presence of: Toothpaste_____ Soap_____ Shampoo_____ Conditioners_____
  Mouthwash_____ Air freshener_____ Bowl deodorizer_____
  Scented toilet paper or tissues_____
- Location of bathroom: _____
- Check for mold: Around the tub_____ On shower curtain/door_____ Under sink_____
  Around toilet_____ Under wall covering_____ Under floor covering_____
- List bathroom items not covered above: _____

  _____

- Closets_____
  Unusual contents _____

- Changes needed: _____
_____
_____
_____

Bedroom

- For each bedroom, note type and age of:

Floor covering _____

Wall covering _____

Curtains/drapes _____

Mattresses _____

Mattress cover (foam back?) _____

Sheets_____

Blankets _____

Bedspread_____

Pillows _____

Furniture _____

- Location in house:_____

- Closets_____

   Unusual contents _____
_____

- Note items not listed above (pets, plants, bookcases, items under bed): _____
_____

- Changes needed: _____
_____
_____
_____

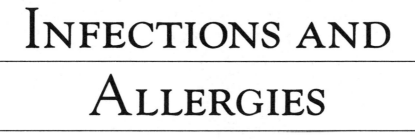

PART 3

INFECTIONS AND
ALLERGIES

THE ROLE OF INFECTIONS IN ALLERGIES

We coexist in our world with millions of microorganisms. Usually the relationship is peaceful. Most organisms live out their lives with little or no interaction with us and some are helpful to us: molds are used in cheese and antibiotics; "good" bacteria in the gut aid digestion, help control disease, and produce vitamins; and yeasts ferment wine and cause bread to rise. If all microorganisms were eliminated, life on earth would cease to exist.

However, sometimes the coexistence is not peaceful, and disease results from our interaction with microorganisms. We may suffer from unwanted symptoms caused by bacteria, viruses, parasites, molds, or yeasts. These organisms can be the primary cause of an attack on the immune system that can exacerbate sensitivities. They may also play a secondary role as a result of lowered immunity caused by other factors, such as chronic stress from allergic reactions.

Microorganisms can affect us in many ways other than the infections themselves. Toxins produced by the organisms as well as sensitivities to them add to the effects of illness. Cell fragments of the organisms, as well as inactive

organisms, can trigger an allergic or hypersensitivity response. As these organisms die, as a result of treatment, further symptoms are caused by the metabolic products released when the cell walls of the organism rupture. Immunotherapy is very helpful in relieving this type of allergic and hypersensitivity symptom.

Latent infections that surface during continued treatment of environmentally ill people are most often not single, primary causes of the symptoms, but rather the result of lowered immunity and resistance to these opportunistic organisms.

Microorganisms may also cause symptoms even when there is no infection. Just their presence in the environment can trigger allergic symptoms. For example, molds in both the indoor and outdoor environment can trigger symptoms in the sensitive person. The presence of viruses or fungi in one person may trigger latent symptoms associated with viruses or fungi in another sensitive person.

In the following chapter, we will look closely at bacteria, Candida (yeastlike fungi), viruses, and parasites and their place in the development and treatment of allergies.

14

COMMON INFECTIONS

Bacteria

Bacteria are single-celled organisms that occur as spheres (cocci), rods (bacilli), curved cells (vibrios), or spiral-shaped cells (spirochetes or spirilla). These organisms reproduce by simple division called binary fission. Some bacteria are motile (able to move by themselves), and have one or more flagella (appendages) for this purpose. Others have creeping mobility, enabled by contractions within their protoplasm.

A few rod-shaped bacteria form spores, also called endospores. The spore is formed within the bacterial cell and is capable of producing one new bacterium. Spore formation is not a part of the reproductive cycle of these bacteria. These spores, probably the most resistant form of life known, help the bacteria survive adverse conditions. Some spores can survive an exposure to steam for more than an hour, and they are highly resistant to chemicals. The endospore will remain in spore form until conditions are favorable for bacterial growth, at which time it will germinate. Some spores can remain viable for many years, complicating sterilization procedures. True bacteria can grow on nonliving as well as living matter.

Bacteria are divided into species on the basis of:

- Size, shape, mode of movement, and resting stage.
- Biochemical and nutritional traits.
- Response to oxygen, temperature, pH, and medications.
- Genetic composition.
- Ecologic traits.

Classifying bacteria can become tedious, when every trait of each bacteria is considered. Our concern with bacteria lies primarily in the diseases they cause. Pathogenicity refers to an organism's ability to cause disease; any organism pathogenic to humans causes disease in humans. However, different strains of the same organism may affect us in different degrees. This difference in pathogenicity is called virulence. The same organism may be highly virulent or nonvirulent, depending on the strain.

The virulence of a bacterial strain is partially determined by its invasiveness. Invasiveness refers to an organism's ability to multiply in the body of the host. Bacteria generally reach our bodies in small numbers. Contact usually takes place on the skin or mucous membranes, where a primary focus of infection is formed. The host's defense mechanisms then attempt to deal with the invading bacteria. The bacteria release substances called aggressins to aid in resisting the defense mechanisms. Some aggressins prevent destruction of foreign matter by our body's phagocytic cells; some defy the efforts of those clean-up cells, and some aggressins actually kill them. If the strain of bacteria is a more virulent one, the body's defense mechanisms will be overcome and a serious infection can result.

Toxicity also contributes to the virulence of a bacteria. A number of pathogenic bacteria produce toxins. One type is called an exotoxin. Exotoxins are heat-liable proteins and are excreted into the fluid around the bacteria. They are also released when the bacteria is destroyed.

Endotoxins are heat-stable complexes containing protein, lipid, and polysaccharide, occurring in the cell wall of most pathogenic bacteria. When injected into experimental animals, endotoxins all produce the same symptoms, regardless of the bacteria of origin. Endotoxins in the bloodstream may cause rapid and irreversible shock. This occurs in massive bacteremias or when contaminated materials are injected intravenously.

Transmission of Bacteria

Bacterial diseases may be transmitted in several ways.

- Bacterial diseases may be spread by fecal contamination of food and drink by persons with poor hygiene, by healthy carriers, or by houseflies. Transmitted diseases include typhoid fever, enteric fevers (bacterial food poisonings), cholera, and bacterial dysentery.
- Diphtheria, tuberculosis, plague, meningococcal meningitis, streptococcal infections, pneumococcal pneumonia, and other respiratory infections are spread by a method called droplet infection. This occurs when pathogenic organisms are spread in drops of saliva released when a person sneezes, coughs, or speaks.

- Diseases spread by direct contact include anthrax, tularemia, brucellosis, gonorrhea, and syphilis. Organisms causing these diseases cannot survive outside their host and require direct mucous membrane contact for transmission.
- Some bacteria are able to live in two or more hosts. There is a vector (a species that transmits the pathogen) and a reservoir of infection from which the vector receives the infection. Disease is spread when an animal host or the vector bites a human. Plague, tularemia, endemic typhus, and Rocky Mountain spotted fever are spread this way.
- Wound infections can be a transmission route for bacteria whenever nonsterile foreign material enters a wound. Tetanus, gas gangrene, pseudomonas and leptospirosis are common wound infections.
- Diseases may also be caused by ingesting bacterial toxins in contaminated food. Food poisoning from the toxins of *Clostridium botulism* or *Staphylococcus aureus* are examples of this type of disease. Only people ingesting the toxin are affected; the disease cannot be spread from person to person.
- Rickettsial diseases are spread by arthropod (insect) bites. Endemic and epidemic typhus, scrub typhus, spotted fevers, rickettsial pox, and Q fever are transmitted this way. Lyme disease, which is caused by a spirochete, is also spread by insect bite.

Bacteria Identification

In human infections, rapidly isolating and accurately identifying the bacterial organism are very important so that effective treatment can be initiated. Specimens for identification may be taken from blood, spinal fluid, stool, sputum, skin, body orifices, and abscesses. In some cases, pure cultures may be obtained. In others, a mixture of organisms is obtained and a subculture must be done to isolate the pathogenic organism. In most cases identification can be made in 12 to 48 hours. However, some organisms, such as the tubercle bacillus, may require two to eight weeks of incubation before the organism appears on the growth media.

The Gram stain, developed by Christian Gram in the early 1800s, is usually the initial step in identifying bacteria. This staining technique divides bacteria into two groups. Gram-positive organisms stain blue, whereas Gram-negative organisms stain red. One half of the bacilli, one third of the cocci, and all of the spiral organisms are Gram-negative.

Tests utilizing metabolic characteristics of the organisms are common, since over 60 percent of human pathogens can be identified by this method. By using specialized culture media that demonstrate various metabolic traits, precious hours can be saved in identifying which pathogen is present.

BACTERIA AND ALLERGIES

Bacterial infections can cause problems other than the disease for us. Some people have an "allergy of infection," where they become allergic to the bacteria or bacterial metabolic products. Their initial response is one of hypersensitivity. In time, antibody formation takes place, and a second exposure to the same antigen will cause a severe reaction.

Within minutes of the second exposure to the antigen, immediate hypersensitivity will cause tissue damage. A dramatic example of immediate hypersensitivity is anaphylactic shock, which causes severe symptoms and even death. Some reactions to a second antigen exposure can be delayed. Reactions peak from 24 to 72 hours after the second exposure, at which time the tissue damage occurs. Dr. D.

Bernard Amos states, in *Zinsser Microbiology*, that an allergic response to bacteria, in addition to the infection itself, should be suspected when symptoms are unusually severe or prolonged, or when they occur in an allergic person.

Another allergic phenomenon that may occur in response to bacterial infection is the Jarisch–Herxheimer reaction seen in syphilis. Chills, fever, headache, muscle pain, and rapid heartbeat may develop two to 24 hours after treatment is begun, apparently due to immune response to antigen released as the syphilis spirochetes are killed.

Because infections contribute to total immune system load, we should be certain all sources of infection have been treated and eliminated. These infections, whether acute or chronic, can make allergies worse. Even after an infection has subsided, one can continue to have an allergic response to the cellular debris from the bacteria and from excess circulating antibodies. Symptoms will be low grade, but over a period of time will contribute significantly to one's total immune system load.

Clinical experience has shown that extracts for the following organisms have helped relieve these chronic, low-grade symptoms.

Chlamydia trachomatis
Enterococcus
Escherichia coli
Gardnerella vaginalis
Hemophilus influenzae
Klebsiella pneumoniae
Mycoplasma pneumoniae
Pseudomonas aruginosa
Salmonella
Shigella
Staphylococcus aureus
Streptococcus

TREATMENT FOR BACTERIAL INFECTION

If antibiotic therapy is indicated, determining antibiotic sensitivity is just as important as identifying pathogenic bacteria. An effective chemotherapeutic agent must be found, as well as determining the concentration level at which it is effective against the bacteria. As high antibiotic usage becomes more common, more and more bacteria are becoming resistant to antibiotics, thus increasing the importance of the sensitivity test. The practice of giving antibiotics to animals in order to reduce disease, speed meat production, and improve meat quality plays a major role in this developing resistance. The meat we eat contains residual antibiotics unless it has been obtained from a special antibiotic-free source.

In addition to treatment with antibiotics and specific immunotherapy extracts, the following will aid recovery from bacterial infections:

- *Lactobacillus acidophilus*: Replaces the helpful bacteria "killed" in the bowel by antibiotic therapy.
- *Colixen:* Contains sialic acid and gum arabic that serve as nutritional support for the body, to reduce pathogenic flora in the intestinal tract.
- *Vitamin C:* Stimulates the immune system.
- *Essential fatty acids:* Aid repair of mucous membranes and deter colonization of harmful organisms.
- *Vitamin A:* Aids repair of mucous membranes.
- *B-complex:* The intestinal mucosa, which produces B-complex, may be damaged by bacterial infections. B-complex supplements serve as replacement until normal bacterial flora can resume vitamin B production.
- *GeOxy 132:* Provides an oxygen medium that will deter the growth of anaerobic organisms (bacteria which live in the absence of oxygen).
- *Echinacea:* An herb that strengthens the immune system.
- *Co-enzyme* Q_{10}: Increases immune defense.

Candida Albicans/Yeast Infection

There are many strains of Candida in our environment, but the two that affect humans the most are *Candida albicans* and *Candida tropicalis.* In our discussion, Candida will refer to *Candida albicans,* and the disease that its overgrowth causes is referred to as candidiasis.

Candida albicans is a body yeast that lives, in small amounts, in all of us. Normally its presence is limited to the skin, the vagina, and the mucous membranes of our gastrointestinal and upper respiratory tracts. In the intestinal tract, the yeast aids in breaking down fibers in our diet. Candida growth is kept in balance by so-called "good" bacteria and our immune system. However, Candida is an opportunistic organism and if our immune system becomes depressed, inefficient, or overwhelmed, the tenuous balance is upset and the good bacteria are destroyed. Candida then multiplies and an overgrowth (chronic infection) results.

Candida albicans is a very complex organism. It releases 79 known toxins that adversely affect our body. If left untreated, a chronic Candida infection and overgrowth can severely debilitate us, leaving us susceptible to more serious diseases. Two chemicals produced by Candida are acetaldehyde and ethanol. Acetaldehyde disrupts cell membrane function and alters protein synthesis. Our metabolism cannot convert these materials into useful compounds and must detoxify them. When the circulating load of these materials is too great, poor memory, lightheadedness, fatigue, inability to concentrate, and depression can result. Acetaldehyde is also a breakdown product of alcohol and is thought to cause the "fuzzy brain" symptoms of a hangover.

Candida normally has a rounded, yeast-like shape. However, it can mutate and develop branching threads called mycelia, which penetrate the mucous membrane of the intestinal tract looking for food. This mycelial form is more difficult to eradicate as it has the ability to change its cell membrane structure in order to escape the effect of single drug therapy. Dr. David Soll of the Department of Biology at the University of Iowa recently demonstrated at least five rapid mutations of the Candida cell membrane. This mechanism is known as switching.

Besides the direct invasion of body tissues that accompanies an overt infection, some people experience hypersensitivity reactions to either surface antigens on the Candida organism or to the metabolic byproducts and toxins released by the organism. These hypersensitivity reactions can occur simultaneously and can set up widespread reactions throughout the body. This increased immune response can create too great a body burden for the hypersensitive person and can worsen already existing reactions to foods, chemicals, molds and other inhalants.

Causes of Candidiasis

Although candidiasis is typically seen as a minor infection of mucous membranes, skin, and nails, Candida overgrowth is not a new problem. The overuse and prolonged use of antibiotics kills the "good" bacteria, allowing Candida to proliferate and to become a chronic intestinal infection. Also, many meats contain high levels of antibiotics. The optimum growth media provided in the moist and dark areas in the gut and the vaginal tract make us excellent "hosts" for Candida overgrowth. Low stomach acid also fosters Candida growth.

Birth control pills, cortisone and other steroids, and nonsteroidal anti-inflammatory drugs cause hormone imbalances in our body, thus encouraging Candida to grow more abundantly. The chemicals produced by the yeast attack our immune system, and if it weakens, the Candida will spread and involve more tissues. As a result of a weakened immune system, membranes swell, germs multiply, and nasal, throat, sinus, ear, bronchial, bladder, vaginal, and other infections develop. Antibiotics are then usually prescribed, promoting further yeast growth. Health problems will continue until this cycle is interrupted by appropriate treatment.

Other conditions that may upset the normal symbiotic relationships of microflora in our body are: prolonged nutritional deficiencies; debility due to other infection, diseases, or aging; drug or alcohol abuse; deliberate chemical suppression of the immune system to avoid organ transplant rejection; and use of chemotherapeutic agents in cancer treatment.

The most common place for Candida growth is the gastrointestinal tract (the entire digestive tube from the mouth to the anus). Its only food source is sugar. A diet with excess refined or simple carbohydrates such as candies, sweets, cookies, and junk food contributes greatly to Candida overgrowth. The average North American eats over 100 pounds of sugar annually.

Candida albicans also interferes with the receptor sites for hormones in our body. The result is disrupted hormone production in the thyroid, adrenal glands, ovaries, pituitary gland, or testes. The entire endocrine system then functions poorly.

Symptoms of Candidiasis

Men, women, and children can have candidiasis. However, since women have more complex hormone systems, candidiasis occurs in them more frequently, and with more severe effects. It strikes children who have received large quantities of antibiotics or who consume excessive sugar and junk food. Candida overgrowth is also suspect in women's infertility problems. Babies can be infected with Candida as they pass through the birth canal if their mother has a yeast vaginitis.

Candida is known as the great masquerader—any symptom is possible, and any organ can be targeted. Many people with severe yeast problems have never described all of their symptoms to their doctors for fear of being labelled neurotic or a hypochondriac.

Candida symptoms fall into several categories:

- Symptoms in the intestinal and genito-urinary tracts include yeast vaginitis; menstrual complaints; bowel problems, such as bloating, constipation, diarrhea, and gas; and inflammations of the prostate, esophagus, stomach lining, colon, and bladder.
- Hypersensitivity reactions to Candida or its byproducts include asthma, headaches, bronchitis, hay fever, earaches, hives, skin rashes, and severe chemical and food sensitivites.
- Emotional and mental problems include severe depression, confusion, extreme irritability, anxiety, memory lapses and short-term memory loss, inability to concentrate, difficulty in reasoning, drowsiness, insomnia, lethargy, and loss of self-confidence.
- Worsening of any existing symptoms can also indicate a Candida overgrowth. Weakness, fatigue, fleeting muscle and joint pains, dizzi-

ness, difficulty in swallowing, acne and other distinctive skin rashes, and sugar cravings can also be indicators. Mock hypoglycemic symptoms are common. Many infected people also have an easily detected body and breath odor.

- Some people have colonies of Candida growing in their nasal passages that can cause severe sinus headaches. The increased sinus congestion and pressure can cause loss of equilibrium and may be confused with a middle-ear infection. A white, "furry" tongue is also a symptom of Candida overgrowth.
- Unrelenting skin itching is an aggravating symptom of *Candida albicans*. The itching occurs deep beneath the surface of the skin with no visible rash. Scratching or rubbing does not relieve the itching. It is perhaps caused by a hypersensitivity reaction either to antibodies produced by our body or to metabolic toxins produced by the yeast.

Candida also seriously interferes with the digestion and absorption of nutrients from the intestinal tract; as a result, prolonged, untreated infection can lead to overt nutrient deficiency. This disruption results strictly from a mechanical process caused by the overgrowth of the organism, covering the microvilli responsible for the last stage of digestion and the absorption of nutrient molecules.

Diagnosis of Candidiasis

A history of exposure to oral contraceptives, steroids, anesthesia, and multiple doses of antibiotics together with these chronic symptoms point to a Candida problem. Positive allergy tests for yeast, mold, and fungus may also indicate candidiasis.

There are several diagnostic blood tests for Candida now available at specialized laboratories. It is possible to detect high levels of

Candida antibodies from three classes of immunoglobulins: IgA, found in mucous membranes in the mouth, vagina, and intestinal tract; and IgG and IgM from the blood. Some laboratories perform blood titers of these specific immunoglobulins against Candida organisms to aid in diagnosis. Diagnostic mold plates for investigation of sputum and nasal discharge are also available.

Other types of culture surveys for *Candida albicans* can be done using smears from the nose, throat, rectal area, genital area, and vagina. Anyone with a positive culture and accompanying symptoms should be treated. In some cases, evidence of the infection cannot be ascertained unless repeated cultures are run. Finally, one's response to treatment confirms the diagnosis of Candida overgrowth.

Treatment of Candidiasis

Treatment for candidiasis is intended to reduce the organism's colonization to a tolerable level. There are several ways to treat yeast overgrowth. A combination of treatment modalities is necessary to prevent cell membrane mutation of the mycelial form mentioned earlier. Treatment should be cumulative; do not stop taking one material when the next is added.

Treatment should:
• Proceed slowly.
• Target all areas in and on the body simultaneously.
• Be persistent.
• Be long term.

If the Candida organisms are killed off too rapidly, our body is flooded with overwhelming amounts of toxins from the ruptured yeast cells. The body immediately reacts with an inflammatory immune response that can cause unbearable symptoms, known as "die-off" or Herxheimer reaction.

Since most Candida infections are long-standing and well-established, treatment must be persistent and continued for as long as necessary to prevent symptoms from returning. Unfortunately, there is no quick fix. Treatment duration will vary—some people may require treatment for only a few months, but most have to be treated for a year or more (more detailed information on treatment approaches is contained in the following pages).

Treatment must be long term because the Candida organism is a very resistant, natural, symbiotic inhabitant of the gut, and our body cannot tolerate the powerful medications it would take to wipe out the overgrowth immediately. Treatment must be consistent and continual. When it is not, the Candida organism is encouraged to bury itself deeper into the tissues by developing the mycelial form. Treatment is complete when there is no relapse after treatment is withdrawn. The immune system must recover sufficiently to keep the Candida under control, since Candida overgrowth will return with a vengeance if therapy is stopped too soon.

When therapy is complete, substances and dosages should be reduced slowly, one at a time, under a physician's care. Watch for a subtle return of symptoms; if they reappear, resume full treatment. When all therapy is discontinued your diet should still remain sugar-free.

Merely destroying the Candida organism does not immediately undo its damage to our immune and endocrine systems. It takes about one to three years for our body to rebuild its immunocompetence against *Candida albicans* infections. Each of us is unique; therefore, treatment programs must be tailored to one's specific needs. Faithfully following a treatment program will speed the rate at which candidiasis is controlled. If Candida overgrowth is not treated, it will continue to spread and break down our body's ability to fight off other serious diseases.

Continued treatment includes sorting out causes and effects of the many and varied symptoms. This can be done more easily as time elapses and as the symptoms of "overload" are whittled away. For this type of treatment, you need a long-term commitment to being fully involved in your recovery. This requires a process of education about our body functions and a willingness to share the responsibility for a return to "wellness."

When one family member has candidiasis, other members are often infected. It is wise to have the whole family checked for infection and treated if necessary. Otherwise, the one who is being treated will be constantly re-exposed, making the treatment less effective.

Facets of Candida Treatment The material later in this chapter, called "Candida Therapy Materials" and "Candidiasis and Diet," provides complete details on treatment of Candida.

- Begin each treatment substance separately and gradually increase your intake at weekly intervals as die-off permits. Build up to top dosage as rapidly as possible so the treatment time will not be prolonged and die-off will not be constant. The speed of therapy varies with the severity of the symptoms and the length of time the infection has been present.
- A low-carbohydrate diet is extremely important in the management of Candida (no more than 60 to 80 grams of carbohydrate should be consumed per day in very severe cases). The yeast feeds only on sugars and simple carbohydrates. Yeast-containing and moldy foods, such as mushrooms and cheeses, must also be avoided as our body cannot distin-

guish between these and Candida organisms. If diet is not improved, progress will be negligible. Your diet should contain proteins, vegetables, some complex carbohydrates, and unsaturated fats and oils. Increase the volume of food intake in order to keep the caloric intake high enough to prevent weight loss.

- A *Lactobacillus acidophilus* preparation will supplement "good" bacteria so that colonies can be reimplanted on the intestinal tract's mucosal lining as the Candida is killed.

Restoring the normal balance of colon flora is essential in maintaining a healthy immune system, reducing allergies, preventing growth of resistant fungal strains, and discouraging the overgrowth of other fungi.

- Fatty acids that have fungicidal properties such as caprylic acid are effective.
- Paramicrocidin, a non-absorbed, broad-spectrum, antimicrobial agent extracted from tropical plants can be used.
- An antifungal prescription drug, Nystatin, is highly effective against Candida and is usually well-tolerated.
- Antifungal prescription medications Nizoral (ketoconazole), or Diflucan (fluconazole) are also effective.
- Garlic and Taheebo or Mathake tea have minor antifungal properties.
- Ointments, lotions, or creams specific for Candida treatment, such as Nystatin Cream, should be used for external rashes to supplement systemic treatment.
- Treating any other suspected illness (including allergies) and infection will lower the total load on the immune system.
- Ask your physician about using Candida and T.O.E. (*Trichophyton, Oidiomycetes, Epidermophyton* —a mixture of common skin fungi) extracts.
- Avoid antibiotics, steroids, and nonsteroidal

anti-inflammatory drugs unless absolutely necessary.

- Seek out immunotherapy treatment for allergies—particularly to yeast and mold—to help build up the ability of the immune system to resist yeast infection and to reduce "cross-reactivity" symptoms between molds and Candida.

- Avoid birth control pills and hormones, particularly progesterone (also known as Provera). Women will have difficulty recovering from candidiasis if they continue to take birth control pills.

- Avoid environmental molds at home and at work. Continued exposure to molds inhibits recovery from candidiasis.

- Avoid chemicals in the environment as much as possible in order to lower the total load of the immune system.

- Take supplements of additional vitamins and minerals, glandulars, and enzymes that will enhance proper functioning of the digestive, immune, and endocrine systems. (See *Nutrition and Allergies*, p. 227.)

- Take detoxification baths or dry saunas to rid the body of toxins produced by the Candida organism. (See *Detoxification*, p. 250.)

- Increase your intake of a "safe" water, up to six to eight, eight-ounce glasses per day, to help flush out the accumulated toxins caused by "die-off."

- A brisk five-minute walk or other tolerated exercise several times daily will help the body rid itself of excess toxins.

- Proper bowel function (at least two soft stools daily) is very important. Increase vitamin C intake to help accomplish this. (See "Vitamin C: A Key Nutrient," p. 242.)

- Exercise stringent hygiene practices in addition to other treatments, including:

  –Careful brushing of teeth and gums, including tongue, three times daily;

  –Using Orithrush mouthwash and gargle;

  –Refraining from oral sex;

  –Cleansing all affected skin areas with soap and water before applying any of the treatment materials;

  –Washing hands with soap and water after using the toilet;

  –Washing hands with soap and water after touching infected areas on skin, scalp, ears, or nose;

  –Wearing only cotton underwear and stockings;

  –Avoiding polyester or nylon clothing, as these fabrics cannot "breathe."

We are in control of our health, and symptoms from Candida are a signal that something in our lifestyle needs to be altered. Exercise, diet improvements, nutritional supplements, and active Candida treatment are necessary to keep Candida under control. Once this has been achieved, our healthier bodies—together with altered lifestyles—will keep the organism suppressed.

For more information about *Candida albicans* and candidiasis, please see *Recommended Books*, p. 304. The more informed you are, the better you will understand your problem and how to fight it.

CANDIDA THERAPY MATERIALS

It is important to change the environment of Candida: deny it food (sugar); provide an acid medium; increase its natural enemy, "good" bacteria; and introduce antifungal agents that our body can tolerate. It is necessary to use two or more different treatment materials simultaneously to prevent the Candida organism from switching its cell membrane, thereby producing resistant strains.

As a reminder, once you begin candidiasis

treatment, you may experience what is called "die-off." You may be slightly dizzy, light-headed, depressed, experience tightness in your chest, have muscle aches, diarrhea, or an upset stomach. These die-off symptoms can also be an exaggerated form of the symptoms you experienced prior to treatment. As each yeast cell dies, the cell ruptures and its toxic contents are released. An accumulation of these toxins produces the symptoms, which will pass within a few days. Although you may feel a little discouraged by temporarily not feeling well, die-off symptoms are a sign that the treatment is working.

Lactobacillus   *Lactobacillus acidophilus* is the name of the friendly bacteria normally present in the lower bowel. It naturally deters over-growth of Candida and other undesirable organisms by competing for nutrients, altering the gastrointestinal tract pH, and by occupying "attachment" sites. As the Candida colonies are destroyed by antifungal agents, other strains of yeast will flourish if "good" bacteria are not recolonized in the intestinal tract. Use of this material is mandatory. Unhealthy flora can lead to ammonia and histamine release, irritating the mucosal lining of the intestinal tract, and causing inflammatory reactions and toxic accumulations.

Use high-quality preparations, containing at least 10 billion viable *lactobacilli* per ¼ teaspoon. Acidophilus preparations are made by culturing good bacteria on milk, soy, carrots, or other plant materials. Food-sensitive persons have a choice of culture media. Acidophilus should be refrigerated at all times.

Acidophilus therapy starts with ¼ teaspoon of acidophilus and gradually increases to one teaspoon, three times daily. An initial die-off period may temporarily increase intestinal gas.

Acidophilus can also be sprinkled on food (it tastes like powdered cream), put on your tongue and swallowed with water, added to beverages, or put into capsules. (A well-packed "00"-size capsule holds ¼ teaspoon.) It is very effective for treating your mouth, throat, and esophagus if it is put under your tongue and left there to dissolve slowly. Acidophilus is also helpful in soothing viral sore throats. It is best to take acidophilus immediately before meals as the food will provide a good medium for continued growth of "good" bacteria.

Acidophilus or yogurt can also be diluted and used as a vaginal douche, as suggested by your physician. Yogurt is not effective orally as a treatment for Candida because it does not contain adequate amounts of acidophilus. Used as a vaginal treatment, however, yogurt can be very soothing as it alters the pH of the vaginal tract, discouraging Candida growth.

Lactobacilli strains also have beneficial effects on vitamin and nutrient synthesis. They aid in lowering blood cholesterol and blood fats; they have antiviral properties; and they produce enzymes which improve digestion and absorption. After Candida problems are under control, Lactobacillus use should be continued as a regular dietary practice.

The following treatments for Candida overgrowth are available at health food stores.

Caprystatin or Candida Guard   Caprystatin is a preparation of caprylic acid, a contact fungicide. It comes in enterically coated tablets that release the caprylic acid slowly throughout the large and small intestines. Swallow the tablet intact to protect the coating.

The total dosage for Caprystatin varies from person to person. Begin with one tablet per day and gradually work up to the dosage suggested by your physician. Usual dosage ranges from six to nine tablets per day, taken in divided doses. When Nystatin is added, Caprystatin can be reduced, but not eliminated. Unless you experience gastrointestinal distress when doing so, take Caprystatin on an empty stomach, one hour before or two hours after a meal, for better absorption. Do not use Caprystatin if you are pregnant, as its effects during pregnancy have not yet been determined.

Other caprylic acid preparations are available, but they may not be as potent or effective. Some contain additional materials that may be allergenic for some people.

Kaprycidin-A A caprylic acid formulation, Kaprycidin-A is packaged in capsules designed to release in the stomach and upper intestine. Next to the esophagus, the stomach is the most common site of Candida infection.

A combination of Caprystatin and Kaprycidin-A is very effective in treating candidiasis because of the distribution of these fatty acid complexes from the stomach throughout the intestinal tract. Usual dosage for Kaprycidin-A is one capsule three times per day. If taken in conjunction with Caprystatin, the dosage of Caprystatin is reduced. Do not use Kaprycidin-A if you are pregnant, as its effects during pregnancy have not yet been determined.

ParaMicrocidin A broad-spectrum, antimicrobial agent extracted from tropical plants, ParaMicrocidin is effective against yeast (Candida) as well as against parasites. It is available from Allergy Research in two strengths, 75 mg or 125 mg. The most effective dosage is two to three capsules three times daily of either dosage, depending on the severity of infection.

The following treatments for Candida overgrowth are available only by prescription.

Mycocidin Mycocidin contains another organic fatty acid (undecylenic acid), which has antifungal activity. It occurs naturally in body perspiration. This product, derived from the castor bean, is contained in an olive oil base. As Mycocidin is gradually released in the digestive tract, it inhibits yeast growth. It is an excellent alternative for those who cannot tolerate caprylic acid preparations, and does not interfere with normal bacterial intestinal flora. There is no drug-nutrient interaction with this material, and it can be used in combination with Nystatin or Nizoral.

Mycocidin must be ordered directly from the manufacturer, Thorne Research. (See *Recommended Sources and Organizations*, p. 299). A prescription form signed by a physician is required to purchase this material. Suggested dosage begins with one perle daily and gradually increases, as die-off permits, to nine to 12 perles daily (three perles three times a day).

Nystatin An antifungal drug that kills yeasts and yeast-like fungi on contact, Nystatin is thought to bind with the yeast cell membrane. This causes changes in cell wall permeability and allows leakage of fluids into the yeast. These excess fluids cause the cell to burst, releasing the intracellular components.

Although Nystatin comes in several forms, produced by several companies, the only one that should be used orally is a chemically pure Nystatin powder that contains no additives. This powder is usually not available at pharmacies unless it has been specially ordered. The Nystatin most pharmacies keep in stock contains talc, and is intended for topical use on a localized area, such as a skin rash. It is *not* for internal use.

Because Nystatin is a "contact" fungicidal agent, it is difficult to attain significant blood levels. Only minor absorption takes place from the gastrointestinal tract, and from sublingual usage if the powder is held under the tongue. For this reason, you must use more than one treatment method—at least one for localized intestinal treatment and one for systemic treatment, depending on the severity and location of the infection.

Nystatin is a yellow, bitter-tasting powder. It has been demonstrated to be safe through more than 30 years of medical application. Nystatin is well-tolerated by all age groups, even on prolonged administration.

Before starting Nystatin treatment, take a warm-water enema to cleanse the lower bowel so the Nystatin can have closer contact with the mucous membranes.

The most effective way to take Nystatin is to stir the powder in $\frac{1}{2}$ to one ounce of water. Hold the Nystatin solution under your tongue for three to five minutes before swallowing. Do not allow the solution to sit after mixing it, as it will become more bitter. Nystatin is also more effective when it is taken on an empty stomach, since its action is enhanced by acid. Avoid food and drink for one to two hours after a dose to receive maximum benefit. Take one to two grams of Vitamin C (ascorbic acid) with your Nystatin to increase the amount of acid in your stomach.

Those who experience nausea may have to take Nystatin with meals. If you cannot tolerate the taste of Nystatin, you can put it into capsules, available at drug or health food stores, but you will not receive the esophageal coating that you do when swallowing the powder. (The lower part of the esophagus is a common site of Candida growth.) Nystatin tablets are also available, but they may contain cornstarch and dye, to which some people are sensitive.

The prescribed amounts for starting doses of Nystatin will vary from person to person, depending on length and severity of the infection and on severity of die-off symptoms. Always divide your daily dose and take partial doses three to four times per day.

A common starting dose of Nystatin is one teaspoon per day between meals. If die-off symptoms are severe, however, you may need to begin with as little as $\frac{1}{16}$ teaspoon per day. Try to struggle through the die-off period as quickly as possible; prolonged insufficient doses may perpetuate these symptoms and create a resistant organism.

When you can tolerate one teaspoon of Nystatin per day between meals, and have had no die-off symptoms for a week, begin taking one teaspoon between meals twice each day. (If die-off is too severe, it may be necessary to increase the amounts by $\frac{1}{4}$-teaspoon increments.) If you experience severe symptoms with a particular dosage level (as a consequence of killing off too many organisms at once), back up one dose and maintain that level until you can take Nystatin without symptoms for several days. At this point, increase your dosage again.

After you have felt well for a week on two teaspoons of Nystatin per day, increase your dosage to three teaspoons: one teaspoon between breakfast and lunch, one teaspoon between lunch and dinner, and one teaspoon before bedtime. At this stage, you probably will not be experiencing many die-off symptoms. In more severe cases, you may need to take a fourth dose at bedtime—consult your physician. If your daily schedule makes taking Nystatin four times a day difficult, increase the amount of the other three doses instead.

Children's doses are half that of the adult dose, or $\frac{1}{2}$ teaspoon three to four times a day. Older teenagers usually require adult dosages.

It is important to refrigerate Nystatin to preserve its potency. If you are going on a long trip, carry it in an ice chest or an insulated soft-side bag, available at sporting goods stores. Nystatin is stable enough to last through only a short trip without refrigeration, but do not leave the medication in a hot car. Carry a small amount with you and leave the remainder at home in the refrigerator.

The length of time you will have to take the oral Nystatin will depend on the severity of your case, and your faithfulness and response to treatment.

If there is a possibility that you have Candida in your sinus cavities, your physician may prescribe Nystatin nose drops. They are used as follows: first, place three drops of the solution into each nostril while holding your head back. Then swing your head forward rapidly and hold it down between your legs for two minutes to force the solution into your sinuses. Finally, sit up and let it trickle down your throat.

Nystatin nose drops are usually taken at least twice a day, and may increase your symptoms for several days due to yeast die-off in your nasal passages. Continue treatment; your symptoms will improve in a short time. Use Nystatin nose drops until you are certain that all of the yeast cells in your nasal passages are dead.

If you have yeast vaginitis, your physician may prescribe Nystatin for vaginal treatment along with other supplemental treatment. For yeast vaginitis, use one or more of the methods listed below.

- Mix one teaspoon Nystatin powder in three to five cc water. Draw the solution into a five-cc syringe (with needle removed) and insert carefully into the vagina. Squeeze the plunger gently to release the solution for retention at night.
- Pack a "00"-sized gelatin capsule with Nystatin powder. Prick both ends of the capsule with a needle and moisten the capsule with water. Insert vaginally (it is usually more convenient to do this procedure at night).
- Commercially prepared Nystatin suppositories are also available from some pharmacies, usually compounded in a cocoa butter base.
- Use Nystatin vaginal treatment every night for two weeks. If severe symptoms have subsided, you may alternate its use with Orithrush Douche or acidophilus suppositories.
- Use a Nystatin douche occasionally, as needed to control symptoms. Use one tablespoon Nystatin per pint of warm water for a slow douche, to provide longer contact with the mucous membranes.

Itching, burning, or excessive discharge may increase temporarily due to die-off, but these symptoms will subside. You may need to repeat this course of treatment several times over several months.

If you have large numbers of Candida organisms in your intestine, your physician may prescribe a Nystatin retention enema. Do not use this enema on yourself or your children unless it has been prescribed by a physician *familiar with your health status*.

1. First take a warm-water cleansing enema before using a Nystatin preparation.

2. Mix ¼ teaspoon sea salt and ¼ teaspoon Nystatin in one cup (eight ounces) of warm, "safe" water.

3. Making sure the mixture is at body temperature, put it into a rectal syringe or enema bag.

4. Lie on your back, insert the nozzle, and squeeze the entire contents into your rectum.

5. Remove the nozzle and roll onto your left side. Lie still for about five minutes to allow the solution to travel to the left side of your colon.

6. Roll over onto your back again (for five minutes), propping up your buttocks to allow the solution to travel up the left side of your colon.

7. Roll over onto your right side and lie still for five minutes to allow the solution to travel across your transverse colon.

8. Get up and walk around, which will allow the solution to travel down the right side of your colon.

9. Retain the solution as long as is comfortable before evacuating.

(Adapted from *The Yeast Syndrome*, by John Trowbridge, MD, and Morton Walker.)

Candida treatment takes perseverance and vigilance—many people require treatment for a year or more. If you stop treatment too soon, your symptoms will come back with increased severity, and your infection will be more difficult to eliminate. Repeatedly starting and stopping treatment for candidiasis also prolongs treatment.

Nizoral   Nizoral is the brand name for a synthetic, broad-spectrum antifungal agent known as ketoconazole. In some cases of deep-seated infection, Nizoral is more effective than Nystatin in eliminating Candida. It is also useful in killing strains of yeast that may be resistant to Nystatin, since Nizoral has a more systemic effect. Its action has been described, by Dr. John Trowbridge in *The Yeast Syndrome*, as "punching holes in the yeast cell wall and letting it slowly bleed to death."

Nystatin remains in the bowel, but Nizoral enters the tissues. Candida must be killed in both places, so both materials should be used simultaneously, if Nizoral is prescribed. Nizoral can cause some side-effects, but most patients tolerate it well. A liver screen blood test to check liver enzyme levels should be performed

before beginning treatment, and these levels must be checked monthly as long as Nizoral is taken.

The usual dosage of Nizoral is one 200-mg tablet daily for approximately six months. However, in some difficult cases, longer treatment and/or two tablets daily may be required. Nizoral should be taken on an empty stomach since it is absorbed better under acid conditions. To ensure adequate acid, take Nizoral with one to two grams of ascorbic acid (vitamin C). While you may experience die-off symptoms with Nizoral, they generally are less severe and of shorter duration than those caused by Nystatin. Also, some men experience lowered sex drive when they take Nizoral.

Nizoral is the most potent known inhibitor of the body's cytochrome P450 detoxification system. There is some speculation that some of the improvement seen in Candida-infected people taking the medication is due to temporary suppression of this important detoxification pathway. If the person is not detoxifying, fewer overt symptoms will be experienced while taking the medication. This also may explain why symptoms may return when the medication course ends. This premise, if true, may account for the rare cases in which liver function is affected while the drug is being used.

Diflucan   Diflucan is the newest available antifungal prescription drug. Its chemical name is fluconozole, and it has a systemic effect on the body similar to that of Nizoral. Early studies claim that its action is more rapid than that of Nystatin or Nizoral. Diflucan specifically inhibits fungal cytochrome P450, an enzyme essential to fungal cell survival.

Diflucan is taken in 50-mg, 100-mg, or 200-mg tablets once daily. Diflucan tablets contain a dye that some people cannot tolerate. Those who demonstrate sensitivity to other azole drugs, such as Terazole or Miconazole, should not use this drug.

OTHER CANDIDA TREATMENTS

Essential Fatty Acids As Candida colonies grow in the small intestine, they interfere with and obliterate the absorptive surface of the bowel. This interference particularly affects absorption of essential fatty acids. Essential fatty acids (EFAS) are special acids which, when combined with glycerine, make various types of fats. They are necessary for normal growth and skin quality. Because our bodies cannot synthesize EFAS, we must consume them in our diets.

Essential fatty acids aid in rebuilding the immune system. They also strengthen cell membranes to prevent the invasion of organisms into the cells. One of the EFAS, oleic acid, helps to prevent conversion of the Candida organism from its yeast form to its invasive, mycelial fungus form. Fish oils, flax oil, evening primrose oil, black currant oil, borage oil, and cold-pressed sunflower or safflower oils are the best sources of EFAS. These nutrients can be used on alternating days for individuals who are on rotation diets.

Mathake and Taheebo Tea (Pau D'Arco or La Pacho) These teas are made from the inner bark of two different species of tropical trees. These materials have been found in clinical studies to have natural antifungal properties. They are best used with other therapeutic agents. While these teas may induce die-off symptoms, they will pass in a few days. The teas can be steeped or ground and put into capsules; they can also be used as a soothing douche. If applied topically, they can deter the growth of athlete's foot and skin rashes. As with other anti-Candida preparations, some people may not be able to tolerate these teas.

Garlic Many people shy away from garlic because of its odor, but garlic has antifungal properties. There are some odorless products that still retain the antifungal ingredient, allicin. In addition to inhibiting Candida growth, garlic also inhibits the conversion of the yeast form to its mycelial form.

A food or chemically sensitive person should exercise care in selecting a garlic supplement, choosing only chemical- and yeast-free products. Garlic is more effective if taken on an empty stomach since it is enhanced by acid.

Germanium Germanium (GeOxy 132) is an organically bound trace mineral that stimulates energy production by providing extra oxygen molecules at the cell level. The immune system is composed of high energy tissue and requires extra oxygen and nutrients during inflammatory and infectious processes, and during periods of stress. Germanium also affects the immune system by stimulating gamma interferon, and macrophage and natural killer-cell functions. Germanium acts as a deterrent to the growth of yeast colonies by providing an oxygen-rich medium. Yeast cells thrive in anaerobic (oxygen-free) conditions.

Coenzyme Q10 Coenzyme Q10 is naturally produced in the body. When used as a supplement, this enzyme stimulates greater energy production in each cell and restores the integrity of all cell membranes, enhancing overall functioning of the immune system. This coenzyme also activates the body's macrophages (specialized killer white blood cells of the immune system).

Orithrush Orithrush (or other specially buffered forms of sorbic acid) is designed to inhibit the proliferation of *Candida albicans.* It can be used on several areas of the body. When diluted, Orithrush can be effective as a mouth-wash or vaginal douche; it can also be used full-strength on infected areas on toes, fingers, the external ear, and skin. When first using the liquid, treat only a small infected area in order to test for allergenicity.

Immunotherapy Testing and treatment with Candida and T.O.E. extracts relieves many of the hypersensitivity symptoms associated with Candida overgrowth. These extracts will also stimulate immune response. Clinical trials have shown that people respond better when treated with both of these antigens, rather than only one or the other.

Testing for T.O.E./Candida should be carried out after you have begun treatment with anti-fungal medications—your health must be stable enough so that testing will not cause an overload. An effective neutralizing dose can then be determined.

Fiber Increase natural fiber in your diet (raw vegetables, fruits and whole grains on a rotated basis). Apple pectin and psyllium seed are also good sources of fiber. When intestinal bacteria work on fiber, they release fatty acids that inhibit yeast growth. Fiber also decreases bowel transit time, decreases toxin absorption from the gut, and stimulates secretion of digestive enzymes.

Thyme Oil Thyme oil (available in health food or herbal shops) is naturally aromatic and has a natural antifungal action on the skin. Thyme oil is very concentrated and should be kept out of reach of children. Do not use it internally. For external use on Candida lesions on the scalp, skin, toes, and fingers, dilute it with oil (one part thyme to three to four parts oil). Thyme oil can be somewhat drying to the skin, so alternate it with Nystatin cream or other tolerated skin lubricants. A phenol-sensitive person may not tolerate thyme oil.

Goldenseal Douche For persistent vaginal itching, the following vaginal douche recipe may be soothing and helpful. Sensitive women should be certain that they can tolerate all of the ingredients.

Mix one cup Golden Seal tincture (available at herb shops) with one cup witchhazel. Use two tablespoons of the mixture in two cups of boiled water. Add ½ teaspoon salt, ½ teaspoon acidophilus, and one tablespoon yogurt. Let stand for 10 minutes. Use as a slow douche, keeping bag at hip level. Use daily for 10 consecutive days, and then only as needed or after intercourse.

Tea Tree Oil Available at health food or herbal shops, tea tree oil is an undiluted plant oil that has antifungal properties. Rub it into rashes on the skin, either diluted or full-strength. Do not use tea tree oil internally. Try it on one small rash area to see if it is tolerated and effective. Its odor is objectionable to some people.

CANDIDIASIS AND DIET

Diet is very important in candidiasis treatment—Nystatin, Caprystatin, Mycocidin, and acidophilus are not enough. You must eliminate or severely limit foods which promote Candida growth to reduce your Candida overgrowth. Everyone is unique, and your dietary requirements may differ in many ways from the requirements of others with candidiasis. Some people will experience symptoms unless they closely adhere to their diets, while others can "cheat" a little without severe symptoms returning. Keep in mind that the less you cheat, the faster you will get well!

An inadequate diet is a major factor in enabling candidiasis to flourish. Nourishment must rebuild your body, rather than encouraging Candida overgrowth. Your diet must restore cells and metabolic systems that are not functioning properly. You cannot eliminate Candida totally from the mouth, vagina, and intestines, but you must reduce it to a minimal level and rebalance the interaction between the yeast and your body.

Eating refined sugars weakens our immune system and promotes yeast growth. Honey (which sometimes contains yeast), molasses, maple syrup, date sugar, turbinado sugar, cane sugar, beet sugar, corn sugar, corn syrup, fructose (found in fruit), lactose (found in milk products), and other refined carbohydrates/sugars are known promoters of yeast growth. Reducing or eliminating these in your diet will help minimize yeast growth.

Some people report strong cravings for carbohydrates during early stages of candidiasis treatment. This "appetite" can be likened to the yeast organisms crying, "feed me, feed me"—but do not succumb to their insistent pressure. Your "sweet tooth" will lessen within a few weeks on your improved diet. A diet this restrictive will be very difficult for those who are accustomed to high-carbohydrate diets. Each day, work toward reducing refined carbohydrates and congratulate yourself as you accomplish more and more.

You may eat any of the complex carbohydrate foods, such as fresh vegetables, limited fruits, and whole grains. If your Candida problem is severe and long-standing you may have to limit even these good carbohydrates. Some people have to restrict their fresh fruit intake during the first few months of treatment. You will be able to tell by the way you feel whether you have consumed too many of these good carbohydrates; an increase in symptoms indicates too many sugars and refined carbohydrates.

Some people also have to restrict their intake of gluten-containing grains. Gluten is found in wheat, oats, rye, and barley, but not in corn, rice, and millet. Observe dietary restrictions if these grains cause proliferation of your Candida and worsen symptoms.

Foods that contain yeasts, molds, or fungi can also cause problems and should be restricted. The cell walls of Candida and baker's and brewer's yeast contain a common carbohydrate; because of this, our bodies cannot distinguish between these two different yeast species, and will produce the same reaction to both. When eaten in foods or even breathed in high concentrations, yeasts will trigger symptoms. (See "Yeast," p. 83, for additional sources of yeast.)

Molds build up on foods while drying, smoking, curing, and fermenting. Avoid pickled, smoked, or dried meats, fish, and poultry, such as bacon, sausage, ham, hot dogs, or luncheon meats. Avoid all cheeses, including Swiss, cottage, and cream cheese. Moldy cheeses such as Roquefort contain the largest amounts of mold. Buttermilk, sour cream, yogurt, and sour milk products can also contain molds. Dried and candied fruits are frequently made from fruit which has molded. Be sure that your condiments are fresh; dry spices, seasonings, and some teas, including herb teas, may mold during the drying process. In damp climates, spices and teas may mold as they sit in the cupboard.

You must avoid all fungi, including all types of mushrooms, morels, and truffles.

You will probably feel less deprived if you concentrate on foods you *can* eat rather than on the avoidance lists.

Allowed Foods   You may eat any meat as long as it is fresh, including fish, chicken, beef, pork, turkey, duck, seafood of all kinds, goat, venison, rabbit, frog legs, pheasant, quail, lamb, and veal.

You may eat vegetables of all kinds, except mushrooms. Eat fresh vegetables as much as possible. Canned, bottled, boxed, and other packaged foods usually contain refined sugar products. Frozen vegetables are sometimes processed with yeast. Mold grows on all vegetables; wash them well before cooking or eating them. Vegetables that grow beneath the soil, such as potatoes, carrots, beets, onions, turnips, and sweet potatoes, should be washed, peeled, and cooked. Do not eat them raw. A potato may be baked with the skin on, but do not eat the skin.

You may eat fresh fruits on a limited basis. However, some people cannot tolerate fruits or juices during the beginning months of their treatment. Even when you can eat them without provoking symptoms, do not overdo them. Bottled, canned, and frozen fruits or juices frequently contain yeast. Also, the fruit used to make juices is frequently moldy. Melons, particularly cantaloupe, often accumulate mold in the rinds as they grow. They can be eaten if they are washed thoroughly and then peeled carefully. Do not cut the fruit in sections while the rind is still intact because the cutting knife will draw mold from the rind across the flesh. Bananas, pears, and apples are fruits that can be reintroduced first because their sugar content is lower.

You may eat limited amounts of whole grains as long as doing so does not worsen your candidiasis symptoms. To avoid yeast, make breads with baking powder or baking soda. Waffles make a good substitute for bread. There are several types of yeast-free crackers, snacks, rice cakes, and oat cakes available at health food stores. These are good bread substitutes.

You may have eggs, milk, and water. (Milk is sometimes restricted during the first part of treatment since it contains lactose, which is a simple sugar.) Also, you may eat unprocessed nuts, seeds, and oils. All nuts and seeds should be roasted; bake at 325°F for 10 to 15 minutes until they are a golden color.

A good rule of thumb for remembering what you may eat is to think of the letters MEVY (meat, eggs, vegetables, and yogurt). Yogurt contains *Lactobacillus acidophilus,* which aids in recolonizing the gut. However, remember that yogurt is a milk product and still a source of lactose, and the acidophilus content is too low for treatment levels.

Begin eating MEVY, and then gradually add fruits in limited amounts. After your immune system has had time to repair—toward the end of your treatment—you may slowly reintroduce a few yeast-containing foods.

The less you eat of the avoidance foods, the faster you will get well. Dr. Trowbridge says, in *The Yeast Syndrome,* that "we provide a luxurious home for yeast colonies and provide 'yeast feasts' for their growth with our poor quality diets." Individual differences may allow some people to eat small to moderate amounts of these avoidance foods without experiencing symptoms. Each person will have to determine tolerance levels, first by total omission of a food from the diet, and later by readmission trials.

If you eat packaged foods of any kind, read the labels carefully. Remember that anything labelled "enriched" usually contains yeast. Manufacturers of such foods have removed nutrients during processing and have attempted to add them back. "Fortified" foods have substances added to make them "better," and may be made from yeast products. Fresh is really best; when reading labels you cannot always be sure of the contents in a product without checking with the food manufacturer.

Be sure to drink at least six to eight, eight-ounce glasses of water daily. This will help to flush out the accumulated toxins from die-off. Also, chew your food well; small, softened amounts of food can be more easily digested.

Your diet is something you control completely, so it is not necessary to feel victimized by Candida. Make your dietary changes gradually so it won't be such a shock, but you must change your dietary lifestyle to starve out the yeast. If you continue to eat simple carbohydrates while taking antifungal agents, you will be on a constant see-saw, feeding the yeast one minute and attempting to eradicate it the next. This action causes the yeast to be drawn more deeply into affected tissues, and it is then much more difficult to eliminate. Continuing sugar intake also makes your treatment more expensive as you will be buying medications to kill the yeast and then eating sugar to feed it.

You may design your own Candida diet, or, as indicated by your physician, you may follow a diet from one of the books listed in *Recommended Books,* p. 304. Of all therapies available to combat Candida, appropriate diet effectively rebalances your body and will lead you back to good health.

The Parasites We Host and Resulting Diseases

Parasitology is the science dealing with organisms that take up residence, either temporarily or permanently, on or within other living organisms for the purpose of obtaining food.

The term parasite applies to the weaker organism that obtains the food, shelter, and benefit from the association. The host is called the harboring organism.

Parasites are classified in several different ways:

- *Ectoparasite:* Lives outside the host on the skin or hair, causing infestation.
- *Endoparasite:* Lives within the body of the host, causing an infection.
- *Facultative:* Lives independently or as a parasite.
- *Obligate:* Is a permanent resident, totally dependent on the host.
- *Incidental:* Is an organism established in a host in which it does not ordinarily live.
- *Temporary:* Is a free-living organism that seeks a host intermittently to obtain nourishment.
- *Permanent:* Remains in or on the host from early life until maturity.
- *Pathogenic:* Causes injury to the host by mechanical, traumatic, or toxic activities.
- *Pseudoparasite:* Is an artifact mistaken for a parasite.
- *Coprozoic or spurious:* Is a foreign species passed through the alimentary tract without infecting the host.

The relationship between a parasite and a host may be symbiotic, a permanent association between two organisms that cannot exist independently. It may be one of mutualism, where both organisms benefit, or it may be commensal, where one partner benefits and the other is unaffected. The host may suffer functional or organic disorders when the parasite is pathogenic. Hosts are classified as:

- *Definitive host:* Harbors the adult or sexual stage of the parasite.
- *Intermediate host:* Harbors the larval or asexual stage and may be a primary or second-

ary intermediate host.

- **Paratenic host:** Harbors the parasite in an arrested stage. Develops in a subsequent suitable host.
- **Incidental host:** Is an infected host not necessary for parasite survival or development.
- **Reservoir host:** Is another animal harboring the same parasite. It ensures continuation of the parasite and is a source of human infection.

Knowing parasite life cycles is important; these cycles tell us how we become infected as well as help in identifying the stages in which preventive measures can be applied. Parasite life cycles can be simple or complex. A more complicated life cycle decreases the organism's chances of survival. Organisms with complex life cycles compensate with increased reproduction and multiplication.

Parasitic disease is believed to be a thing of the past in the more industrialized parts of the world, but this is untrue. Parasitic diseases are among the major causes of human misery and death in the world today. They represent enormous obstacles to the development of countries that are economically poor and that have inadequate sanitation.

Medical parasites include protozoa (one-celled animals); helminths (worms); and arthropods (insects—bugs, flies, ticks, mites, spiders, and scorpions). Parasitic diseases caused by these organisms have no geographical boundaries or class distinction. Parasites have been carried all over the world by travellers and immigrants. For example, hookworm and schistosomiasis were brought to this continent by the early slaves. The fish tapeworm was introduced to the United States by immigrants from the Baltic region. With today's extensive travel, parasites are regularly transported all over the world. Diagnosis is complicated be-

cause of the wide range of possibilities produced by travel.

Although parasites are distributed worldwide, they abound in the moisture and humidity of the tropics. Short summers in the temperate zones prevent the growth of species that require higher temperatures in their larval stage. Low temperatures arrest the development of larvae and eggs. Moisture is essential for parasites with free-living stages.

In some parts of the world, you cannot walk barefooted because of the risk of getting hookworms in your feet. Many insects, such as mosquitoes, black flies, and tsetse flies, carry developmental forms of parasites that are spread when these insects bite humans. Streams and rivers can be polluted with several types of parasites, and infection can result from any contact with the water, including drinking, wading, and bathing. In Africa, the rate of parasite transmission is so high that control measures seem to be ineffective.

Economic and social conditions affect the prevalence of parasites. Low standards of living, lack of information, and inadequate personal and community sanitation play a large role in the spread of parasites. The use of human feces in agriculture in some Third World countries constitutes a major factor in the spread of parasitic infections. This becomes a problem for us when we ingest produce imported from these countries.

The spread of parasites depends on the source of the infection, the mode of transmission, and the presence of a suitable host. Humans may be the only host, the principal host (together with animals), or an incidental host, with animals as the principal host. Transmission takes place through direct contact, indirect contact, contaminated food or water, soil, vertebrate and invertebrate vectors (a living carrier that transports the parasite to the host), and in rare cases, from mother to offspring.

Pathology due to parasites depends on the number of parasites, their tissue specificity, and their mechanisms of tissue damage. Damage to the host is caused by:

- Sheer numbers of the parasites as they multiply.
- Mechanical damage by obstructing vessels.
- Destruction of host cells by parasite invasion.
- Inflammatory reaction to the parasite or its metabolic products, causing symptoms affecting many systems of the body.
- Competition for nutrients, depleting the host body.

Several factors affect resistance to parasites. Some people have innate or natural resistance; genetic factors may give us resistance to parasitic infections. Remaining parasite-free as we age may represent either an acquired or a natural resistance. Being nutritionally deficient may increase the severity of a parasitic infection. On the other hand, good nutrition can decrease the severity of an infection.

SOURCES OF PARASITIC INFECTION

Sources of parasitic infection are many and varied. Contaminated water, food, dirt, and dust are primary sources of infection. Wild animals as well as household pets are infected with parasites, and can transmit these parasites to humans.

Observing the following guidelines can aid in preventing parasitic infections:

- Drink only safe water. If there is any doubt concerning the water, boil it for 20 minutes.
- Wash all fruits and vegetables. Use Clorox if tolerated. Clorox-sensitive people may substitute hydrogen peroxide, NeoLife Green, or soap and water. Rinse thoroughly in a fresh bath of plain water, then store or cook.

Whenever possible, peel fruits and vegetables.

- Rinse meat, fish, and poultry thoroughly in cold water before cooking. Be sure to cook well. Tapeworms and other parasites may be transmitted by improperly cooked or raw meat, fish, and poultry.
- Do not allow children to play in sand or dirt where cats and dogs relieve themselves.
- Change cat litter daily and keep your pets wormed.
- Keep your immune system strong, and your intestines healthy.
- Minimize your sugar intake; parasites thrive on high-sugar diets.
- Be aware of sexual risk factors: oral sex, rectal sex, and multiple sex partners.

SYMPTOMS OF PARASITIC INFECTION

In some people, infection is chronic with few or no symptoms. These people are carriers and represent the normal state of infection, in which there is an equilibrium between host and parasite, or infection without disease. In others, infection is acute.

Parasitic infections can cause:

- Diarrhea, colitis, dysentery.
- Tissue damage from parasitic invasion.
- Nonspecific gastrointestinal distress, such as bloating and gas.
- Alternating diarrhea and constipation.
- Nutrient malabsorption and metabolism disruption.
- Stimulation of the mixed-functions oxidase system cytochrome P450 (a complex system of enzymes that processes chemicals).
- Eosinophilia (an increase in specific white blood cells).
- Immune suppression.
- Increased food intolerance.
- Allergic responses.

- Rheumatologic symptoms (an immunologic response in the joints from intestinal parasites).
- Chronic fatigue.
- Night sweats.
- Fever.
- Asthma.
- Specific dysfunction of neuroendocrine function.

Even when infection has been long term, many of these effects are reversible with treatment. In sensitive people, there are three main areas in which symptoms manifest:

- Chronic gastrointestinal distress including irritable bowel, malabsorption, nonspecific symptoms, and severe food allergies.
- Fatigue resembling Epstein-Barr virus (EBV). Intestinal symptoms are not the major presenting symptoms.
- Allergy and inflammatory symptoms linked with chronic immune dysfunction. These include allergy symptoms that have nothing to do with the intestinal tract, such as aching joints and muscles and chronic asthma.

COMMON PARASITIC ORGANISMS

The most common parasitic infections causing symptoms are those caused by protozoa, or one-celled microscopic animals. Although most are free-living, some are parasitic. They have anaerobic metabolisms, allowing them to live without oxygen in the lumen (interior space) of the intestines. Their presence constitutes intestinal contamination and contributes to immune dysfunction.

These pathogenic protozoa secrete:

- Proteolytic enzymes that decompose protein.
- Hemolysins that rupture red blood cells.
- Cytolysins that destroy cell membranes.
- Toxic and antigenic substances.

Intestinal parasites obtain their nutrition through liquids absorbed from the intestine of the host. Some ingest solids, and many utilize both solids and liquids. Several species ingest red blood cells and bacteria.

All protozoa have a trophozoite form (which is the vegetative form) and a cyst form (which is the inactive state). The cysts are able to resist more environmental insults and are the infective stage. Methods of locomotion and reproduction divide protozoa into four major classes:

- *Rhizopods* (amebas).
- *Flagellates.*
- *Ciliates.*
- *Sporozoa.*

Rhizopods   Amebas are *Rhizopods*, the most primitive protozoa. They move by forcing liquid endoplasm into projections called pseudopodia (false feet). These move the organism forward and engulf food sources in its path. Amebas multiply by simple binary fission (dividing in half).

Amebas are a common human parasite, and the following species have been established as parasites in humans. All of these live in the intestine, except *Entamoeba gingivalis*, found in the mouth.

- *Entamoeba histolytia.*
- *Entamoeba coli.*
- *Entamoeba gingivalis.*
- *Entamoeba hartmanii.*
- *Dientamoeba fragilis.*
- *Endolimax nana.*
- *Iodamoeba butschlii.*

ENTAMOEBA HISTOLYTICA   A tissue-invading ameba, and the second most common protozoan infection in North America, *Entamoeba histolytica* is the cause of amebiasis, amebic dysentery, and amebic hepatitis. The wall and the lumen of the colon is the area of the body inhabited by *Entamoeba histolytica*. The organism is 10 to 60 microns in size and has remarkable locomotion that enables it to crawl up the sides of culture tubes. It is considered an anaerobe, but it can consume oxygen. Its distribution is world wide, but *Entamoeba histolytica* infections are prevalent in the tropics.

Entamoeba histolytica's mature cysts contain four nuclei, which are very hardy and are resistant to the acid of the stomach. The cysts disintegrate in the alkaline medium of the small intestine. Infected people shed large numbers of infective cysts every seven days.

Cysts enter our bodies through:

- Wells, springs, and other water supplies contaminated by feces.
- Vegetables and fruits contaminated with feces.
- Food contaminated by houseflies.
- Food contaminated by infected food handlers.
- Direct transmission by cyst carriers.
- Carelessness in personal hygiene in asylums, hospitals, children's homes, and prisons.

At particular risk are travellers, college students, homosexuals, prisoners, and patients in mental institutions and long-term medical facilities.

Entamoeba histolytica uses its cell-destroying enzymes to leach nourishment from host tissues. After tissue invasion, this ameba no longer depends on the bowel nutrients, ingesting red blood cells, tissue fragments, bacteria, and intestinal contents.

In the large intestine, *Entamoeba histolytica* causes lesions that become ulcerous, forming nodules of inflamed tissue. Damage done depends on the resistance of the host, the virulence of the ameba, and the conditions in the intestinal tract. There are some nonvirulent strains that can cause diarrhea in those with impaired immune function. They may also cause ulcerative colitis or irritable bowel syndrome.

If the *Entamoeba histolytica* organisms leave the intestine, every organ can be affected. Some people develop systemic amebiasis, or amebic infection. The liver can then be invaded and diagnosis becomes difficult. Lung amebiasis accompanied by fever and chills may develop; brain abscess, although rare, can also occur. Infected people can have ulcerative vaginitis, cervicitis, and lesions on the penis. Secondary bacterial infections frequently follow the amebic invasion.

Entamoeba histolytica infections can be impossible to distinguish from ulcerative colitis. Appropriate tests for amebiasis should be performed on all persons with ulcerative colitis because steroids, a common treatment for ulcerative colitis, can cause death if the patient has amebiasis.

Prevention includes:

- Maintaining sanitary conditions both in the home and the community.
- Using filtered and treated water.
- Controlling insects, particularly houseflies.
- Maintaining adequate personal hygiene.

ENTAMOEBA COLI   This ameba has a life cycle similar to that of *Entamoeba histolytica,* and is often mistaken for it. While *Entamoeba coli* is not considered a pathogen, it can cause a difficulties to those with immune system problems. It occurs with a 10 to 30 percent frequency in America; it is even more prevalent in Europe.

The ripe cyst of *Entamoeba coli* contains eight nuclei, which are an identifying feature, enabling differentiation from *Entamoeba histolytica.* This ameba is transmitted by ingesting the cysts in food, in drink, on the fingers, and on other objects.

When *Entamoeba coli* is found in the stools, this indicates ingestion of fecal contaminants.

It lives in the intestine in the same area as does *Entamoeba histolytica*, and feeds on enteric bacteria and possibly red blood cells.

ENTAMOEBA GINGIVALIS   An inhabitant of the mouth, this ameba is found in the tartar and gingival pockets. While *Entamoeba gingivalis* is considered a nonpathogen, it is found in 10 percent of people with healthy mouths and in 95 percent of those with diseased teeth and gums. The presence of this ameba suggests the need for better oral hygiene. *Entamoeba gingivalis* transmission takes place through droplet spray from the mouth and through contaminated drinking glasses or dishes.

ENTAMOEBA HARTMANII   Transmitted by ingesting contaminated food or water, this ameba can cause diarrhea in otherwise healthy people.

DIENTAMOEBA FRAGILIS   A small amoeboflagellate, *Dientamoeba fragilis* is 5 to 12 microns in size. It has been identified worldwide and has a 4 percent incidence of infection. *Dientamoeba fragilis* lives in the human intestine, causing moderate, persistent diarrhea, gastrointestinal symptoms, some low-grade fever and vomiting.

ENDOLIMAX NANA   Formerly classified as a commensal organism, this ameba is now believed to be the fifth most common pathogen, living in the lumen of the intestine. Six to 15 microns in size, *Endolimax nana* is identified by its small size, sluggish movements, and four-nuclei cyst. It feeds on bacteria and has a 10 to 20 percent prevalence rate. Methods of infection include ingesting viable cysts in polluted water, contaminated food, contaminated objects, or poor personal hygiene.

IODAMOEBA BUTSCHLII   Another ameba that was formerly believed to be only commensal, *Iodamoeba butschlii* has a prevalence rate of 8 percent. It is distributed worldwide, with a higher incidence in tropical regions. Its charac-

teristic nucleus and the large glycogen body of its single-nucleus cyst are identifying properties. *Iodamoeba butschlii* lives in the lumen of the large intestine and feeds on enteric bacteria. It is transmitted by contaminated food, drink, and soiled objects.

BLASTOCYSTIS HOMINIS   There has been much controversy over the classification of *Blastocystis hominis*, and at one time it was thought to be a fungus. Now classified as a protozoan, and by most authorities as an ameba, it is 10 to 15 microns in size. *Blastocystis hominis* is frequently mistaken for the cyst form of other protozoa because of its spherical central mass, thick outer protoplasm, and thin cell membrane. It is now recognized as a pathogen that causes diarrhea in humans, and has been reported in epidemics of gastrointestinal disease in subtropical areas. It is frequently found in the bowel with *Candida albicans*. Symptoms accompanying infection by this ameba include diarrhea, pain, cramps, nausea, fever, vomiting, headaches, gas, chills, and malaise.

Flagellates   A second class of protozoa, *Flagellates* are one-celled animals that have developed special organs to enable them to withstand the peristaltic (contraction) action of the intestine. *Flagellates* have both a trophozoite and cyst form, but unlike the ameba, the trophozoite is also infective in some species. *Flagellates* infect both humans and lower animals; however, it is difficult to determine whether the species are the same in animals and humans.

GIARDIA LAMBLIA   The most widespread protozoan intestinal parasite in North America is the *flagellate, Giardia lamblia*. It lives in the duodenum and jejunum (parts of the small intestine), and possibly in the bile ducts and gallbladder. This parasite causes increased permeability of the gut and allows larger food particles to pass through the gastrointestinal mucosa into circulating blood. The immune system does not recognize these particles as food, and so allergic responses develop. These allergies resist treatment until the Giardia infection is treated. Giardiasis is a problem in 30 to 40 percent of allergy patients.

Giardia has both trophozoite and cyst forms. The trophozoite form has four pairs of flagella (whiplike structures that aid in propulsion) and a concave sucking disk that attaches to the intestine. By attaching itself to the intestine, Giardia is able to maintain its position in spite of the peristaltic action. It obtains food from the intestinal contents and from the intestinal wall through the sucking disk.

Giardia proliferates in an alkaline environment. Hypochlorhydria and achlorhydria (low or no acid in the stomach) and a carbohydrate-rich diet enhance multiplication. Multiplication occurs by mitotic (complex) division during the cyst stage. The cysts, which make up the infective stage, are very resistant and may remain viable for months outside the host.

Giardia is transmitted by food and water contaminated by sewage, food handlers, flies, and from hand to mouth in cases of poor hygiene. It is prevalent in the mountains, and persons can become infected from swimming in contaminated water. Infection is more common in children than adults; outbreaks are frequently reported in day care centers and nurseries. Giardia incidence is highest in areas with poor sanitation and among populations unable to maintain adequate hygiene.

Wild animals are thought to be capable of infecting humans and to be one of the causes of water contamination in the wild. Beavers are natural reservoirs and leading contributors to contamination. Household pets can also be reservoirs for the parasite. Campers should be particularly careful, since even chlorine treatment does not always kill Giardia. There have been reported cases of Giardia in campers who obtained their water from ice runoff.

Some authorities believe over half of our water supply is contaminated by *Giardia lamblia*. Travellers should also be careful—for example since 1970, 23 percent of all tourists to the USSR have acquired giardiasis there.

Some people may become infected without having symptoms. Others may suffer diarrhea, total malabsorption, steatorrhea (excess stool fat), or irritable bowel syndrome. Chronic infection with *Giardia lamblia* resembles an Epstein-Barr virus infection because of the persistent, chronic fatigue. Anyone suffering from fatigue should be checked for Giardia. A Giardia infection also promotes small intestine bacterial overgrowth. While bowel symptoms are common in giardiasis, it is possible to have a serious Giardia infection and experience no intestinal symptoms at all.

The following factors increase the risk of giardiasis:

- Hypochlorhydria or achlorhydria.
- IgA deficiency.
- Candidiasis.
- Homosexuality.
- Type A blood.

Ciliates These *protozoa* are distinguished by threadlike cilia that cover their bodies and are appendages of locomotion. *Ciliates* reproduce by binary fission (dividing in half).

BALANTIDIUM COLI The only pathogenic parasite of the *Ciliate* class, *Balantidium coli* is the largest of the intestinal protozoa. Its trophozoite ranges in size from 30 by 25 microns up to 150 by 120 microns. The cysts average 52 to 55 microns.

Balantidium coli trophozoites live in the lumen, mucosa, and submucosa of the upper region of the large intestine, and in the terminal portion of the small intestine. Its thread-like cilia allow rapid propulsion. This parasite also has a boring action, allowing it to invade the mucosa and submucosa of the intestine with the aid of a cell-destroying enzyme. There it divides rapidly and forms "nests" containing many organisms.

There is a high incidence of *Balantidium coli* in hogs, which, together with their contaminated feces, are an important source of human infection. Infection causes liquid stools containing blood and pus, sometimes alternating with constipation. Although a *Balantidium coli* infection can be present without symptoms, in someone who is debilitated it can be fatal. Sanitary control is probably the best means of prevention.

Sporozoa   The species of this fourth class of *Protozoa* have no method of locomotion, and have both sexual and asexual reproduction.

CRYPTOSPORIDEA   The third most common protozoan intestinal pathogen, *Cryptosporidea* parasites infect the stomach and small bowel, causing enterocolitis (intestinal inflammation) and diarrhea in humans. *Cryptosporidea* have been documented as causing disease in male homosexuals, and have also been found in preschoolers attending daycare. A fecal-oral method of transmission is suspected, and there is no known treatment.

DIAGNOSIS OF PARASITES

Recent improvements in diagnostic techniques have shown that gastrointestinal and systemic parasites are more significant in immune system suppression than previously recognized. In the past, parasites were diagnosed after demonstration of ova and parasites in a stool specimen. This method, however, posed many problems. Stool examination, even with purged specimens, is frequently negative even when a person has an active parasitic infection. Parasites typically grow in the intestinal mucosa. Unless the parasite breaks off from the mucosa into the stool on the day the specimen is obtained, it will not be visible on examination. Sometimes the specimen is too old when it reaches the laboratory, and there is excess material to deal with, calling for complicated concentration techniques.

New diagnostic techniques involve examining smears taken from the rectal mucosa. This specimen is then stained with immunofluorescent stains for examination with specialized microscopy. It is a highly sensitive and specific test.

Those with the following symptoms should be tested for parasites:
- Unexplained fatigue.
- Chronic bowel symptoms (diarrhea, alternating diarrhea and constipation, excessive gas, abnormal stool formation and appearance—frothy, floating, blood-tinged, mucus-laden, crumbling).
- Malabsorption.
- Immune suppression.
- Food intolerances.
- Soft tissue rheumatoid-like pain.
- Night sweats.
- Chronic asthma.
- Disorders of the endocrine or nervous system.

You do not have to be experiencing bowel symptoms for a parasite infection to be a problem. Anyone who has camped extensively or who has travelled outside of North America should be tested for parasites. University or preschool students should be tested if they suddenly develop any of the above symptoms, since they are often in contact with many people from other areas of the world.

TREATMENT OF PARASITES

There have been significant advances in parasitic infection treatment. Powerful drugs are not necessary except in extremely resistant cases. Previously used drugs, such as Flagyl, Atabrin, arsenic, and Furoxone, are toxic to the liver and can be used only for a short time.

Present treatment is twofold, involving the use of ParaMicrocidin and Par-Qing, distributed by Allergy Research Group and available at health stores. ParaMicrocidin is an antimicrobial agent extracted from tropical plants or citrus seeds. It comes in two forms—Paracan Liquid 144 and ParaMicrocidin, the capsule form. Both contain an identical material that is effective against intestinal parasites and that has significant antifungal activity. ParaMicrocidin comes in 75- and 125-mg capsules.

Paracan Liquid 144 is a strong-tasting liquid reminiscent of grapefruit rind. It is not absorbed through the intestinal wall, and studies show it has a very low toxicity. The usual dosage is two drops (25 mg/drop) two times per day. It must be diluted in four to eight ounces of liquid since it is irritating to the mucosa at full strength. It tastes better in orange or grapefruit juice. Paracan is also available in topical and spray preparations.

Par-Qing is a non-toxic, non-carcinogenic, generally well-tolerated herbal product. Its major ingredient is *Artemesia annua,* which is presently being studied as an anti-malarial agent. This form of *Artemesia* has become available only recently in North America; other species of *Artemesia* are not effective. Par-Qing contains 50 percent *Artemesia annua* and 50 percent cinnamon-anise, *Yerba buena,* *Valeriance officinalis,* and *Mejorana.* No alcohol should be consumed during treatment with this herbal product.

You may experience some die-off symptoms (Herxheimer reaction) when you begin treatment as the body reabsorbs protein from the dead parasitic cells. These proteins are toxic to the body, and will cause die-off symptoms such as fever, chills, sweating, diarrhea or constipation, headaches, irritation, muscle aches, memory loss, poor concentration, hormonal imbalances, or depression. Die-off may also include a worsening of symptoms already present; these symptoms will subside as treatment progresses.

Begin all treatment gradually—increase the dosage slowly and in increments. Never begin any medication program at full strength. This helps minimize die-off and lessens the shock to the body, since our bodies respond poorly to sudden or large changes. If a particular dosage causes die-off symptoms, remain at that level of treatment until you can take the medication without experiencing symptoms, and then increase your dosage. Hypersensitive people should be checked for material compatibility before starting the use of either ParaMicrocidin or Par-Qing because they are derived from plant material.

Begin your treatment as follows:

ParaMicrocidin

1. Begin with one capsule per day, taken with meals.

2. When you can tolerate this dosage with no symptoms, add the second capsule at another meal.

3. Gradually increase the dosage to two capsules three times daily (as die-off permits). Resistant cases may require a larger dosage.

When you are able to take two capsules of ParaMicrocidin three times daily, and when you have had no die-off symptoms for two weeks, add the Par-Qing. The treatment is cumulative—you must continue to take the ParaMicrocidin.

Par-Qing

1. Start with one capsule per day, taken with meals.

2. When you can take one capsule per day with no symptoms, add the second capsule at another meal.

3. Gradually increase the dosage to three capsules three times daily (as directed and as die-off permits).

4. The minimum length of treatment will be a full dosage of Par-Qing for 20 days.

Because there is a very high relapse rate in parasitic infections, treatment must be continued long enough to ensure that the infection is gone. Repeat mucosal smears must be used to confirm this.

- The first repeat test should be performed if symptoms have disappeared after a full dosage of Par-Qing has been taken for 20 days. Continue to take Par-Qing and ParaMicrocidin until negative parasite test results are received.

- If symptoms are still present, continue treatment and delay the repeat test until they are gone.

- If the repeat test is negative, continue treatment for three more weeks.

- Then suspend treatment for one month. After that time, have a third repeat parasite test.

- If any of the repeat tests are positive, treatment will be continued or changed as determined by your physician.

Children's doses are dependent upon body weight; your physician will determine the dose for each child. For everyone, however, treatment will vary depending on the following factors:

- Progress of the individual.
- Severity of the infection.
- Duration of the infection.
- Organism(s) causing the infection.

Multiple organism infections and infections by more virulent organisms are more difficult to treat. Treatment requires consistency, and stringent personal hygiene is essential in order to prevent reinfection.

It is also important to take an acidophilus supplement both during and after treatment. This encourages "good" bacteria growth on the intestinal mucosa to prevent reinfection of fungi or parasites. Consuming fluids and exercising are also important during treatment, to flush out toxins. Vitamin C can relieve symptoms caused by toxins released during die-off. Coenzyme Q10 (30 mg) and organic Germanium (GeOxy 132) aid in restoring immune function.

A treatment regimen combining ParaMicrocidin and Par-Qing has a failure rate of less than 10 percent. Drugs should be considered only for the few who do not respond to this treatment. One effective medication that is much less toxic than previously available drugs is Yodoxin, available only by prescription. Because some parasitic infections can be transmitted throughout a family, all family members must be treated. Even symptom-free members should be treated to prevent reinfections, since person-to-person contact is the most important factor in the spread of parasites.

PARASITES AND ALLERGIES

As is the case with viral and bacterial infections, our body responds with allergic reactions to parasitic infections. This response is twofold: reaction to the parasite itself and reaction to the parasite's metabolic products. Parasites stimulate the production of antibodies (IgE, IgG, and IgM) by the B-cells. High levels of parasite-specific antibodies are useful in diagnosis for some cases. The histamine and other mediators released when these antibodies attach to basophils or tissue mast cells contribute to the pathogenicity of the parasites.

Treating parasites may temporarily worsen die-off symptoms. As the parasites die, the host is exposed to greater levels of parasitic antigens, which exacerbate symptoms. Exposure to parasitic antigens also increases when egg deposition begins in egg-producing parasites. Severe systemic symptoms may result.

Antigenic responses to parasites may continue long after the parasitic infection has subsided, because of remaining cellular debris. Allergy extracts for the specific organism will help relieve these symptoms and reduce the total immune system load of the infected person.

Viruses

For those with immune system problems, a viral infection can tip the scale toward extreme hypersensitivity, chronic fatigue syndrome, or an autoimmune disease spiral.

This tiny, opportunistic invader has ravaged humans, plants, and animals for centuries. Viruses were unknown by sight prior to the invention of the electron microscope in 1931. However, victims of viruses were well aware of the effects of disease they caused, even though the viruses could not be seen. The face of Ramses V provided evidence that he had succumbed to the smallpox virus 3,000 years ago. Spanish conquistadors provided contaminated blankets to the South American Aztecs and Incas. The blankets had been taken from homes in Europe whose inhabitants had died from smallpox, and

the unsuspecting natives died by the thousands. The first antiviral treatment was given in 1798 in England, when Edward Jenner inoculated a patient with cowpox exudate in an attempt to prevent the dreaded smallpox. Jenner took this drastic measure after observing that farmhands who contracted the milder cowpox did not contract smallpox.

Scientists in the late 19th century were able to observe bacteria under their microscopes, but there were other infectious organisms that they could not see. Viruses were small enough to pass through porcelain filters that would trap the smallest known bacteria. They can be as small as 16/1000 the size of a pin head, yet their potential for devastation cannot be correlated with their miniscule size. Any living cell is susceptible to a viral invasion. Viruses are not complete cells, but rather consist of double-layered shells of protein, lipids, and carbohydrates surrounding strands of either DNA or RNA. They do not need nor can they metabolize nutrients; they do not grow, nor can they replicate without host cells. They are the true essence of a parasite.

Viruses can remain in a limbo state between living and inanimate for long periods of time. They mutate into many shapes that are both species and type specific. A particular virus can attach itself to only one type of cell—either bacterium, plant, animal, or human. It must attach to a specific receptor site on a specific cell. The hepatitis virus finds its way to the liver; the AIDS virus meshes with a T-cell; the polio virus seeks out an exact subset of nerve cells in the spinal column; and the rabies virus makes its way to particular cells in the brain. Clever mutations have allowed viruses to adapt to pre-existing receptor sites for hormones and other substances vital to the cell's function.

Some viruses look like soccer balls with triangular facets while others resemble space vehicles, with angular appendages. The influenza virus, for example, looks like a Roman mace, complete with spikes extending in all directions; the AIDS virus is spherical.

Our body is a tremendous repository for both bacterial and viral organisms, but only about four percent of these organisms cause illness. They enter through every portal in our body (nose, mouth, sexual organs, eyes), they live in our blood and nerves, and they invade every organ. We transmit them on our fingers and with our breath and saliva. They can be carried by insects and in animal saliva.

When the specific shape of the virus meshes with its counterpart on a cell, like a lock and key mechanism, the cell welcomes the virus as if it is a well-known friend, unaware it is welcoming its own death. The cell membrane envelops the virus, which proceeds to exploit and alter the cellular machinery to its own advantage in order to replicate.

Some viruses gain access to the cell by synthesizing an enzyme that dissolves a portion of the cell membrane. After entry, the viral shells or coats are dissolved, leaving the viral RNA or DNA free to suppress the RNA or DNA of the host cell. The virus then proceeds to control the cell function with its own nucleic acid pattern. It reprograms the cell to use its own raw materials and machinery to make new virus particles. Some viruses can assemble these parts like a jigsaw puzzle, while others produce enzymes to aid in the assembly into virons. There are thousands of virons manufactured in each single cell of the host.

These replicated viruses are then shed from the host cell in two ways—one is a "budding" mechanism through the cell membrane, while the other causes the death of the cell by rupturing its membrane and leaking the virons and cell contents. A clever virus is one that uses its host in a long-term symbiotic or cooperative relationship. If the virus is poorly adapted to its host and destroys it, it also destroys itself and all of its clones.

EFFECTS OF VIRAL INFECTION

Some viruses can live in cells over a long period of time without replicating, and do not produce classic viral syndromes. Research done by Michael Oldstone and his colleagues at Scripps Clinic and Research Foundation in La Jolla, California, has demonstrated that these insidious viruses alter a specialized cell function, such as production or secretion of a hormone. The affected cell is not in danger of rupture or death, but the overall function and health of the host organism is greatly affected. The invaded cells do not show any abnormality or inflammation when seen under a microscope. This mode of viral activity is suspected to be a factor in such diseases as neuropsychiatric disorders, diabetes, growth retardation, hypothyroidism, and some autoimmune diseases.

The many and varied symptoms accompanying a viral infection are caused by cell alteration and the resulting effects of the overstimulated or underfunctioning immune system. Many viruses increase cytokines from the immune cascade, causing unpleasant symptoms associated with viral infections. (Cytokines are chemicals produced by the T-cells during an infection as our immune system's second line of defense.) Interleukin-2 levels (one of the cytokines) have been shown to be 40 times greater in people with chronic fatigue syndrome than in healthy people. Another series of studies have identified lower levels of gamma interferon (another cytokine) in affected persons.

Research is being conducted worldwide to show that many forms of cancer are linked to a variety of viruses. Viruses have been tied to liver cancer, Burkitt's lymphoma, leukemia, and cervical cancer. It is believed that viruses further damage the DNA of some cells that are already stressed, and weaken a host immunity that is already compromised.

Oldstone and his colleagues found in recent research that only a small number of viruses are needed to cripple immune function to a state of immune suppression. The research also demonstrated that incomplete viruses may also be effective in suppressing lymphocyte (disease-fighting) function. Researchers believe it is possible that this form of immune suppression may be present in cytomegalovirus, hepatitis B, and HIV, since these diseases all include the infected lymphocyte phenomenon.

Latent viruses may be reactivated when the balance between host and virus is upset. Some factors in upsetting this balance are prolonged stress; hormonal or immunological shifts; sudden temperature changes (either extreme cold or the sun's ultraviolet rays); overgrowth of other pathogens; nutritional deficiency; age; drug, alcohol, or tobacco over-use; deterioration of the environment; lack of rest; genetic and hereditary factors; changes in diet; and excesses of anything, even exercise.

TYPES OF VIRUSES

The diversity of viruses is evident in acute diseases such as the common cold or poliomyelitis, where there is rapid cell death. Another form is the latent virus, which can lie undetected and dormant for long periods between flare-ups. Each successive viral burst weakens the host's immune defenses. Yet another type of virus causes a slow viral infection, which builds up over a long period of time and causes a form of progressive dementia. Some viruses mutate rapidly by changing their surface antigens. By the time the immune system produces an antibody to one form, the virus has already changed the antigen beyond recognition.

Some viruses lie dormant in nerve centers or ganglia, where no drug or antibody can reach them. This occurs with such viruses as *Herpes simplex*, which causes genital or mouth sores; and *Herpes zoster*, which causes chicken pox, and which may surface from nerve cells later in life to cause shingles. Epstein-Barr virus hides in B-cells, the very cells that make antibodies to viruses. The virus associated with AIDS (HIV) makes its home in T-cells and the DNA of other cells to await a lowering of the host's immunity before replicating and eventually causing cell death. The Hepatitis B virus continues to multiply slowly in the liver and surfaces 20 to 30 years later to cause extensive liver damage. A less lethal virus, the papilloma virus, causes warts on the skin. Recently, however, this virus has been linked to some forms of cervical cancer. Still another strain known as a retrovirus (such as HIV) can produce an enzyme that converts the cell's RNA to DNA. It then lies dormant, hidden away from the functions of the immune system to wait for an opportune time to resurface and cause disease.

Some of the more well-adapted forms of viruses were probably classed as "flu" in past decades. With today's sophisticated diagnostic methods, the viruses now take on specific personalities that can be recognized.

Cytomegalo virus (CMV) has been implicated in learning disabilities. Like its close cousin EBV, it can amplify an already existing problem and cause a variety of neurological symptoms. Specific antibody titers indicate the presence of cytomegalo virus. It is a member of the Herpes family, characterized by a double strand of DNA. When the host's immune system overcomes the virus, the immunity prevents further outbreaks. However, excessive antibodies or viral debris can remain, causing a chronic stimulation of the immune system.

Herpes zoster (Varicella) is the culprit that causes chicken pox. After the initial infection, the virus can lie dormant in nerve cells. If the host is overly stressed for any reason, the virus can re-emerge in the form of painful "shingles." During early days of exploration sailors carried this rather mild infection to people of the New World. Since they had never encountered the disease and had no immunity, the natives experienced severe symptoms and died within days.

Another virus in the Herpes family is *Herpes simplex I*; this organism causes the familiar cold sores that plague many people. It, too, will become dormant and hide in facial nerves, only to reappear when the host becomes stressed. It has been implicated in ulcerations of the corneas, damage to nerves in the eyes, and swelling of the brain (encephalitis).

In the initial stages of another Herpes virus, EBV (Epstein-Barr virus), antibodies are almost undetectable. As the immune system recovers from the early invasion, the antibodies can be detected. Debilitating fatigue; sore throat; headaches; muscle and joint pains; swollen lymph tissue, spleen, and liver; and elevated liver enzyme levels are but a few of the possible symptoms of this chronic, cyclic infection.

Herpes simplex II is a new type of sexually transmitted disease. It is highly resistant and contagious and also tends to recur at times of high stress. Infants can be infected as they pass through the birth canal.

The Coxsackie virus strains belong to the family of enteroviruses (intestinal). Most cases of this virus occur in Europe and England. With global travel, however, the incidence of this virus is rapidly spreading. The symptoms are similar to EBV and appear to affect muscle function. When first identified, Coxsackie virus strains were thought to be polio.

Influenza viruses hardly need description, since most of us have experienced them. Symptoms can range from minor two- to three-day upper respiratory problems to a severe, fatal syndrome. Influenza virus mutates rapidly, creating new strains each year to which we must adapt. Epidemics of virulent new strains also appear from time to time, causing worldwide fatalities.

Lymphotrophic viruses, HTLV-1 (human T lymphotrophic virus), attach themselves to T-cells and central nervous system cells. Some studies suggest that it may play a role in multiple sclerosis.

The most dreaded of this class of viruses is HIV (human immunodeficiency virus). Concentrated research efforts are being made to learn more about this virus. As its name suggests, it creates a rapidly mutating form that debilitates the immune system and often leads to death. HIV mutates by changing the structure of its surface protein markers (antigen). It attaches itself to the T-cells of the immune system and changes the host RNA to DNA (the master molecule of life). More than 20,000 North Americans have succumbed to this tiny invader, and it occurs throughout the world. HIV is contagious only through intimate contact or by exposure to contaminated body fluids. At this time, prevention is the best weapon against HIV.

TREATMENT OF VIRAL INFECTIONS

In treating viral infections, the goal is to stop viral replication as quickly as possible in order to prevent the spread of infection to other host cells. Many viral diseases result from a series of growth cycles. Unfortunately, symptoms do not occur until after a number of viruses have entered host cells and altered cell function and machinery enough to start rapid replication.

Treatment with drugs is extremely difficult, considering the evasion tactics the viruses employ. It is virtually impossible to kill a virus hidden in lymphocytes or nerve cells without also destroying the host cells.

Inoculations for some viruses are very effective. Most of us, at one time in our lives, have had vaccination for measles, rubella, mumps, and polio. Because of vaccines, smallpox and yellow fever are almost eradicated. When people are at high risk, hepatitis B or influenza vaccines are administered. However, some physicians fear that the viral antigens and debris from vaccines may adversely affect the immune systems of hypersensitive people.

Donor immunoglobulin is used to prevent extreme symptoms in some infections. Human serum containing specific antibodies is the preferred source of this artificially acquired immunity; however, this method provides only temporary protection.

Cytoimmunotherapy, with injections of virus-specific T-cells into infected mice, has been tried recently by Oldstone and his associates. Killer T-cells were taken from the spleens of healthy mice that had been immunized against a specific virus. The results were very encouraging—the infected mice became free of infection.

Two years ago, Doctors Hafler and Weiner from Brigham and Women's Hospital in Boston, Massachusetts, did a small clinical study with four multiple sclerosis patients. A similar study is now being done on rheumatoid arthritis patients by Rene de Vries of the University Hospital in Leiden, The Netherlands. In this expensive study, clones of T-cells taken from the inflamed joints of patients are being used for injections.

While drug therapy is limited in treating viral infections, a drug named Acyclovir (Zovirax) is being used to control some forms of the Herpes virus with effective results. Amantadine, a synthetic drug, has been used as a preventative agent in Influenza A; a small therapeutic effect was noted in early trials. However, it is a very selective drug, which appears to interfere with the viral nucleic acid injection of the host cell.

Doctors Cathcart and Pauling have used large dosages of vitamin C to control a number of viruses. Vitamin C is known to have active antiviral properties as well as being an important nutrient for immune system repair. Dr. Cathcart uses up to 150,000 mg each 24 hours over a period of time to effect a remission in severe viral infections. During infection, our body uses up to four times more than normal amounts of vitamin C. The indicator introduced by Dr. Cathcart for optimal intake is known as the bowel tolerance level, the point just short of the amount that produces a liquid type of stool. (See "Vitamin C: A Key Nutrient," p. 242.)

A nontoxic material, Monolaurin, has also been found to be effective against a number of viruses. Its action is two-fold; it disintegrates the virus envelope or shell, and it also stimulates the host immune response by augmenting the effect of lymphokines (molecules of the immune system that send messages between immune system cells) and mitogens (molecules that induce cell division). Monolaurin is most effective if started early in a viral infection, before viral injection of host cells.

Another effective nontoxic viral treatment is lysine (an amino acid). It, too, should be started as early as possible when a viral infection begins. Viruses change the host cell's metabolism to demand more arginine (also an amino acid) in order to replicate within the cell. Arginine is found in nuts, beans, and chocolate; it is wise to reduce or even eliminate these foods during a viral infection. Lysine is effective because it has a similar chemical structure and is taken into an infected cell in place of arginine. The virus uses lysine for food but cannot use it for replication.

There are several homeopathic remedies that also aid in relief of symptoms from viral infections. Glycyron is available in intravenous or oral preparations. This material detoxifies the host from the harmful effects of the virus. Engystol, another homeopathic preparation, is taken by injection. This material stimulates immune system function and detoxification pathways. It has no direct effect on the virus.

Viruses and Allergies

Because many viral infection symptoms are caused by allergic responses to viral antigens or debris, viral extracts can be helpful to relieve symptoms. Several types of extracts are available and neutralizing dosages can be determined by provocative neutralization testing (see p. 70). Some extracts are made from influenza vaccine material, which controls fever blisters from *Herpes simplex* types I and II, as well as symptoms of infectious mononucleosis and *Herpes zoster*. Some people use the extract only when experiencing acute symptoms, while others with chronic symptoms use it daily.

The best treatment for any disease process—especially a chronic viral disease state—considers the whole person, including mental, emotional, and spiritual aspects as well as physical. Holistic medicine pays attention to improving immune function; achieving healthy diet and nutrient supplementation; making changes in lifestyle, environment, and occupation as needed; getting adequate exercise; and investigating past and present emotional or spiritual issues followed by appropriate therapy. (See *The Emotional and Psychological Impact of Environmental Illness*, p. 282.)

An excellent reference for additional effective programs for recovery from chronic viral illness is *Chronic Fatigue Syndrome*, by Jesse A. Stoff, MD, and Charles Pellegrino, PhD.

PART 4

NUTRITION AND ALLERGIES

WHY NUTRITIONAL SUPPLEMENTATION IS CRUCIAL

As an active participant in your own health care, it is important to understand the relationship between nutrition and good health. Our body contains trillions of cells, each with its own biochemical function. Numerous enzymes within each cell control its chemical processes, and each enzyme has specific nutrient requirements.

Vitamins, minerals, amino acids, and fatty acids are the "building blocks" used by all cells and body functions to affect growth, repair damaged tissues, and keep our bodies in a healthy state. When the "right molecules" are in short supply, or are in greater demand, we need to provide additional nutrients through supplementation. This is known as nutritional biochemistry or orthomolecular medicine.

Consider the constant readjustment taking place within each cell for it to maintain adequate numbers of "building blocks." To keep this internal environment functioning properly, correct replacements for damaged or missing parts must be provided. We do not substitute parts from a waffle iron or toaster when a washing machine is broken.

At one time it was thought that a balanced diet provided all the nutritional factors our body required; only the elderly and infants who did not eat a balanced diet needed nutritional supplementation. Whether this was ever true is debatable and certainly is not true today.

Unless we grow it ourselves or obtain it from special sources, our food is of inferior quality for the following reasons:

- The soil in which it is grown is depleted because of poor agricultural practices.
- High-nitrogen fertilizers are used rather than organic replacement fertilizers that contain essential minerals.
- Some hybrid seeds produce inferior plants with high productivity, but with low nutrient levels.
- Fruits and vegetables are harvested before they are ripe, and may then be ripened artificially.
- Many foods are not fresh, due to long periods of storage and transport.
- Some foods are stored improperly, often with inadequate refrigeration.
- Produce is contaminated by herbicides, insecticides, and fungicides.

When the food reaches us, its quality is further degraded:

- Foods are overprocessed (heat and chemicals used in processing destroy nutrients).
- Improper cooking methods, reheating, or

keeping food warm rob it of nutrients.
- Vitamins and minerals are lost when food is soaked.
- Preservatives, colorings, and flavor enhancers are added to foods.
- Fast food and refined foods have lost most of their nutrients during processing.
- Some produce is coated with paraffin (which has a petrochemical base) to slow deterioration.

Besides poor food quality, other factors also affect our nutritional status, such as:
- Dietary restrictions.
- Environmental pollution.
- Stress.
- Economic status.
- Personal food preference.
- Ethnic influences.
- Chronic infections.

It is clear that a variety of factors affect the balance and quality of our nutrition. Nearly everyone needs some supplementation, and those with special health problems or allergies may need extensive supplementation.

Diet is the most important factor in our nutritional status. Once we have a nutrient deficiency, the highest quality diet is not sufficient to meet our increased needs. However, poor eating habits cannot be corrected even by the finest vitamin and mineral supplements.

Nutritional Deficiency Symptoms

You may have a nutritional deficiency if you are:
- Constantly aware of your body.
- Excessively worried.
- Unhappy without cause.
- Unable to cope with stress.
- Depressed.
- Sensitive to foods, inhalants, and chemicals.

You may have a nutritional deficiency if you have:
- A poor work output.
- Aches and pains.
- No tolerance for noise, flashing lights, or variations in temperature or altitude.
- Headaches, gastric distress, muscle soreness, joint pains.
- Problem skin.
- Dental caries.
- Poor eyesight.
- No reserve energy.
- A poor self-image.
- Metabolic insufficiency.
- Frequent infections.
- Lowered mental acuity and memory.
- Varying stages of digestive problems.
- Lowered sexual interest and performance.

Your Own Nutritional Needs

Dr. Roger Williams writes that there are five levels of nutrition: starvation, poor diet, fair diet, good diet, and super nutrition. Super nutrition is the level we should all strive for. It consists of diet and nutritional supplementation for optimum health and performance.

You should determine your nutritional needs with the help of your physician or a nutritional counselor. Because of biochemical individuality, your needs will not be the same as those of your spouse, siblings, children, friends, or other environmentally ill persons. Each of us has specific requirements or deficiencies that must be addressed.

Factors Affecting Nutritional Requirements for Allergic People

Stress Demand for all nutrients is greater during times of stress caused by allergic reactions;

infections; physiological, psychological, emotional, and environmental problems; or disease states.

Incomplete Digestion   Many of us who are sensitive to chemicals, foods, or inhalants have low levels of hydrochloric acid in our stomachs or low levels of digestive enzymes in our gastrointestinal tracts. This causes incomplete digestion of food, resulting in poor absorption and assimilation of nutrients. A vicious cycle is created because there are then too few nutrients available to manufacture adequate amounts of hydrochloric acid, regulating hormones, digestive enzymes, and immune factors.

As offending foods pass through our intestinal tract, they inflame and irritate the intestinal lining. Histamine and serotonin are released in the gastrointestinal tract during an allergic episode, further irritating the mucosal lining. This causes the microvilli to swell and flatten. The villi (microscopic hair-like fingers that line the small intestine) are responsible for enzyme function to help break down food particles, and for nutrient absorption. Loss of this two-fold function contributes to vitamin, mineral, essential fatty acid, and amino acid deficiencies.

Allergic Reactions   When food is not digested properly, larger molecules of food material are absorbed into the bloodstream and become allergens. Systemic inflammatory responses will result, and a greater demand for additional nutrients is created to repair the resultant tissue damage.

Lack of nutrients also heightens sensitivity reactions. Magnesium deficiency increases the histamine release during an allergic reaction. Calcium helps to neutralize the effect of histamine, but if body calcium is deficient, the ex-cess histamine will circulate in body fluids, creating greater damage from the immune cascade. While our bodies are in the reactive state, they may become overly acidic, which affects the balance of nutrients. Specific nutrients are necessary to correct this problem.

Restricted Diets   Nutrients may be low and unbalanced as a result of restricted diets for some food-sensitive people, or as a result of personal choices. A rotation diet offers a great variety of untried, balanced food choices.

Lowered Endocrine Function   Many allergic or sensitive people have impaired endocrine system functioning (pituitary, thyroid, adrenal glands, thymus, pancreas, pineal gland, and gonads). The adrenal and thyroid glands are always the first parts of the endocrine system to suffer; as they underfunction, our body requires more nutrients. Specific nutrient supplements will help the endocrine system regain much of its normal function.

Overworked Immune Function   Our body's defense system, the immune system, is overworked in those with allergies or sensitivities. Continued overstimulation leads to an eventual dysregulation of the immune system. This causes a special demand for additional, specific nutrients to protect against frequent infections and to rebuild defenses against other foreign invaders (allergens, antibodies, debris from inactivated organisms, toxins).

Nervous system support   The nervous system is under assault in a hypersensitive person as it regulates all body functions involved in a reactive state. Many inflammatory responses affect neurotransmitter functions in the brain. Neural tissue needs amino acids, minerals (calcium, phosphorus, magnesium, potassium), and B vitamins, while neurotransmitter production requires all nutrients.

Environmental Pollutant Exposures Each of us is continually exposed to environmental pollutants. If cell membranes are not protected against these pollutants, tissue damage will occur. Specific nutrients known as antioxidants, and free radical scavengers, are essential to protect the cells, tissues, and organs against chemical pollutants. These nutrients are also needed to help the body detoxify after either acute or prolonged exposure to chemicals, pesticides, fungicides, and industrial pollutants.

How to Assess Your Nutritional Deficiencies

Begin with a detailed history, including genetic and hereditary information, your dietary habits and major food intake, chemical or inhalant exposures, trauma, present symptoms or diseases, and your current nutrient supplement intake. Carefully observe physical signs that indicate nutritional deficiencies. A few examples are diminished eyesight; ringing in the ears; dry scaly skin and scalp; poor connective tissue quality; misshapen nails; spots on nails; inadequate musculature; acne; grooved, scalloped, and reddened tongue; edema; and swollen, tender joints. (For additional symptoms, see "Nutritional Deficiency Symptoms, above.)

Levels of many nutrients, however, cannot be determined without laboratory evaluation.

- Blood or urine analysis of amino acid levels determines possible deficiencies of vitamins and minerals required for proper amino acid metabolism.
- Blood evaluation of enzymes required for detoxification, and urine evaluation of liver enzyme function, may indicate a need for increased antioxidant/detoxification nutrients.
- Hair, serum, and blood analyses for mineral levels are useful. Hair analysis can also indicate high levels of toxic, heavy metals, requiring specific nutrients to reduce them.
- Tests should be done for specific diseases that increase the demand for specific nutrients.
- Testing with nitrazine paper will determine alkalinity or acidity of saliva and urine, indicating a need for specific nutrients.
- C-stixs indicate spilled vitamin C in the urine. If none is spilled, it may indicate the need for vitamin C supplementation.

All test results should be evaluated along with your history and symptoms. In our body's effort to maintain a homeostatic state (a stable balance), nutrients are moved from one type of tissue to another as needed. Examining only one type of tissue will not give a true picture of our body's state or needs. Hair samples show levels of stored nutrients, blood and serum samples show circulating nutrients, and urine and fecal samples show levels of excreted nutrients.

Guidelines for Nutrient Supplementation

For allergic or hypersensitive people, the entire cell metabolism needs to be supplemented with nutrients. Supplements are an important part of a recovery program that also includes diet changes, moderate exercise, environmental clean-up, immunotherapy, and elimination of infection.

Take nutritional supplements, vitamins, minerals, and amino acids throughout the day for best utilization. Choose brands that are free of all common allergens, and pay attention to the form in which they are supplied:

- *Powders* are rapidly absorbed and contain no fillers or binders. They can provide a higher potency, and are cheaper than tablets. However, their taste and texture bother some people. They are an excellent form for those who have difficulty swallowing tablets or capsules.
- *Liquids* are also useful for people who have difficulty swallowing pills and for children. They are rapidly absorbed, but may contain sugars, additives, and colorings.
- *Chewables* are suitable for children, but be aware of sugar, additive, and coloring contents.
- *Time-release tablets* contain a water-soluble vitamin released over a period of time. Allergic people frequently lack adequate stomach acid to dissolve the tablet coatings to release the vitamin.
- *Tablets* have a longer shelf-life. Sensitive people should be cautious of the binders and fillers used in tablets. Tablets are not absorbed as rapidly as powders, liquids, or capsules.
- *Capsules* are easier to swallow. They generally contain fewer binders and fillers than tablets, but are not absorbed as rapidly as liquids or powders. While most capsules are made from pork or beef gelatin, vegetable-based capsules have recently become available at health food stores.

Each brand of nutritional supplement varies in bio-availability (absorptive properties) depending on its fillers, coatings, or binders. The quality of the nutrient itself depends on the source material from which it is extracted, the ratio of ingredients, and the chelating materials (substances which aid in absorption).

While you should choose hypoallergenic brands of vitamins and minerals as much as possible, there is no such thing as a completely hypoallergenic material for everyone. If possible, have supplements tested to see which you tolerate before you begin using them.

It is best to start your nutritional supplementation program gradually. When the body is stressed, it is unable to readily adjust to sudden changes. Introduce one new supplement every two days, unless otherwise instructed. If you experience any adverse symptoms, it will be easier to trace the cause if you start each supplement separately. Most symptoms last only a short time. Drinking more fluids and taking a brisk walk will reduce symptoms quickly. If problems do arise, contact your nutritional counsellor or physician so minor adjustments can be made to your program.

Do not become discouraged and discard the whole program if you have problems with one nutrient. Other brands are available that may be more compatible with your metabolism. Take most of your supplements with a meal unless otherwise instructed, since supplements taken on an empty stomach sometimes cause slight nausea or other abdominal discomfort. These nutrients are very concentrated, and mixing with food dilutes their potency. Some people also experience a temporary increase in gas and bloating when a different nutritional program is introduced. This usually subsides in several weeks—however, if it persists, inform your nutritional counsellor or physician.

Think of supplements as concentrated food, not as medicine. Just as food is more readily absorbed when eaten in small, more frequent amounts, so are your nutritional supplements. Divide supplements into smaller doses taken throughout the day. This will ensure adequate absorption and will not overload your digestive system. Since these materials are food substances, they will be slower acting, and visible results will not appear in a short time. Nutritional therapy should be given a fair trial of consistent use for at least six months. Use beyond that period will bring continued improvement.

ADVANTAGES OF NUTRITIONAL SUPPLEMENTATION

- Nutrients are not taken singly, as are drugs. There are over 40 vitamins and minerals that work together as a team, needed every day in balanced amounts. One nutrient cannot effect a change unless all of the other nutrients are present either in food, reserves, or supplements.
- Vitamins act slowly; drugs act rapidly.
- Vitamins are food; drugs are chemicals.
- Vitamins have a wide action; drugs are narrow in their effects.
- Side-effects from vitamins are low, minor, and usually reversible; side-effects from drugs are more serious. Symptoms will disappear within one to two days after stopping a vitamin supplement.

TREATING ALLERGIES
WITH NUTRIENT SUPPLEMENTS

The following discussion of nutrients applies specifically to the effects and treatment of allergy and environmental illness. Each of the nutrients listed has many additional functions in our body.

Remember that each nutrient functions not as a single unit, but only in the presence of all other nutrients. Our body requires all of these nutrients, operating by multiple interaction. In *The Advancement of Nutrition*, Dr. Roger Williams states:

> If the available amount of any essential nutrient is inadequate, the body as a whole may be afflicted with generalized cytopathy, a condition in which every cell in the body is deficient and the whole body may be said to suffer from "cell sickness."

Vitamins

VITAMIN A

- Drops sharply in serum level tests of chronically stressed people. If adequate supplements are not taken, the body tries to maintain homeostasis by taking vitamin A from mucous membranes, increasing vulnerability to infection and allergies.
- Used in mucous cell membranes, which are the first sites of penetration by antigens, viruses, bacteria, fungi, and chemicals.
- Essential to suppressor cell, B-cell, T-cell, and killer lymphocyte activity.
- Enhances our body's immunological response to both DNA and RNA viruses.
- Is needed by the liver to anabolize (build) protein, and stabilizes protein in epithelial structures (skin, mucous membrane).
- Acts as an essential co-factor in the metabolism of essential fatty acids.
- Protects the lipid portion of cell membranes from oxidation. Damage to the cell membrane can also harm receptor sites for hormones and neurotransmitters.

BETA-CAROTENE

- Converts to vitamin A, but is not readily converted by diabetics and hypothyroid persons.
- Acts as an excellent antioxidant, especially for free radicals (a highly reactive form of oxygen).
- Prevents damage to cellular components, especially DNA, and cell membranes.

VITAMIN B₁ (THIAMINE)

- Maintains normal carbohydrate metabolism.

- Acts as a co-factor in many enzyme functions in the nervous system. In deficiency states, nerve cells become swollen, impairing transmission of messages from one nerve cell to another.
- Stimulates immune function.
- Works with other antioxidants, vitamin C, and cysteine to combat the effects of acetaldehyde and free radicals.
- Is needed to prevent shrinkage of the thymus and lowered antibody response.
- Is essential to hydrochloric acid production in the stomach.
- Improves muscle tone in the gastrointestinal tract.
- Helps the body absorb and utilize magnesium.

Vitamin B₂ (Riboflavin)

- With a group of enzymes, helps to break down proteins, carbohydrates, and some fats.
- Utilizes oxygen to liberate energy within the cell. Vitamin B_2 is known as an electron transfer vitamin.
- Needed for protein synthesis.
- Is used by the adrenal glands in cortisol production.
- Transports hydrogen ions by enzyme action.
- Is involved with vitamin A in synthesizing muco-proteins.

Vitamin B₃ (Niacin/Niacinamide)

- Operates in coenzyme forms to carry hydrogen ions in all cells. Vitamin B_3 also acts as a coenzyme in the energy cycle of the cell.
- Helps to control blood lipid levels.
- Is essential to all enzyme functions in the nervous system.
- Increases flow to blood capillaries in epithelial tissue. This function is helpful if niacin is used during detoxification baths or dry saunas.

- Helps in glucose metabolism to stabilize blood glucose levels.
- Is needed for histamine production. However, large dosages are helpful in controlling histamine release during an allergic reaction.
- Deficiency can cause irritation of the entire gastrointestinal tract.

Vitamin B₅ (Pantothenic Acid)

- Is necessary for antibody production.
- Helps in synthesis of anti-inflammatory substances (cortisol) produced by the adrenal glands.
- Aids in synthesis of cholesterol and fatty acids.
- Stimulates movement of the gastrointestinal tract.
- Helps in production of hydrochloric acid in the stomach.
- Is essential for adrenal support and prevention of adrenal exhaustion during any type of stress.
- Is helpful in large doses in reducing allergic reactions (has an antihistamine effect).
- Has antioxidant properties.
- Is needed for conversion of choline to acetylcholine (an important neurotransmitter).
- Is a precursor for synthesis of coenzyme A (an enzyme needed for various cellular functions).

Vitamin B₆ (Pyridoxine)

- Is essential for proper metabolism and utilization of protein.
- Aids in transportation of amino acids across cell membranes.
- Is necessary for proper nervous system function.
- Facilitates magnesium and B_{12} absorption.
- Regulates sodium and potassium balance

(useful in some types of edema).

- Helps with production of protein-based antibodies.
- Facilitates glycogen conversion in the liver.
- Is essential to DNA and RNA synthesis.
- Helps with degradation of estrogen to estriol in the liver.
- Is needed in synthesis of hydrochloric acid.
- Heightens T- and B-cell function.
- Increases thymic hormone production. Deficiencies cause immune tissue to shrink, diminishing activity of the thymus and spleen.

Vitamin B_{12} (Cobalamin)

- Helps in formation of DNA and RNA in cells.
- Is essential for maintenance of myelin sheath (lipid covering on nerve fibers).
- Is deficient in some vegetarian diets and in people with digestive problems. Hydrochloric acid, pepsin, and the intrinsic factor (a substance produced by normal gastrointestinal mucosa) are all required for its extraction from food.
- Is necessary for B-cell maturation.
- Helps in histamine production in persons with gluten allergies. Used in conjunction with folic acid.
- Is most effective when given as an injection.
- Is used as an injection with success in some cases of fatigue and unresponsive asthma.

Vitamin B_{15} (Dimethylglycine or DMG)

- Acts as an antioxidant.
- Lessens lactic acid accumulation in muscles.
- Increases tissue oxygenation.
- Stimulates glucose oxidation, which increases energy and prevents rapid fatigue.
- Increases antibody production to provide anti-allergenic properties.

Other B Vitamins

Biotin

- Assists in synthesis of essential fatty acids.
- Improves colonization of intestinal flora.

Choline

- Helps in transportation and utilization of fats and cholesterol.
- Aids elimination of toxins from the liver.
- Is essential to the integrity of the myelin sheath structure covering nerve fibers.
- Helps in thyroid hormone production.
- Assists the function of vitamin E.
- Is a component of the neurotransmitter acetylcholine chloride.

Folic Acid

- Works in conjunction with vitamin B_{12}.
- Is essential for red blood cell formation.
- Stimulates hydrochloric acid production in the stomach.
- Is required for DNA and RNA formation in the cells.
- Is produced in the large intestine if adequate bacterial flora is present. The major food source of folic acid is green leafy vegetables.
- Is required in larger quantities during periods of stress or disease.
- Is absorbed at a diminished rate with aging.
- Is essential to the metabolism of tyrosine, a precursor for the neurotransmitters dopamine, epinephrine, and norepinephrine.
- Raises blood histamine levels.

Inositol

- Stimulates the musculature of the intestinal tract.
- Aids brain cell function.
- Helps to induce sleep.

VITAMIN D

- Acts on intestinal mucosa to synthesize enzymes needed to transport calcium and phosphorus into the blood.
- Is necessary for deposition of calcium and phosphorus into bones and teeth.
- Helps the thyroid gland to produce the hormone thyroxin.
- Helps to maintain a healthy nervous system.

VITAMIN E

- Prevents oxidation of ingested fats, of lipids in the cell membranes and other cell structures, of the vitamins A and K, and of fat-soluble hormones by joining with the lipid molecule.
- Acts as a scavenger by joining with harmful oil-based chemicals, ozone, and nitrous oxide.
- Is found in large amounts in the brain, pituitary gland, and adrenal glands.
- Activates the immune system. Its function is enhanced with the addition of selenium.
- Affects prostaglandin (chemical messenger) functions.

ESSENTIAL FATTY ACIDS (VITAMIN F)

- Is essential for oxygen transport to cells.
- Aids absorption of fat-soluble vitamins, lipids, and minerals.
- Is an essential part of the lipid layers in cell membranes and other structures.
- Stimulates conversion of carotene to vitamin A.
- Is essential to the formation of enzymes, steroid hormones, and lipoproteins.
- Aids in prostaglandin synthesis. Prostaglandins regulate immunity, cell recognition, and inflammation.
- Helps to slow down peristalsis of the intestinal tract, thereby relieving some cases of diarrhea.
- Suppresses the formation of leukotrienes, which are 1,000 times more inflammatory than histamine.
- Modulates pain, water retention, and mucus secretion in inflamed tissues.

Minerals

CALCIUM

- Is essential for the proper function of magnesium and phosphorus.
- Acts as a catalyst for some enzyme synthesis.
- Acts, together with magnesium, as a natural tranquilizer.
- Aids in displacement of lead in tissues.
- Helps maintain a proper acid/alkaline (pH) balance in tissues.
- Regulates movement of nutrients and waste products in and out of cell membranes in its exchange with magnesium, sodium, and potassium.
- Absorbs excess stomach acid.
- Reduces histamine production.
- Discourages cell uptake of toxic metals such as lead, cadmium, and mercury.
- Is prevented by high sugar intake from being reabsorbed (together with magnesium) in the kidneys.
- Is essential to neuromotor impulses.
- May contribute to migraines if not metabolized properly.
- See "Non-Dairy Sources of Calcium and Magnesium," p. 94.

CHROMIUM

- Stimulates enzymes involved in metabolizing glucose, thereby stabilizing blood sugar levels at either end of the spectrum (both hypoglycemia and hyperglycemia).

- Is essential to the synthesis of fatty acids, cholesterol, and high-density lipoproteins (HDL).
- Aids metabolism and transport of amino acids.
- Is removed from foods in processing.
- Is required in larger quantities if diet is high in sugar and refined foods.
- Moderates effectiveness of insulin.

COBALT

- Activates a number of enzymes.
- Is needed for proper utilization of vitamin E.
- Works in concert with copper.
- Aids in mucous membrane repair.
- Is a mineral component of vitamin B_{12}.

COPPER

- Activates synthesis of a number of enzymes.
- Is essential to synthesis of thyroid-stimulating hormone (TSH) produced by the pituitary gland.
- Is essential to the metabolism and utilization of some amino acids.
- Is a component of superoxide dismutase (SOD), which protects against free radical damage to the mitochondria (energy-producing portion of the cell).
- Aids enzymes needed for neurotransmitter production in the tyrosine-to-dopamine pathway.
- Is essential to vitamin C utilization in collagen tissue formation.
- Is required for the formation of phospholipids in cell membranes.
- Is required by the liver to degrade estrogen.
- Aids regulation of essential fatty acid metabolism.
- Is required for the movement of calcium from the blood into bone tissue.

- Is crucial to the formation of helper T-cells.

GERMANIUM

- Increases serum levels of gamma interferon, which increases killer cells, T-suppressor cells, and macrophages.
- Acts as a free radical scavenger.
- Aids in heavy metal detoxification.
- Has oxygen-enrichment properties.
- Raises levels of glutathione (a peptide that activates some enzymes).

IODINE

- Is essential, along with the amino acid tyrosine, for the formation of thyroxin (a thyroid hormone).
- Keeps mucous lining of the body healthy.
- Affects tone of smooth muscle, including intestinal tract and lungs.
- Facilitates passage of nutrients into the cell mitochondria (energy producer).
- Helps to thin mucous membrane secretions.

IRON

- Binds quickly to protein molecules during an infection in order to prevent bacteria from using it for their growth metabolism.
- Energizes T-cells and macrophages when they are needed for inflammatory processes.
- Is a constituent of chemicals produced by T-cells to destroy organisms.
- Is required for the production of hemoglobin, which carries oxygen in the blood.

MAGNESIUM

- Aids in the production of antibodies.
- Affects permeability of cell membranes to allow for transport of nutrients.
- Is essential to protein metabolism and to the energy cycle of the cell.
- Is an essential component in over 300 enzy-

matic reactions.
- Maintains the electrical potential of cells.
- Is essential for the proper function of calcium by activating the release of parathyroid hormone.
- Has a calming effect on the nervous system.
- Regulates the body's acid/alkaline (pH) balance. Buffers the acidic stage of an allergic reaction along with calcium and potassium.
- Is required in converting glycogen (sugar stored in liver and muscles) to glucose (body fuel).
- Helps the body metabolize essential fatty acids into prostaglandins, which regulate many body functions.
- Deficiency causes mast cells to increase histamine secretion.
- Is usually used in a ratio of two parts calcium to one part magnesium. In immuno-compromised or hypersensitive people, this ratio often must be 1:1 or greater in order to alleviate symptoms.
- Is required for many detoxification pathways.

MANGANESE

- Is essential in synthesis of glutathione, a peptide used in the body's detoxification functions.
- Is needed for synthesis of three neurotransmitters (glutamine, gamma-aminobutyric acid, and acetylcholine).
- Aids production of superoxide dismutase.
- Works in balance with molybdenum.
- Acts as a catalyst for synthesis of fatty acids and cholesterol.
- Aids enzymes used in digestion and absorption of proteins, fats, and carbohydrates.
- Is essential for synthesis of insulin needed for glucose utilization.
- Is essential for some hormone production.

MOLYBDENUM

- Enhances the use of sulfur amino acids by the body. Sulfur is critical to immune system function, to antioxidant activity, and to detoxification pathways.
- Is a component of enzymes that regulate hormone and neurotransmitter functions.
- Is a component of enzymes that detoxify sulfites and aldehydes.
- Is essential for cell utilization of vitamin C.

PHOSPHORUS

- Works in multiple interactions with calcium.
- Is an important component of phospholipids in cell membranes and the brain.
- Is essential to many chemical reactions in the body.
- Leads to calcium loss if consumed in excess.

POTASSIUM

- Acts with sodium, calcium, and magnesium on cell membrane permeability to allow transport of nutrients and waste products in and out of the cells.
- Aids many enzyme functions.
- Supports the adrenal glands.
- Is required for synthesis of structural protein within the cells.
- Helps ensure function of smooth involuntary muscles (heart, lung, intestinal tract). Relieves arrhythmia and intestinal and uterine cramping.
- Is necessary for neuromuscular interaction.

SELENIUM

- Acts as an antioxidant, protecting cell membranes.
- Aids synthesis of glutathione peroxidase for detoxification pathways in the cells.
- Enhances the function of vitamin C.

- Is essential for protein synthesis and antibody formation.
- Stimulates immune functions.
- Increases B-cell antibody response.
- Neutralizes the effects of cadmium (a heavy metal).
- Is essential to the production of coenzyme Q10.
- Dosage must not exceed 500 micrograms (mcg) daily.

Sodium

- Is essential for cell permeability to provide for nutrient and waste exchange across cell membranes.
- Affects nerve cell excitation.
- Keeps other minerals in a soluble state.
- Aids in hydrochloric acid production.
- Is necessary, along with potassium, for muscle contraction.
- Is excreted at a greater rate if taken in excess. Excessive consumption also increases potassium excretion, which can lead to adrenal exhaustion.

Zinc

- Is essential to protein synthesis.
- Is essential to RNA and DNA production
- Is an essential ingredient in 90 metalloenzymes.
- Keeps mucous membranes intact and aids in their healing.
- Is needed for alkaline phosphotase, the enzyme in white blood cells that destroys bacteria.
- Is needed for alcohol dehydrogenase, the enzyme that detoxifies aldehydes.
- Is necessary for neurotransmitter synthesis.
- Is necessary for insulin storage.
- Is essential for white cell differentiation.
- Maintains the balance between fighter and suppressor cells and increases the number of T-cells.
- Is depleted during chronic infections and inflammatory diseases.

Other Nutrients

Coenzyme Q_{10}

- Is an enzyme normally manufactured in each cell of the body.
- Enhances phagocytosis (foreign matter destruction) by the lymphocytes.
- Induces energy in the immune cells, increasing immunocompetence.
- Reverses cell immunosuppression.
- Acts as an antioxidant to protect cell membranes.

Quercitin C (a Bioflavonoid)

- Has a strong affinity for mast cells and basophils. It stabilizes their cell membranes, thus preventing them from spilling histamine.
- Inhibits two enzymes that regulate release of leukotrienes, which are implicated in asthmatic-type reactions.
- Reduces spontaneous bruising, along with vitamin C.

Amino Acids

The base components of protein are amino acids, sometimes called building blocks. While the importance of these materials in animal studies has been understood for about 50 years, the application of this knowledge to human health has only recently been explored. Amino acids interact with all of the other groups of nutrients: minerals, trace elements, fats, vitamins, and carbohydrates. Amino acids are involved in most body functions:

- Building, repairing, and maintaining all cells.
- Degrading and excreting damaged protein material.
- Aiding all chemical reactions within the cell.
- Producing hormones, enzymes, and antibodies.
- Joining with vitamins and minerals to carry these cofactors to the cells.
- Detoxifying cells and protecting them from foreign invaders.

All 22 of the amino acids are essential for proper body function, and there must be a balance between them. Taking single amino acid supplements is sometimes desirable in order to correct imbalances or to satisfy a temporary demand.

Individual amino acids are being used in clinical practice to correct some genetic problems, to repair damaged health, to support metabolism in chronic illness, and to promote optimum health. Individual assessments must be made to consider the symptoms, diagnosis, diet, genetic factors, nutritional imbalances, and relationships between various amino acids and specific body functions. Diagnostic tests can determine amino acid levels in the urine or blood to aid you, together with your physician or health practitioner, in planning therapy.

Only those amino acids that pertain to treating environmental illness and allergy will be discussed here; and all of these have many functions other than the ones listed.

ARGININE

- Initiates release of growth hormone, an immune system stimulant.
- Stimulates white blood cell production in the thymus gland.
- Aids detoxification of ammonia in the liver.

ASPARTIC ACID

- Helps to detoxify ammonia that results from improperly degraded, damaged, or unwanted protein in the body. The brain is especially sensitive to ammonia.

CYSTEINE

- Is a sulfur-based amino acid needed for detoxification in the cell.
- Is a necessary component of the peptide glutathione, a reducing agent that protects the body against oxidizing chemicals. Glutathione contains the amino acids glutamic acid and glycine.
- Detoxifies aldehydes produced by consumption of alcohol or foreign chemicals, or produced by the Candida organism.
- Is a component of mercapturic acid, a detoxification end product.

GLUTAMIC ACID

- Lessens the seesaw effect of fluctuations in insulin production in hypoglycemia or diabetes.
- Helps reduce mental symptoms resulting from some types of allergic reactions.

GLUTAMINE

- Changes into glutamic acid by combining with ammonia, thus reducing excess amounts of ammonia, which accumulate in those people who cannot convert ammonia into urea for excretion.

GLYCINE

- Helps to reduce excess secretion of hydrochloric acid in the stomach.
- Is an important component of the antioxidant glutathione.

HISTIDINE

- Is a precursor to histamine.
- Reduces excess stomach acid secretion.
- Binds with excess copper when copper levels become toxic.

LYSINE

- Acts as a deterrent to viral replication while the immune system mounts its defense; must be initiated quickly in the course of infection.
- Is essential to carbohydrate metabolism.
- Is required in increased amounts during stress.

METHIONINE

- Offers up a methyl group that combines with free radicals to deactivate them.
- Lowers histamine levels if used together with calcium. Detoxifies histamine.
- Is essential to collagen formation.
- Stimulates bile production.
- Is necessary for production of heparin, which can modulate allergic reactions.
- Is used to make choline, a precursor to the neurotransmitter acetylcholine.
- All other sulfur-containing amino acids used in detoxification pathways can be synthesized from methionine.
- Protects cell membranes against lipid peroxidation.

ORNITHINE

- Stimulates growth hormone production in the pituitary gland, thereby stimulating the immune system.
- Helpful for people with insomnia.

PHENYLALANINE

- Affects the tyrosine-dopamine-norepineph-rine pathway, which increases vitality, mental acuity, learning ability and attention span.
- Stimulates the production of cholecystokinin, which is helpful in reducing inflammatory responses in allergic people.

TAURINE

- Acts as a detoxifying material.
- Combines with bile acids from the liver to aid in absorption and metabolism of lipids (cholesterol and triglycerides).

TRYPTOPHAN

- Is a precursor to serotonin, required during the sleep process.
- Is necessary to antibody production by the bone marrow (B-cells).
- Raises pain threshold.
- Converts to niacin in the presence of vitamin B_6.

TYROSINE

- Is used by the thyroid gland along with iodine to produce the hormone thyroxin.
- Is a precursor to norepinephrine (a neurotransmitter) and to some adrenal hormones.

Vitamin C: A Key Nutrient

Ascorbic acid (vitamin C) is one of the most important, protective, biochemical substances in all life processes. It is essential to a large number of biochemical functions, yet humans, guinea pigs, apes, and monkeys cannot synthesize vitamin C in their bodies. Obtaining adequate amounts of vitamin C from food is difficult, so supplementing this vital nutrient is important. Ascorbic acid and the various ascorbates are all classified as vitamin C. Ascorbic acid and ascorbate are used interchangeably in this discussion.

Vitamin C's Role in Allergy Treatment

- Helps relieve allergic symptoms and prevents local inflammatory reactions.
- Provides an antihistamine-like effect (without the side-effects of antihistamines).
- As an antioxidant, it protects our body from the effects of pollutants by joining with oxygen and enzymes to convert toxic substances into non-toxic derivatives (which are then excreted in the urine).
- Assists in the manufacturing of adrenal hormone, needed to combat the stress imposed by allergic reactions.
- Enhances T-cell and phagocyte function.
- Increases immunoglobulin production by the lymphocytes.
- Improves tissue oxygenation.
- Promotes wound healing.
- Is a natural laxative when optimum dosage is taken.
- Is rapidly expended during any infection.
- Has active antiviral properties.

Vitamin C has many additional physiological benefits, but those mentioned are of the most help to people with food, chemical, and inhalant sensitivities. Ascorbate is found in these tissues, in order of decreasing concentration: adrenal glands, white blood cells, pituitary gland, brain, pancreas, liver, cardiac muscle, and plasma. Because it is required by so many body tissues, it is extremely important for the allergic person.

Large amounts of ascorbate will have additional benefits by increasing mental acuity and reducing symptoms of stress. Vitamin C is an important component of collagen, the material which "cements" our cells together. It is also a component of cell membranes throughout the body.

Safety of Vitamin C

Vitamin C is very safe to use; it is one of the least toxic substances known. Even at high levels, there has been no evidence of toxicity. There has been much discussion in the media about the possibility that a high vitamin C intake could cause the development of oxalate kidney stones. Physicians like Dr. Robert Cathcart in California, have found that the slight increase in acidity and flow of urine prompted by vitamin C use causes the calcium salts associated with kidney stones to dissolve. High concentrations of ascorbate—which is bacteriostatic (inhibits bacteria growth) in the urine—prevent the infectious residues around which stones frequently form. Vitamin B_6 and magnesium in adequate amounts have been found to prevent the formation of calcium oxalate kidney stones.

Victor Herbert claimed that supplementary vitamin C taken with a meal destroys 95 percent of the B_{12} contained in the food. These claims were researched by two other teams of investigators, who found that improper analysis methods led to erroneous conclusions in the original study.

A small number of people with a G-6-PD deficiency (Glucose-6-phosphate dehydrogenase) are found in groups of Asian and Mediterranean extraction. Large doses of ascorbate in these people may cause hemolysis (dissolution of red blood cells). Research is being conducted to see if this condition can be reversed.

Vitamin C Supplementation— Bowel Tolerance

Because of its action on the immune system, vitamin C should be taken daily by allergic people. Reactivity will be lessened if a daily level of vitamin C is maintained. It is impossible to recommend an exact amount of vitamin C for everyone—the amount needed will vary depending on age, stress, exposure to allergens or infection, absorption rate, and other factors. Bowel tolerance is a good indicator of your need.

As an effective vitamin C requirement indicator, bowel tolerance level was introduced by Dr. Cathcart. Dr. Cathcart states the maximum relief of symptoms that can be expected with oral doses of ascorbic acid is obtained at a point just short of the amount that produces diarrhea. The timing and amount of the doses is usually sensed by the individual.

Diarrhea at bowel tolerance level occurs when adequate amounts of ascorbate accomplish detoxification, free radical scavenging, and repair. The level of vitamin C in the blood then rises, slowing ascorbate absorption from the intestinal tract. The excess reaches the rectum and produces diarrhea. Diarrhea can also occur when a buffered form of vitamin C is used. This material can be irritating to the gut and can cause diarrhea because of its magnesium content. This does not represent a true bowel tolerance level—you should try a different form of vitamin C, such as ascorbic acid or ascorbate forms, or ascorbic acid plus a sodium/potassium buffer. (Do not take more than 500 milligrams of potassium per day unless you check with your physician or nutritionist. Some buffered forms of vitamin C contain potassium.)

The degree of toxicity in your body will dictate the amount of vitamin C you can tolerate before bowel tolerance is achieved. We cannot stress enough the importance of consistently using your bowel tolerance level of vitamin C to improve health. Best results can be achieved only if bowel tolerance levels are reached and maintained. Most people err in taking too small rather than too large an amount of vitamin C. Remember, too, that other nutrients are equally important to balance the vitamin C and to enhance its action in the body.

BEGINNING YOUR VITAMIN C THERAPY

When starting your vitamin C therapy, begin with one gram of the ascorbic acid form (nonbuffered) per day, taken at mealtime. Then increase that amount by one gram daily, spacing the doses evenly throughout the day, until you have reached your bowel tolerance level. This will be your maintenance level. Test this level periodically, since exposures may change your need from time to time. For children, start with 500 milligrams (mg) rather than one gram (1,000 mg = 1 gram).

If you experience diarrhea when you are taking only two to three grams daily, try again after a few days to increase your bowel tolerance level. When diarrhea does occur, it will subside in a few hours. Drink additional tolerated water to flush out the excess vitamin C causing the diarrhea. You may experience a small amount of bladder irritation or burning in the stomach when increasing your vitamin C; however, this is not a sign of toxicity or reactivity to the vitamin. These symptoms usually subside if a different form or source is used.

You may also experience gas as you increase your vitamin C consumption to your maintenance level. This may temporarily be uncomfortable, but it usually subsides. If you do develop gas, you may want to time your increases to coincide with the weekend so you will be more comfortable at work. You can also divide your doses into smaller amounts and spread them out over a longer period of time. Patients who have candidiasis may experience more bloating and gas, and sometimes diarrhea, when increasing vitamin C levels. The Candida organism ferments the vitamin C in the lower bowel, forming gas bubbles.

When nearing your correct level, you will develop a sense of well-being. Dosages below this level will not relieve your symptoms. When the sense of well-being lessens, it is always a good indicator of the need for more vitamin C. This is no more difficult to discern than knowing how much water you need to quench your thirst. At first, the mechanics of spacing your intake will seem very cumbersome, but in a short while it will become more routine.

Another important aspect of vitamin C therapy is consistency. Once you have achieved a daily maintenance level, you should keep your consumption at that level in order to keep inflammation and cell damage caused by allergies to a minimum. If taking more than 20 to 30 grams per day, you should supplement with additional minerals, because vitamin C at that level will act as a diuretic (increase urine flow) and will rinse out some of your minerals.

Vitamin C is water-soluble; it is not stored in our body. Excess is usually excreted within two to three hours, so you need to space your intake evenly throughout the day. If you awaken at night, take vitamin C at that time; your body repairs itself most during rest periods. If you have difficulty remembering to take your vitamin C every hour or two, carry a small timer to remind you. Since most of your exposure to allergens will be during the day, it is essential to keep a high concentration of the vitamin in your bloodstream at all times.

When you are exposed to unusually high amounts of allergens or to infection, you will need to increase your dosage above your maintenance level as soon as possible after the exposure. Quick action will prevent the cascade effect of adverse symptoms that accompany inflammatory reactions. You may be able to tolerate as much as three to four grams every half-hour without experiencing diarrhea. Your body will utilize that increased amount of vitamin C in the presence of a virus, an infection, an allergic reaction, or an increased stress level. You will soon learn to reach for vitamin C whenever a sensitivity reaction begins, and the benefits will be evident.

If you have temporarily increased your intake of vitamin C above your maintenance level, return to maintenance dose gradually over a period of several days to avoid a "rebound" effect, which is a rapid return of your symptoms or infection. If consumption of the vitamin is reduced too rapidly, a scurvy-like condition can result.

FORMS OF VITAMIN C

If you experience problems (other than irritating gas formation) with vitamin C, it is usually attributable to the substance from which the vitamin has been extracted. Problems may also result from the chemicals used in the manufacturing process. Vitamin C is currently extracted from sago palm, tapioca, corn, potato, and carrots. (See *Recommended Sources and Organizations*, p. 299.) An allergy to any of these substances may prevent you from being able to use vitamin C extracted from that source unless it is highly purified. Consider rotating vitamin C extracted from different sources so that you will not develop a sensitivity to any one source.

Use only hypoallergenic forms of vitamin C. Some less expensive brands may have allergenic binders, fillers, or coatings, or may not have been adequately refined. Do not use time-released or chewable vitamin C. Most sensitive people do not have enough hydrochloric acid production in their stomachs to properly pro-

production in their stomachs to properly process the time-released form. Chewables always contain some type of sugar or sweetener as well as flavorings to conceal the "vitamin" taste.

There are several different forms of vitamin C, ascorbic acid being the most common. Vitamin C is also available as sodium ascorbate and calcium ascorbate, which are considered to be a type of buffered C since they are not acidic. Those on salt-restricted diets should avoid the sodium ascorbate form; use the ascorbic acid form to make up the major portion of your vitamin C intake. Both the ascorbic acid and ascorbate forms of vitamin C should be rinsed off the teeth, since prolonged exposure can cause damage to the enamel.

Ascorbic acid is available in both crystalline form (powder) and capsule form. The crystals have a "tart" taste and can be added to either juice or water. One-quarter teaspoon of the crystalline form contains 1,000 mg or one gram of ascorbic acid. The capsule form is easier to use, particularly when travelling, but the capsule is made from either beef or pork gelatin. Do not add vitamin C to hot liquids; the heat decreases its effectiveness.

BUFFERED VITAMIN C

Several companies manufacture a product called "Buffered C," which is ascorbic acid in combination with a buffer of calcium carbonate, magnesium carbonate, and potassium bicarbonate. Buffered C is an excellent aid for stopping reactions to many substances. (See "Temporary Relief During an Allergic Reaction," p. 262.)

Take Buffered C routinely one hour after meals. During the digestive process, the pancreas releases bicarbonate to neutralize the acidic food from the stomach as it passes into the small intestine; the Buffered C will aid in this process. You should not take Buffered C less than one hour before or one hour after a meal since the buffers interfere with the stomach acid necessary to start digestion. However, if you are experiencing an allergic reaction and need the Buffered C to stop the reaction, take it promptly, regardless of proximity to a meal.

When taking Buffered C, do not exceed more than five teaspoons or 20 capsules daily (10 grams) because potassium, calcium, and magnesium intake will exceed safe levels for some people. Each teaspoon contains 450 mg calcium, 250 mg magnesium, and 99 mg potassium. These amounts should also be considered if you are taking other calcium, magnesium, or potassium supplements. If you feel better with some buffering, and want to increase intake of vitamin C, you can add some ascorbic acid to your Buffered C powder, or take one capsule of ascorbic acid and one to two capsules of Buffered C.

You can make an inexpensive form of sodium ascorbate and mix it with fruit juice or water. Mix together 100 grams (g) ascorbic acid (crystalline form) and 48 g sodium bicarbonate and store in an airtight bottle. Mix the powder with juice or water immediately before ingestion to prevent the oxidation of vitamin C.

One teaspoon of this mixture will equal 2.5 g sodium ascorbate. This form should be taken only occasionally during a 24-hour period because of the sodium ion content.

Like ascorbic acid, Buffered C is available in both powder and capsule form. The powder acts more quickly than the capsule, and one teaspoon equals about four capsules. One teaspoon of Buffered C powder contains 2.4 g or 2400 mg of vitamin C. Stir one teaspoon of Buffered C into a small amount of water and follow it with a water "chaser." Some brands of Buffered C dissolve more easily than others. If water, add it to juice—however, the acidity of the juice inhibits some of the buffering action. If you are experiencing a reaction that is particularly severe, you can dissolve the Buffered C in a very small amount of water and hold it under your tongue. In a situation where there is no water, a capsule of Buffered C held under the tongue will dissolve and act in the same way. If the magnesium content of Buffered C is irritating to your intestinal tract, you can hold the solution under your tongue for five minutes and then spit out the solution, rather than swallowing it.

It is wise to take other nutrients along with vitamin C in order to enhance its action in your body. Each of the more than 40 essential nutrients is linked to all of the others. Because of this, special attention should be paid to providing adequate amounts of all vitamins and minerals so that your body will have the materials needed for repair and proper cell functioning.

Vitamin C will help control many symptoms a sensitive person experiences. It will not cure allergies, but it will help to control them and to repair all body tissues.

Vitamin C Summary

1. Take your bowel tolerance level of vitamin C daily. Use mainly the ascorbic acid form.

- To determine your bowel tolerance level, add one gram daily until you develop diarrhea.
- When you develop diarrhea, back up one increment. This will be your daily level except when you are experiencing increased stress, infection, or allergic reaction.
- Spread your vitamin C doses throughout the day to maintain a constant level in your body. It is excreted rapidly.

2. Take Buffered C one hour after each meal to aid digestion unless you are experiencing an allergic reaction.

3. If you are in reaction, take Buffered C immediately, regardless of proximity to a meal.

- Take one to two grams every 15 to 30 minutes until your reaction clears.
- Take one gram each of Buffered C and ascorbic acid so that you will not exceed the mineral safety level of calcium, magnesium, and potassium.
- As long as you do not have diarrhea, your body is using both the vitamin C and the buffers to stop your reaction and to repair and protect your body.
- Because most people think poorly when they are in reaction, instruct your family or friends to give you Buffered C whenever they see you experiencing symptoms.

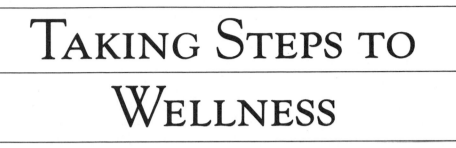

PART 5

TAKING STEPS TO WELLNESS

CHAPTER 17

DETOXIFICATION

Many people are burdened with so many symptoms that they are unable to separate one from another, or to trace any single symptom to a single cause. Early warning symptoms have been ignored or suppressed for so long that vital body functions start to deteriorate.

Underlying this complicated end result is a complicated cause. However, many of these people have been treated with "band-aid" approaches, and the use of masking drugs such as antidepressants, tranquilizers, calcium channel blockers, analgesics, vasodilators, or vasoconstrictors. Instead of helping, these drugs add to an already heavy body burden. A new and more effective approach to medicine is emerging, attempting to slowly and carefully identify and correct the underlying causes of inferior health.

One of the insidious causes of symptoms is an overload of toxins, chemicals, and biochemical debris that our body is unable to properly discharge. This cumulative toxicity has developed as a direct result of our 20th century demand for "better living through chemistry."

The adaptive capability of our biochemistry is amazing, but it has limits. When the detoxification pathways in our body are too heavily bombarded, they are unable to complete their task, and the remaining chemical load will damage the normal functions of each cell, leading to end organ damage (disease).

As the body becomes increasingly burdened with both exogenous (external) and endogenous (internal) chemicals, it becomes more reactive to smaller and smaller amounts of a greater variety of foods, chemicals, and inhalants. This eventually leads to a condition called pan-reactivity. Depending on one's genetic target organs and individual susceptibility, a wide variety of symptoms or syndromes are possible. (See the *Index* under "Symptoms.")

In her book, *Tired or Toxic*, Dr. Sherry Rogers likens the detoxification pathways to a janitorial service, which has the job of ridding our body of daily accumulations of unwanted dirt and stains (biochemical debris). When the janitorial service works properly and efficiently, the debris is swept along a biochemical transformation pathway, changed into a less toxic form, and prepared for dumping (excretion). We are all familiar with our body's dumping areas—skin, lungs, intestinal tract, kidneys, liver, and bladder. When the workload for the janitorial service is too great, some of the debris (toxins or chemicals) is not transformed properly, and more potent toxic chemicals are created. The new chemicals will continue to damage our body, causing intoxication (too high a level of chemical debris).

Xenobiotics is a term recently coined to describe foreign chemicals in the body. These undesirable foreign materials enter our body through direct skin contact, through the lungs as we breathe, and through the intestinal tract as we eat and drink. After entry, they are absorbed through the capillaries into the bloodstream.

However, external sources of injurious chemicals are not the only problem that overloads the detox system. Our own bodies also add to the load when processing chemicals produced by: normal metabolic functions; attempts to fight off acute or chronic infections; malfunction of any body system; and release of chemicals from amalgam fillings. Water-soluble chemicals are not difficult to excrete. However, fat-soluble chemicals pose a real threat to our health. These chemicals accumulate in our fat cells, where they remain indefinitely. This is known as toxic bioaccumulation, occurring in most organs and body systems, including all cell membranes, the brain, nerve sheaths, endocrine system, and in human milk.

Fat molecules are very mobile when our body is stressed. The molecules, along with their toxic burdens, are released into the bloodstream to circulate freely, causing damage and symptoms. Over 300 chemicals have been identified in human fat tissue.

Fat cells can be mobilized by heat exposure, exercise, emotional stress, illness, and fasting (including the fast during sleep). This mobilization during sleep may explain the severe morning symptoms experienced by some sensitive people. The intermittent, internal release of chemicals can also account for "unexplained" worsening of symptoms during recovery, even while the sensitive person is minimizing exposures to external chemicals.

How Our Body Detoxifies

The detoxification system works to convert toxic chemicals into less toxic metabolites to excrete them as quickly as possible. Several mechanisms of detoxification in our body have been identified. The first occurs on the cellular level in a ripply network of fibers known as the endoplasmic reticulum. This processing of foreign particles (xenobiotics) is accomplished by a system (cytochrome P-450) using specialized liver enzymes. The enzymes aid in destroying or transforming harmful chemicals by oxidation (loss of an electron), reduction (addition of an electron), or hydrolyzation (removal of a hydrogen atom). One or more of these reactions take place before the end product (metabolite) is prepared for excretion. The enzymes that catalyze these functions are greatly dependent on specific vitamins and minerals.

The second stage of detoxification, also performed within the cell, is accomplished by coupling two molecules—the xenobiotic molecule and an amino acid (protein) molecule. This process is called conjugation. The resultant, larger molecule is more electrically charged, more soluble in water, and easier for our body to excrete in either bile or urine. Several amino acids that conjugate easily are cysteine, glutathione, glycine, glucuronic acid, and PAPS (phosphoadenosine-5-phosphosulfate). All of these amino acids contain sulfur, and when joined to another chemical, the process is called sulfonation. Another form of coupling takes place when an acetyl group is joined to a xenobiotic to prepare the chemical for excretion (acetylation) through the kidney.

The third phase in detoxification can give rise to chemical compounds which injure our body. When these compounds are formed it is more a biotransformation (changing a chemical structure) than a detoxification (creation of a less toxic material). These new toxic compounds circulate in the bloodstream and lodge in various body tissues, where they can cause irreparable damage. The formation of these harmful chemicals can occur when the first two systems are either overloaded, nonfunctioning, or blocked.

Detoxification Inhibitors

There are a number of factors that can disrupt or cause a malfunction in the various detoxification pathways. Many chemicals that make their way into our body are transformed into alcohols. A problem can occur in the subsequent change of alcohols to aldehydes. The enzyme, alcohol dehydrogenase, required in this biochemical exchange is dependent upon an adequate supply of zinc. The next step in the process is initiated by another enzyme, aldehyde oxidase, which is dependent upon an adequate supply of molybdenum and iron. The enzyme changes the aldehyde into an acid that can be excreted in the urine. If there is a breakdown in these two chemical transformations, the resultant free-radical, highly reactive chemicals (classed as epoxides) can damage the immune system, initiate cancer, and damage cell genetics. One can begin to see the end result of deficiencies of vital minerals and vitamins coupled with a chemical overload. The aldehyde detox system can also be overloaded with a high intake of sugar or alcohol, exposure to chemical aldehydes (formaldehyde), or formation of aldehyde by Candida overgrowth in the intestinal tract.

In the cytochrome P-450 pathway, a deficiency of nutrients (co-factors) essential for the synthesis of critical enzyme components can severely inhibit our body's detoxification efforts. Damage can be done to the P-450 system by direct action of specific chemicals entering the body. Dry cleaning or copy machine fluid (trichlorethylene) and plastics (vinyl chloride) are two such common chemicals. Vinyl chloride overexposure is a known cause of angiosarcoma of the liver. This chemical also damages cell membranes and enters cells to further damage the mitochondria (energy-producing portion of the cell). Highly reactive, unstable molecules are also formed when an oxygen molecule is added to some of the ingested chemicals. These molecules (epoxides) are very damaging to cell membranes.

Our body's detox systems can be overwhelmed by the sheer volume of chemical intake, plus intermittent release of chemicals stored in fat tissues of the body. Our detox systems cannot process this deluge of material. Heavy metals like cadmium, mercury, or aluminum can cause damage to detox enzymes.

Detoxification enzymes have specific affinities for specific chemicals; they cannot substitute in other pathways that may be overburdened. Problems can arise if a person is missing specific enzymes because of genetic or hereditary factors. Metabolites then build up to toxic levels. Clinical studies by Dr. Jean Munro and Dr. Jonathan Brostaff in England have shown that inefficient or defective enzyme systems are a major cause of food intolerance.

Nutrients for Detoxification

Some of the vitamins, minerals, and amino acids essential for the detoxification system to function properly are:

Riboflavin (Vitamin B_2)	Zinc
Pyridoxine (Vitamin B_6)	Magnesium
Vitamin A	Selenium
Vitamin E	Copper

Vitamin C

Niacin (Vitamin B$_3$)

Pantothenic acid

Cysteine

Taurine

Molybdenum

Iron

Manganese

Glutathione

Many of these nutrients are attached to the xenobiotic during the detoxification process and are lost when the resulting metabolite is excreted. It is important to replenish the supply of these nutrients so that body systems can continue to function adequately. Many of these nutrients are also essential for repairing damaged cell components.

Testing for Detoxification Effectiveness

Biochemists and physicians working together have recently developed sophisticated diagnostic procedures. Blood, urine, tissue, and sweat analyses can now determine levels of specific chemicals (pesticides, heavy metal). Urine tests can determine the effectiveness of the detox systems. Blood, urine, and hair analyses are done to measure levels of vitamins, minerals, and amino acids.

When mercapturic acid, a metabolite of glutathione conjugation, is found in the urine, it indicates that organophosphate pesticides, benzene, and toluene are being detoxified. Low levels of the enzyme superoxide dismutase (SOD) indicate the possibility of damage by free-radical, reactive chemicals, because SOD is a free-radical quencher.

Elevated urine levels of D-glucaric acid signify that liver pathways for detox are actively working, and that significant levels of xenobiotics are present in the body. If the D-glucaric acid levels are low, this indicates that the cytochrome P-450 enzyme system is exhausted and almost ready to shut down. By contrast, standard liver function tests will show an abnormal result only after about 70 percent of the liver is damaged.

Increased lipid peroxides in the blood are a sign that cell membranes are being damaged by free-radicals and chemicals. Lipid peroxides are breakdown products of cell membranes.

If formic acid levels are normal or low, this indicates that the detoxification pathway for aldehydes is functioning. If elevated, this is evidence that there is a backlog of this formaldehyde metabolite and that the detoxification pathway is either overloaded or failing to function adequately.

When any one of these detox mechanisms is malfunctioning, the chemicals that should be detoxified are then free to circulate in our bloodstream and wreak havoc on cell membranes and tissues.

A careful, detailed history and close monitoring of your changing symptoms and progress are also important tools. They can help in diagnosing the competence level of your body's detox systems, the extent of your past and present chemical exposures, and your total body burden. It may be possible to differentiate between external exposure to chemicals (exogenous), both past and present, and internal chemical load (endogenous). Both factors are important in planning proper detoxification treatment.

Guidelines for Detoxification Programs

During even a moderate detoxification regimen, your symptoms will worsen temporarily as the chemicals are released from storage in fat tissue. As the chemicals circulate in the blood-stream being readied for excretion, they will once again cause a variety of symptoms.

Here are some measures to follow in starting a detoxification program.

- Do not attempt complex detoxification pro-grams without the help of a physician who is knowledgeable about the biochemistry of de-toxification pathways, nutrient and electro-lyte management, and symptoms accompa-nying detox procedures.

- First of all, present and past exposures to xenobiotics should be evaluated. Then clean up your present environment (work and home) as much as possible in order to lessen your toxic body burden (See "Keeping a Chemically Clean Home Environment," p. 156.)

- Drink large amounts (eight to 10, eight-ounce glasses) of water each day to flush detoxification waste products into the urine for excretion.

- Adjust your diet to remove all sugars, and eat a balance of proteins, vegetables, and whole grains. As much as possible, eat chemically uncontaminated foods in a rotated, diversi-fied diet.

- Include three tablespoons of unsaturated oils daily in your diet. Use cold-pressed oils from nuts, vegetables, fish, evening primrose, black currant, flaxseed, or borage. The oils slow down the assimilation of toxic chemicals from the intestinal tract.

- Take a high-quality vitamin/mineral supple-ment or plan a detailed supplement program with your physician.

- Start a mild exercise program depending on your limitations. Exercise in a "clean" envi-ronment.

- Reduce and manage stress. This will reduce

the number of metabolic byproducts and is an important part of any detoxification process. Stress also creates demand for additional nu-trients needed in the detoxification process.

- Maintaining proper bowel function is impor-tant for your detox program. At least two semi-soft stools per day are necessary to rid your body of accumulated toxins. Adequate water, fiber, and vitamin C will help to ac-complish this. If excreted toxins are not con-tinually moved through the bowel, they can be reabsorbed into the bloodstream and add to the already loaded detoxification path-ways. Maintain bowel tolerance levels of vi-tamin C. (See "Vitamin C: A Key Nutrient," p. 242.)

- Take detoxification baths (see p. 255) to begin the mobilization of chemicals from fat cells, bringing them to the skin for excretion.

- Maintain a proper electrolyte balance with use of potassium and sodium salts. The dos-age should be regulated by your physician.

- Get help in evaluating vitamin and mineral levels and designing a supplement program to include all of the antioxidants and specific minerals which stimulate detox pathways.

- Monitor cardiovascular levels during exercise sessions in order to avoid risk and stress. Increased doses of niacin (vitamin B_3) should be taken before each exercise session to in-crease skin capillary activity, enhancing toxin excretion.

- Obtain regular massage by a physiotherapist, massage therapist, or rolfer. An important detox tool, massage increases circulation in the blood and lymph systems to help carry processed toxins to the proper organs for ex-cretion.

- Use a dry sauna—but only with **extreme cau-tion**, starting with five-minute sessions and increasing gradually to 20 to 30 minutes. Scrub your skin well before and immediately following the sauna. (See the preliminary instructions for detox baths, p. 256.) Saunas at health clubs are usually wet saunas or are too hot. They have inadequate levels of available oxygen, and are made of environmentally unsafe materials. Sauna temperatures should not exceed 150°F. Use saunas only on the advice of your physician, as the resulting detox symptoms can be severe and possibly life-threatening.

DETOXIFICATION CENTERS

Environmentally ill people with severe symptoms may consider using the services of detoxification centers. Presently, there are detox units in California, South Carolina, and Texas. Their programs are very carefully monitored, and some of them are specially constructed for environmental safety. Continual laboratory tests and evaluations are carried out.

You may consider this concentrated approach if:

- You have severe, debilitating symptoms of environmental illness.
- You continue to experience acute symptoms after receiving standard treatment from an environmental medical specialist and cleaning up your environment.
- You have a high exposure to toxic chemicals, both now and in the past.
- You have continued high levels of toxic chemicals in your blood, urine, fat tissue, or sweat.
- You have continued malfunction of detoxification pathways.

After you complete a detoxification program, it is important that you continue a careful lifestyle. Your home environment must be chemically free. Your workplace should not contain heavy occupational exposures. Continue diet, nutrient supplement, and other treatments for environmental illness, and maintain general lifestyle and health habit improvements. Together, these factors should lead to your return to optimum health.

Detoxification Baths

Detoxification baths are very helpful for those who have toxic, chemical bioaccumulations. The hot bath water increases blood capillary action near the skin surface for faster release of toxins. Heat expands the pores in the skin and increases perspiration carrying toxins to the skin surface. Heat also raises pulse rate (an indicator of increased blood circulation).

Scrubbing your skin with a loofa sponge or rough washcloth stimulates capillary action, while removing a layer of dead skin and excess skin oils to allow closer contact with the vinegar or Epsom salts.

Vinegar or Epsom salts work as counter-irritants on the skin to increase blood supply and activate fluid movement in the tissues. These solutions change the pH on the skin surface, which also tends to facilitate fluid movement. The sulfur component of Epsom salts is a good detoxifying agent. Sulfur springs throughout the world are well known for their palliative properties.

However, do not attempt these baths unless they are prescribed by your physician. You may experience detoxification symptoms during and after your bath. If your chemical load is extremely high, the baths can make you feel very ill. An alternative treatment may be necessary.

If you have been advised to take a detoxification bath, follow your physician's instructions carefully. Do not try another method on your own. Be sure someone is in the house with you when you take your detoxification bath; you may need help if your symptoms become severe. Terminate your bath early if symptoms—possibly including dizziness, headache, exhaustion, nausea, weakness, and fatigue—become too uncomfortable.

PRELIMINARY BATH INSTRUCTIONS

Your bathtub should be spotlessly clean for a detoxification bath.

A trial series of hot water baths should be taken three times per week until you have no symptoms. Then begin taking the detox bath described below as directed by your physician.

- Take your tolerated dose of Buffered vitamin C before and after each bath to help removal of toxins released into your bloodstream. If you are using antioxidant vitamin therapy, take these materials before your bath.
- Wash thoroughly with tolerated soap in the tub or shower before your detox bath to remove excess body oil. Scrub your skin with a loofa sponge or a rough washcloth. Rinse thoroughly.
- Fill your tub with water as hot as you can tolerate without burning your skin and high enough so you can immerse your body up to your neck. (Overflow drain covers can be obtained at a hardware store to allow for deeper filling of your tub.)
- Drink an eight-ounce glass of water during all detox baths.
- Soak in the hot bath for only five minutes for the first bath. You may experience delayed detoxification symptoms the following day. Gradually increase the time for subsequent baths to 30 minutes.

- If immediate symptoms become intolerable, release the stopper and allow the water to drain from the tub. Sit until you feel you can safely get out of the tub. If you feel weak, you can easily fall.
- Scrub your skin thoroughly in a tub of clean water or in a shower to remove any accumulated toxins deposited on your skin during the detoxification bath. (Toxins left on the skin will be reabsorbed.)
- Continue to take detox baths until your general health has improved significantly. Then use the baths once or twice weekly.
- If you have an unusual chemical exposure, take your baths more frequently.
- Detoxification baths may need to be repeated in several series because detox in some people occurs in a cyclic fashion, sometimes with months between episodes.

DETOXIFICATION BATHS
(WITH EPSOM SALTS, VINEGAR, OR CLOROX)

Refer to the Preliminary Bath Instructions above. You can choose one of three materials for your detoxification bath: Epsom salts, apple cider vinegar, or liquid Clorox.

If you choose Epsom salts, add one cup to a full tub of clean bath water. Those who are very sensitive may have to begin with ¼ cup. Over time, you will need to gradually increase the Epsom salts until you are using four cups in a tub of water. Or, add one cup of apple cider vinegar to a full tub of clean bath water. Sensitive people may have to start with ¼ cup vinegar. Or, add two tablespoons Clorox (liquid only) to a full tub of clean bath water. Chlorine-sensitive people should not use Clorox.

- Use water as hot as you can tolerate and fill the tub so that you can submerge up to your neck.

- Soak for five minutes for the first bath, depending on the level of your detox symptoms. Gradually increase the time for subsequent baths to 30 minutes.
- Scrub thoroughly in a tub of clean bath water or in a shower to remove any accumulated toxins deposited on your skin during the detox bath.
- If you continue to perspire, you may need to repeat a cleansing bath or shower.
- Take a detox bath every other day or three times weekly.

18

SOLVING EVERYDAY PROBLEMS

The Importance of Water Quality

We do not usually consider water as a nutrient, but it provides our bodies with oxygen and hydrogen—two materials essential for proper metabolism. The average adult is made up of approximately 45 quarts of water, accounting for roughly two-thirds of body weight. Our body loses about three quarts of water each day through excretion and perspiration. The rate of water loss depends on activity level and environmental conditions—it may range from less than a quart, for a sedentary person in a mild or cold climate, to 10 quarts per day in a desert.

Water is involved in every body process, including digestion, absorption, circulation, and excretion. Water is the primary transporter of nutrients to every cell in our body. It diffuses rapidly across membranes and also carries waste products out of the cells. Each cell not only contains fluid (intracellular), but is also bathed in fluid (extracellular). Water supplies the fluid for secretions and serves as a medium for chemical reactions taking place in each cell.

Water modulates temperature by evaporating from the skin and respiratory passages. Very little water is absorbed in the stomach; some is absorbed in the small intestine, and the greatest amount is absorbed in the large intestine.

Water is excreted in the urine, feces, skin, and lungs. It is kept at an almost constant level in our body by precise regulatory mechanisms in the kidneys. However, continuous replacement is essential to prevent dehydration and salt depletion.

Organically grown fruits and vegetables are good sources of chemically pure water. Our water intake should balance the usual daily excretion:
- 1,300 cc in urine;
- 500 cc through the skin;
- 500 cc through respiration in the lungs;
- 100 cc in the feces;
- total of 2,400 cc.

(Menstrual flow in women adds to this amount.)

About 500 cc of water is derived in the body from organic nutrient oxidation. This source of water is involved in energy and heat exchanges in the cells. Our water intake from food and fluids should then be about 1,900 cc, or approximately 2½ quarts, to make up the 2,400 cc required.

WATER AND ALLERGIES

Adequate water intake is very important for the allergic person.
- All nutrients are kept in solution, available for cell repair and nourishment.
- An adequate water level is required to flush toxins (chemical and biological) and waste products from cells. This flushing helps to

reduce the total overload of the allergic person.

• Positive and negative ions require adequate fluid levels in order to flow and function as good electrical conductors and to help maintain a state of equilibrium in the body.

Water retention in extracellular spaces is referred to as edema. This can occur as a result of trauma, disease, allergic reactions, stress, malfunction of certain organs (heart, lungs, kidneys, adrenal glands, thyroid), and ingestion of drugs.

As a result of this excess fluid build-up, nutrients cannot be transported as easily to the cells. Cells then do not function well and waste products accumulate within them, causing cell damage. Early evidence of this process is evident in swollen tissues in the hands, feet, or ankles; swollen tissue under the eyes; or swollen nasal membranes. Later signs include swollen legs and abdomen, and headache (caused by swelling of brain tissue). For edema treatment, see "Natural Remedies for Common Complaints," p. 261.

WATER SUPPLIES AND STANDARDS

Available water supplies differ greatly in different areas of the world. The water that is most beneficial contains balanced amounts of minerals. Hard water is a good source of mineral nutrients needed by our body for proper cell metabolism; water that rushes over rock or water from deep wells is usually hard water. Excessive hardness, however, can cause mineral imbalances, leading to poor health or sensitivity. Soft water (such as rain water) contains very few dissolved minerals. Water can be softened by using specific salts that react with minerals, causing a precipitate that is filtered out.

In the past, most water sources were safe for drinking. As populations increased, however, drinking lake water, stream water, and water from common wells became increasingly hazardous. Epidemics of diseases, such as diphtheria and cholera, became more commonplace as water supplies became contaminated with human waste. Attention had to be directed toward providing clean drinking water. Today, we have even more problems finding safe sources of water. Water supplies on this continent may be relatively free of bacterial contamination, but many other hazardous materials and parasites may be present in the water you consume. Lake water may contain algae growth that can cause allergic reactions in plant-sensitive people.

Water standards, regulated by public health departments, cover only the following:

• Bacteriologic quality (number of coliform organisms).

• Physical characteristics (turbidity, color, odor).

• Radioactivity.

• Chemical characteristics—maximum permissible limits are set for:

Alkylbenzene sulfonate	Manganese
Arsenic	Nitrates
Cadmium	Phenol
Chlorides	Selenium
Chromium	Silver
Cyanide	Sulfates
Fluorides	Total dissolved
Iron	solids
Lead	Zinc

These standards fail to address other hazardous, manmade chemicals. Contamination of ground and surface water supplies may occur in many ways. Chemicals do not readily break down before they enter the ground water supplies. In England, recently dug wells were found to be severely contaminated by whale oil that was dumped in 1815.

SOURCES OF WATER CONTAMINATION

- Agricultural contamination from runoff containing residues of pesticides, herbicides, nitrites, and chemical fertilizers.
- Household contamination from detergents, phosphates, petroleum products, and hexachlorophene.
- Industrial contamination from dumping of hazardous chemical wastes into surface water; seeping of chemicals into ground water waste dumps; and brine from oil and gas drilling.
- Old, inadequate water purification plants in many communities that are unable to handle increased populations and industrial contaminants.
- Natural contamination from excess mineral deposits in the ground (such as molybdenum, lead, copper).
- Leaching of excess minerals from old lead or copper water pipes.
- Plastic piping or containers, to which some people are sensitive.
- Chlorine added to public water supplies for bacterial contamination control, to which a number of people are sensitive.
- Fluorides added to water supplies to help control dental caries. Fluoride also liberates aluminum from cookware when heated, and poses a problem for some allergic people.
- Nitrates and bacteria from leaky septic tanks, or from community dumping of raw sewage into surface waterways.

SAFER WATER SOURCES

There are sources of water other than public supplies that may be considered safe, but even some of these may pose problems for the sensitive person.

- In the past, well water was considered relatively safe if the well was situated away from septic tanks or other human waste disposal systems. However, in some communities the deep ground water has begun to show chemical contamination. Some well water contains high levels of minerals from the soil and is not tolerated by some sensitive people.
- Bottled waters can be obtained from spring water or distilled water. Exercise caution in looking for a reputable supplier, since some companies have been known to bottle tap water and sell it as spring water. The sensitive person should enquire about the source of the spring water since ground water in some areas is chemically contaminated.

Triple-distilled water may be safe for some sensitive people, but its distilling process removes minerals needed for good metabolic function. Supplementing trace minerals and macrominerals is important for anyone using triple-distilled water. Store water in glass or ceramic bottles rather than plastic containers—soft plastic containers leak plastic components into the water.

- Some brands of mineral water are tolerated by some people with chemical sensitivities.
- Boiling water will destroy bacteria and will remove chlorine and volatile chemicals in the steam. Heavy metals or nitrates, however, will remain in the water.
- Rain water, previously considered safe, can be contaminated with atmospheric pollution.
- Filtered water is relatively safe for many environmentally ill people. Many types of filters are available, from whole-house filters to portable filters or single-faucet filters.

In choosing a filter, you must evaluate the

severity of your illness, your finances, and the availability of various systems. Mineral supplementation is wise when filter systems are used. In addition, some people are sensitive to the charcoal medium used in the filters. Clean and check your filter system regularly for effectiveness and to prevent mold growth.

To determine which water source causes the least problem, an environmentally sensitive person must test varieties of water. This can be done by rotating various waters, just as with food on a rotation diet. Safe water should be used for drinking, cooking, brushing teeth, and washing fresh foods. Some very sensitive people may also need filtered water for bathing if chlorine or fluoride is a severe problem.

Considering the importance of water to our body functions, we should evaluate our water sources and take appropriate steps to ensure a pure supply.

Home Water Purification Systems

(adapted with permission of Dr. William Rea)

Distillation   These systems are somewhat noisy and give off heat. The units must have sediment and scale removed periodically.

Removes	Does Not Remove
Salts	Chlorine
Asbestos	All organic chemicals
Bacteria	
Viruses	
Fluorides	
Heavy metals	
Minerals	
Nitrates	

Reverse Osmosis   Three filters are arranged in a series (sediment filter, reverse osmosis filter, activated carbon cartridge).

Removes	Does Not Remove
Large particulate matter	Chlorine
Some organic chemicals	All chemicals
Some organic pesticides	All pesticides
Nitrates	All bacteria
Fluorides	All viruses
Asbestos	All minerals
Heavy metals	
Chlorine compounds	

Carbon Block   The filters must be changed regularly in order to prevent breeding bacteria or molds in the carbon medium. Some people are sensitive to the carbon medium.

Removes	Does Not Remove
Chloroform	Heavy metals
Chlorine	Minerals
Pesticides	Salts
Organic chemicals	Nitrates
Bad taste and odor	All fluorides
Bacteria	
Giardia	

Natural Remedies for Common Complaints

Problems with Medications

Many sensitive people cannot tolerate chemical exposures from medications commonly prescribed by most physicians. There are a number of reasons for this.

- Medications are chemicals that can cause sensitivities in many people.
- Medications are processed in our body by detoxification pathways, which process all chemicals (endogenous and exogenous) to which we are exposed. In most sensitive people, one or more of these pathways do not function well.
- Extra nutrients are required so that the detox

pathways in the liver can process the medications. Adequate amounts of these nutrients are frequently lacking in sensitive people.

- Some medications are manufactured from by-products of mold metabolism. Mold-sensitive people may have difficulty tolerating this type of preparation.
- Fillers, binders, dyes, flavorings, coatings, shellacs, and inks in tablets may be allergenic and are poorly tolerated by most sensitive people.
- Some liquid medications contain sweeteners, dyes, preservatives, and flavorings that may be allergenic.
- Most injectable medications contain preservatives to which many people are sensitive.
- Medications given to alleviate one condition may create other problems. For example, antibiotics may cause candidiasis to flare. Cyclosporin, which prevents rejection of transplanted organs, can make one susceptible to infection.

A sensitive person should have any medication tested before beginning a course of treatment. Medications taken regularly should be tested periodically to be sure an intolerance has not developed. Many sensitive people cannot tolerate any over-the-counter medications for relief of minor symptoms.

Temporary Relief During An Allergic Reaction

The following natural remedies are intended to help provide immediate, temporary relief of the symptoms accompanying an allergic reaction, whether it is caused by food, chemical, or inhalant exposures. These remedies do not, of course, address the specific underlying causes of an allergic reaction.

If you know what substance is causing your reaction and you have extracts for that substance, take your recommended dosage immediately. Then use the following methods to further aid in clearing your reaction. Speed of treatment is the most important factor in stopping an allergic reaction. Some reactions cannot be reversed if there is a delay in starting treatment.

You may want to post this section so that you and your family can find it quickly. If you feel ill and are thinking poorly, it is a good idea for another person to check whether you are taking the proper substances at the proper times.

Vitamin C

- Buffered C is the most effective form of vitamin C for stopping reactions. It works because allergic reactions may cause our bodies to become acidic; a substance that reverses this condition will help stop the reaction. The buffer (calcium carbonate, magnesium carbonate, and potassium bicarbonate) will aid in eliminating excess acidity, restoring the proper pH balance. The vitamin C content also aids in reversing or stopping allergic reactions, but by a different mechanism.
- Many reactions can be "turned off" with Buffered C if it is taken promptly, before the reaction progresses to the point where the cascade effect makes it no longer reversible.
- Some people become more alkaline when they have an allergic reaction. This can be determined with the use of nitrazine paper or litmus paper (available at your pharmacy). Both saliva and urine must be tested to determine the pH. These people will need to take the ascorbic acid form to stop their reaction.
- For dosage amounts and additional information, see "Vitamin C: A Key Nutrient," p. 242.

Magic Brew

- "Magic Brew" helps to stop reactions by reducing acidity and correcting pH imbalance. You may alternate "Magic Brew" with Buffered C.
- Mix one teaspoon salt and one teaspoon baking soda with one quart of water. Take two to four ounces (two to four large mouthfuls) at least every 15 minutes the day you have the reaction, and every hour the next day. (It will taste better cold until you become accustomed to the taste.)
- If you have high blood pressure, you will want to take this preparation in limited amounts because of its sodium content.

Alka Seltzer Gold

- The "Gold" version of Alka Seltzer has a buffering action to reduce acidity; however, it does contain corn. Corn-sensitive individuals should not use this remedy.
- A dose of Alka Seltzer Gold may be repeated every 45 minutes to an hour until symptoms lessen.
- Alka Seltzer Gold is available only in the U.S., or through Miles Consumer Healthcare Division. (See *Recommended Sources and Organizations*, p. 299.)

Tri-Salts

- Cardiovascular Research Ltd. produces this formula, which contains carbonate and bicarbonate sources of calcium, magnesium, and potassium. (See *Recommended Sources and Organizations*, p. 299.) It is the same buffer used in Buffered vitamin C.
- Take ¼ teaspoon of Tri-Salts with each gram of vitamin C. You may stir Tri-Salts into water or juice, but because juice is acidic the buffering effect will be reduced.
- This is an excellent buffer to combine with nonbuffered vitamin C, or to use alone.

Bi-Carb Formula

- Vital Life produces this formula, which is a combination of sodium and potassium bicarbonates. (See *Recommended Sources and Organizations*, p. 299.) It is an excellent buffer and will help to lower acid levels.
- Take two to four capsules at a time. This dose may be repeated every 15 to 30 minutes if necessary, depending on your symptoms.
- You may combine Bi-Carb Formula with any nonbuffered vitamin C (ascorbic acid) that you can tolerate.
- If you have high blood pressure, you will want to take this preparation in limited amounts because of its sodium content.

Proteolytic Enzymes

- Proteolytic enzymes, such as papain from papaya, bromelain from pineapple, and pancreatic enzymes, can be used to reduce the inflammatory processes that accompany allergic reactions. Inflammatory reactions, when allowed to proceed unchecked, will cause damage to mucous membranes, arteries, capillaries, brain tissue, and other organ tissue.

Exercise

- A brisk walk or other moderate exercise will sometimes clear an allergic reaction.

Oxygen

- You can obtain an oxygen tank for emergency use by prescription from a physician familiar with your condition.
- Oxygen is an excellent aid in clearing an allergic reaction. In reactive or inflammatory processes, hemoglobin releases more oxygen to the cells actively involved in combating

foreign substances. This creates a greater demand for oxygen. By providing an increased supply of oxygen to these active cells, energy in the form of adenosine triphosphate (ATP) is increased to help maintain proper cell function and accelerate the metabolic process of detoxification.

- Oxygen should be used in conjunction with the alkaline salts found in Tri-Salts, Buffered C, or Bi-Carb Formula. Most people tend to be acidic during reactions, and in this medium the hemoglobin has less affinity for oxygen.
- Ceramic masks and special tubing are available for people who do not tolerate plastic masks and tubing. (See *Recommended Sources and Organizations,* p. 299.)

Other Reaction Stoppers

Histamine and heparin extracts, and adrenalin are all very effective in stopping allergic reactions, but they must be prescribed by a physician familiar with your condition.

COMMON COMPLAINTS

The following are some simple, nontoxic remedies for relief of common symptoms. Dosages listed are adult dosage suggestions only. Check with your physician for recommendations for children.

Bad Breath

- Maintain proper dental hygiene with brushing and flossing. Keep your toothbrush disinfected so as not to reinfect your mouth. Use hydrogen peroxide or Zephiran (benzalkonium chloride, a germicide and disinfectant) soaks for your brush. Rinse the brush well afterward. Buy a new brush every one to two months.
- Undesirable bacterial growth in your mouth

or esophagus can cause bad breath. Place ½ teaspoon acidophilus underneath your tongue and allow the sweet liquid to trickle down your throat. This will help to recolonize the oral mucous membranes with "friendly" bacteria.
- A magnesium deficiency can sometimes be the cause. Take a high-quality magnesium supplement.

Bee or Insect Stings

- Apply a paste made of a small amount of papain meat tenderizer and water.
- Proteolytic enzymes (papain, bromelain, pancreas) can be mixed in a small amount of water and applied to the sting site.
- Apply baking soda paste or witch hazel.
- Buffered vitamin C paste applied to the sting can be soothing.
- A homeopathic preparation called Apis is very helpful for any type of insect sting or bite.
- Taking a combination of vitamin C, potassium, and zinc (in appropriate dosages) will help to alleviate the systemic reactions from a sting.
- Cold compresses will keep toxins and inflammatory byproducts from spreading to a larger area, and will also lessen the pain.
- Histamine and/or heparin extracts will reduce systemic effects of the sting.
- Raw, cut onion placed on the sting site will help to draw out the venom. This method was used in the past by North American Indians.

Bloating

- Bloating pain is caused by a stretching of the bowel, and can be relieved if you move some of the gas forward. Gently press on the lower right abdomen, and gradually work your finger pressure up to the rib cage. Move your hand across the upper abdomen and proceed downward on the left side. Repeat this procedure several times until the gas "bubble" moves forward.

- Buffered vitamin C (one teaspoon dissolved in water and held under the tongue) will be absorbed rapidly and will help stimulate intestinal tract peristalsis to move the bloating forward.
- A hot water bottle (placed on the abdomen) or a hot bath will help relieve intestinal spasm and allow the gas to move.

Burns (minor)
- Apply ice to the burn as soon as possible.
- Vinegar applied to burns will help reduce pain.
- Aloe vera not only lessens pain, but aids in healing.
- Vitamin E oil lessens pain, aids in healing, and prevents scarring if it is applied faithfully.

Colds
Begin the following as soon as symptoms appear to prevent the virus from growing in body cells.
- Vitamin C (one to two grams taken every 30 minutes to an hour) will speed recovery.
- Take Viricidin or Monolaurin, and lysine. (See "Treatment of Viral Infections," p. 224, for additional help).
- Drink lots of water.
- Zinc lozenges taken at the first sign of a cold can prevent it from developing, and will relieve sore throats.
- Vitamin C nosedrops will ease a drippy or stuffy nose.
- Na Sal (a saline nose spray) will help to clear clogged nasal passages and keep mucous

membranes moistened. You can make a homemade spray using ½ teaspoon salt in eight ounces water.
- Do not consume dairy products during a cold because they may tend to thicken mucus.
- Sleep with your head elevated on pillows or a wedge so your nasal passages will drain more easily.

Constipation
- Constipation can be prevented by taking vitamin C to your bowel tolerance level every day. One gram of vitamin C every 30 mintues to an hour will eventually loosen bowels.
- Taking extra magnesium will help relieve constipation.
- Obtaining increased fiber and fluid from dietary sources is helpful.
- Exercise as much as possible. Walking is an excellent form of exercise.

Cough
- Lemon juice with enough honey to cut the tartness will help soothe a cough. It can be used hot or cold; sip slowly.
- Slippery elm lozenges, available at health stores, will help a cough.
- Dissolve vitamin C crystals in a small amount of water and sip slowly.
- Breathe steam from hot water in a basin or bowl to help relieve coughing spasms.
- The BHI Cough preparation (homeopathic) will control a cough.
- Do not eat dairy products as they can increase and thicken mucus.
- Postural drainage helps to reduce bronchial congestion. Lie across a bed on your stomach with your head, shoulders, and chest bent downward at the waist over the edge of the bed. Rest your elbows on a pillow on the floor. While in this position, force yourself to

cough. Hold this position for five minutes, three to four times daily.
- Remember, coughing is a natural reflex to keep your throat clear of mucus.

Diarrhea (if occasional)
- Small amounts of vitamin C taken over several hours will help stop diarrhea. A small amount of buffering—containing calcium, magnesium, and potassium (Tri-Salts)—taken at the same time may also help. The buffering will also replace minerals lost during excess bowel evacuation. Mix the buffered vitamin C in a small amount of water and hold under your tongue for five minutes so the minerals will be absorbed; then spit out the remainder of the solution.
- Water and electrolyte replacement is important during a bout of diarrhea since fluid is being excreted at a greater rate. Warm water or liquid will help to slow peristaltic bowel action. Pedialyte and Ricelyte may be used to replace fluids and electrolytes.
- Check to see if your diet includes any sorbitol, an artificial sweetener. It has a strong laxative effect.
- During a bout of diarrhea, adopt a temporary liquid diet in order to prevent bowel irritation.
- If diarrhea persists, dehydration can occur. The cause should be isolated with the help of your physician.

Edema (swelling, if intermittent)
- Exercise followed by a 20-minute rest, lying down, will help ease edema. The kidneys work more efficiently when the body is at rest.
- Eating foods high in potassium (bananas, watercress, strawberries, spinach, chicken, and tuna) will help lessen edema. Potassium sup-

plements are another alternative, but do not exceed daily dosage recommendations.
- Taking bowel tolerance level of vitamin C, a natural diuretic, will reduce edema.
- Vitamin B_6 is also a natural diuretic.
- Swelling of hands and feet may be caused by a vitamin B_1 deficiency.
- Reducing salt (sodium chloride) consumption is helpful in heart disease, pregnancy, and premenstrual edema.
- Causes of prolonged edema should be diagnosed by a physician.

Eye Fatigue
- For a quick refresher while reading for prolonged periods: move your eyes to the extreme left, hold for 30 seconds, then close your eyes and relax for 10 seconds. Repeat, moving them to the right.
- Vitamin C eye drops soothe tired or itchy eyes.
- Deficiencies of vitamins A or B_2 can cause eye fatigue.

Fever Blisters
- Neutralizing doses of fluogen extract will help relieve the pain of fever blisters.
- Buffered C paste applied to a fever blister lessens pain and encourages healing.
- Fever blisters are caused by a virus (*Herpes simplex*). (See suggestions under "Treatment of Viral Infections," p. 224.)
- Coenzyme Q10 and organic germanium can be taken daily to prevent fever blisters.
- Taking Lysine and Monolaurin daily will lessen your tendency toward cold sores. When sores first appear, immediately increase dosages of both substances.
- Vitamin E applied directly on the lesions will reduce pain and help them heal faster.
- Ice applied before a blister forms will shorten

its duration and lessen pain.

Foot Odor

- Fungal infections of the feet are often a cause. Wear shoes that "breathe," such as canvas, leather, or sandals. Wear only cotton or wool socks and avoid plastic or rubber footwear. Change socks frequently.
- Some brands of anti-odor shoe liners contain antibacterial agents and activated charcoal to destroy odor and absorb perspiration.
- Wash feet daily and soak in a mixture of ½ cup vinegar in two quarts water.
- Placing powder (talc) or baking soda in the socks will help absorb some moisture.

Headache

SIMPLE

- White willow bark, available at health stores, contains salicin, a mild pain remedy similar to aspirin, and without its cornstarch filler.
- The buffering action of "Magic Brew" (p. 263) will reduce acidity and correct pH imbalance, which often causes headache.
- Organic germanium (two to three GeOxy 132 capsules) will help relieve a mild headache.
- DLPA (DL-Phenylalanine) taken alone or with a pain reliever will help reduce or eliminate headache pain. DLPA causes the body's endorphins, as well as the pain killer, to be metabolized more slowly.
- Vitamin C, both buffered C and ascorbic acid, will help relieve a headache.
- Applying either an ice pack or a heat source (hot water bottle or heating pad) depending on your response will help relieve a headache.
- Avoid any offending substance that triggers your headache.

- Eat regular meals in order to avoid fluctuations in blood sugar levels.
- Feverfew herb (a member of the chrysanthemum family) is considered a good pain reliever. Be sure that you tolerate this plant material before using it.

MIGRAINE

- Initiate treatment methods immediately when the first signs of migraine appear.
- Organic germanium (six to 10 GeOxy 132 capsules) will sometimes stop a migraine if taken when the aura or warning symptoms first appear.
- "Magic Brew" (p. 263), sipped over a period of time, will help reestablish your body's proper pH, relieving headache pain.
- Taking two to four grams of Buffered C at the first sign of a migraine will sometimes prevent a headache. Two to four grams of vitamin C every 15 to 30 minutes, as bowel tolerance will allow, will also help clear a migraine. Alternate with Buffered C on the hour.
- Two 500-mg capsules of DLPA every 4 hours will help control the pain.
- A bath, as hot as you can tolerate, will reduce head pain. Be sure your hands and feet and as much of your body as possible are submerged. Soak until the water cools; repeat several times. Each soaking will lessen the pain.
- Applying either an ice pack or a heat source (hot water bottle or heating pad), depending on your response, will help relieve migraine headache pain.
- Avoid any offending substance that triggers your migraine.
- Sleeping for an hour or more with a heating pad (set on low) over your head may help to relieve the pain. Some people prefer cold; an ice bag can be substituted.
- Taking six to eight Bi-carb Formula capsules

at the first sign of a headache followed by two to four capsules every 15 to 30 minutes sometimes helps prevent a headache.

- Avoid foods containing tyramine (wine, beer, cheese, avocado, chicken livers, nuts, and pork).
- Avoid foods containing monosodium glutamate (MSG, a flavor enhancer), or dyes.
- Eating more fish or taking omega-3 fatty acid supplements is helpful for some migraine sufferers. The fish oil inhibits prostaglandin secretion, which occurs during a migraine episode.
- Take Feverfew herb to prevent migraine headaches, if you tolerate the herb.

Insomnia

- Taking 1,000 to 1,500 mg of Tryptophan at bedtime will help induce sleep (not currently available in the U.S.).
- Taking two to three calcium/magnesium supplements (Cal-Mag) at bedtime will help you to relax. These can be repeated during the night.
- Buffered C (containing calcium, magnesium, and potassium) will aid sleep. This may be repeated during the night.
- Check any medication or beverages you may be taking to see if it contains caffeine, which can cause insomnia.
- Two 500-mg capsules of Ornithine taken at bedtime can also be effective against insomnia.

Menstrual Cramps

- Taking neutralizing doses of hormone extracts—progesterone or estrogen—will help relieve or control cramps.
- Taking two calcium and magnesium capsules (Cal-Mag) every four hours may help relieve cramps.

- Essential fatty acids, such as evening primrose oil or black currant oil, taken consistently will help lessen menstrual cramps.
- Vitamin B_6 (100 to 150 mg per day) will help relieve cramps and PMS symptoms. It should be taken with a nonyeast source of B-complex.
- Increase your Buffered vitamin C intake to five teaspoons daily about three days prior to your period. The increase in calcium, magnesium, and potassium will encourage smooth uterine contractions rather than the spasmodic, cramping contractions experienced during menses.
- Doing pelvic strengthening exercises daily will help to relieve cramping during menses.

Muscle and Joint Pain

- DLPA—taken with a tolerated pain killer gives more, and longer lasting, pain relief.
- Applying heat will help lower pain levels. Hot baths, heating pads, or wet towels can be used.
- Increase your vitamin C intake to bowel tolerance level.
- Magnesium is essential for proper functioning of muscle tissue. It will relieve muscle spasms and pain.
- Potassium in small amounts will help to relieve muscle cramping, especially premenstrually.
- Tryptophan 1000 mg to 1500 mg is useful for chronic pain (but is not currently available in the U.S.).
- Zeel, a BHI homeopathic cream, is soothing for joint pain.
- White willow bark is a source of salicin, a mild pain remedy similar to aspirin.
- GeOxy 132, taken with pain medications, will enhance their effectiveness.

Muscle Pulls and Mild Sprains

- Applying ice immediately will help reduce swelling. Continue using ice packs for 36 to 48 hours, depending on the severity of the injury.
- Traumeel, a homeopathic cream, helps reduce muscle pain or trauma.

Nausea or Stomachache

- "Magic Brew" (p. 263), sipped warm or cold, helps ease nausea and stomachache.
- Two to four Bi-Carb Formula capsules will help ease a stomachache.
- BHI Stomach (homeopathic) tablets help relieve stomach pains, cramps, indigestion, and nausea.

Sinus Pain and Congestion

- Applying heat helps soothe sinus pain. Wet heat or a heating pad on low setting, applied directly to the sinus area will help.
- Slight pressure applied with the fingertips for two to three minutes on the brow line above the eye near the nose may help to relieve pain.
- Vitamin C nose drops are helpful in reducing sinus congestion.
- Euphorbium Compositum nose drops (a homeopathic mixture) drain the sinuses, reducing swelling of inflamed mucous membranes.
- BHI Sinus (homeopathic) tablets help to drain sinuses and relieve pain.
- Na Sal nose drops help to moisturize the nasal passages.
- Regular exercise keeps nasal mucus flowing so it cannot back up, creating congestion. Walking up a flight of stairs twice will help clear simple congestion.
- Salt Water Rinse (Snuffluphagus) adapted from *The Yeast Syndrome* by Dr. John Trowbridge, can be used to help moisturize dried

nasal passages, reduce nasal mucous secretions, and relieve sore throat caused by postnasal drainage. The mixture is inexpensive, and can be used throughout the day as often as needed, since it has no side-effects. It is especially helpful for infants and small children who cannot blow out mucus accumulation.

1. Mix a solution using ½ teaspoon sea salt or table salt to one cup warm water. Cool the solution to body temperature.

2. Fill an infant bulb syringe (available at pharmacies) with the solution.

3. Insert the narrow tip of the syringe into your right nostril first. Lean over a sink with your face downward and gently and slowly squeeze the solution well back into the nostril. Do not take a breath while the solution is in your nose. Gently blow out the solution into a tissue.

4. Gently sniff the solution remaining in your nose well back into the sinuses.

5. Repeat steps 3 and 4 with your left nostril.

6. The remaining solution can be kept refrigerated for later use, or can be used as a gargle to relieve a sore throat.

Sore Throat

- Gargling with warm saline solution every 30 minutes to an hour will help ease sore throats. (Use the proportions listed under Salt Water Rinse, above.) Keeping the throat moist is the best way to soothe pain.
- Acidophilus powder placed under your tongue and allowed to trickle down your throat will ease sore throat pain.
- Zinc lozenges will reduce pain.
- BHI Throat (homeopathic) will reduce pain and aid in healing.
- If your sore throat becomes more severe or

continues for longer than two to three days, you should contact your physician for diagnosis and treatment.

Tension and Stress

- Buffered C contains two ingredients (potassium and vitamin C) that aid in adrenal gland repair. The adrenal glands are overworked during episodes of stress and demand extra nutrients. Use one teaspoon dissolved in water. Pantothenic Acid (vitamin B$_5$) is also important for proper adrenal function.
- Running water helps reduce tension. The negative ions given off by water movement restores your body's electrical balance. The rhythm and sound of moving water (a stream, a fountain, rain, surf) is very soothing to the nervous system. Taking a shower or running water over your lower arms and hands are simple aids to reduce tension.
- With your fingertips, gently stroke your forehead from the center outward toward a point above the ears. Repeat in a slow rhythm.
- Magnesium reduces muscle tension and is used by neurotransmitter pathways in the brain. During stress, mental activity is usually very active, and magnesium can be calming.
- Use relaxation techniques daily. Remember that repeated allergic reactions are perceived by the body as stress.
- Practice deep breathing and exercise frequently during the day to help your body cope with both exogenous and endogenous forms of stress.
- Talking with an understanding person helps put any problem into proper perspective and releases stress.
- Crying is a good physiological tension release. The tears release endorphins, which

help our body cope with the stimuli of stress.

Viral Infections

- Taking six to eight capsules of Viricidin per day will help control a viral infection, but it must be continued for two weeks beyond the end of the infection. If taken when symptoms first appear, infection can sometimes be prevented. Viricidin will at least reduce the infection's duration and severity.
- Taking three to six capsules of Monolaurin per day will help control a viral infection, but it also must be continued for two weeks after the infection subsides. If taken when symptoms first appear, the infection can sometimes be prevented. (Take either Viricidin or Monolaurin, but not both.)
- Taking 3,000 to 4,000 mg of lysine in divided doses during the day will help control a viral infection.
- Neutralizing doses of fluogen extract will help relieve flu symptoms.
- Drink larger amounts of water.
- Cut back on foods containing arginine. Arginine feeds viruses and is contained in nuts, chocolate, barley, corn, gluten, oats, and coconut.
- Oscillococcinum (a homeopathic preparation available in health stores) stimulates the body's natural defense mechanism and helps relieve flu symptoms, such as fever, chills, body aches, and pains.
- Refer to "Viruses," p. 221, for additional help.

Wheezing and Tight Chest

- Wheezing or a tightening in your chest due to an allergic reaction will be helped by taking repeated doses of vitamin C.
- Taking magnesium in oral, sublingual, or in-

tramuscular preparations helps reduce wheezing. Magnesium relaxes smooth muscle.

- Avoid the offending allergens as much as possible.
- BHI Asthma or Bronchitis (homeopathic) tablets help to relieve wheezing.
- Vitamin A and manganese strengthen mucous membranes and enhance cilia function in the bronchial area.
- Taking pyridoxine (vitamin B_6), about 100–200 mg daily for four weeks, is helpful in reducing bronchospasms. Take a high-potency B-complex along with vitamin B_6.
- Sipping warm liquids will help to relax your throat and bronchial muscles.
- Make a conscious effort to relax your throat and chest muscles. Breathe deeply and exhale completely in a slow rhythm; this helps alleviate the sensation of panic associated with breathing difficulties.
- Avoid breathing cold air. Wear a scarf that can be quickly pulled up over your nose and mouth when you are suddenly exposed to cold air.

Choosing Your Physician

We all need a primary care physician to monitor our health, to care for us when we are ill, and to turn to in case of emergency. In addition, the sensitive person needs a physician who has training in clinical ecology or environmental medicine. Ideally, your physician should be both a primary care and an environmental medicine physician. However, this is not always possible because of the limited numbers of physicians practicing an environmental medicine specialty.

If there is not an environmental medicine specialist in your community or in a town near you, you will have to choose a local doctor to be your primary care physician. Ask your friends, relatives, and other health professionals to determine whether there is an open-minded, innovative physician available in your area. You will want this person to be willing to continue as your primary care physician even if you receive care from physicians in other facilities or cities.

Once you find a likely candidate, go to the office to make your appointment. This will give you the chance to determine whether you will be able to tolerate the exposures there. If you are chemically sensitive you will need to determine the following:

- Is the office clean and well-maintained?
- Does it have an odor of cleaning supplies?
- Is there a strong smell of personal care products, room deodorizers, or other substances generally used in medical offices?
- Is the doctor approximately on schedule, or is the waiting room full of people? This could mean you would have more exposures if you stay in the office for longer periods of time.
- Is smoking allowed in the building?

If the office seems tolerable, make an appointment for a consultation with the doctor. Ask the receptionist if the doctor treats other patients with chemical sensitivities. If so, this will be a help to you. If not, the interest and sympathy expressed by the reception staff may indicate whether this office will be cooperative.

When you have your consultation, explain that you need a primary care physician to oversee your routine medical care, and to care for you when you are ill. It would also be helpful if you have a brief letter from your environmental medicine physician outlining the pertinent details of your condition. Invite the doctor to call your environmental medicine physician at any time to receive additional information to help with your care.

You will need to pay particular attention to determining whether you can easily talk to this physician. Is he or she truly listening to what you say? You want the doctor to treat you with courtesy and to be open enough to accept what you say about your condition as being true. If the physician immediately refutes your statements, argues with you over your present treatment, or appears uninterested in cooperating, you will know that this person is not the best physician for you.

A physician with whom you can talk freely and develop a rapport is the person who can best help you. Even if he or she knows little about allergies or chemical sensitivities, you can, over time, share information so that the doctor can learn more about helping you.

Be aware that any physician who is not an environmental medicine physician will treat you with standard pharmacological medications. People with chemical sensitivities frequently do not tolerate these medications because of poorly functioning detoxification pathways. Those with food allergies or sensitivities may also have difficulty with some medications. Try to be knowledgeable about tolerated alternatives in order to avoid a medication crisis.

CHOOSING AN ENVIRONMENTAL MEDICINE PHYSICIAN

Your environmental medicine physician should be able to answer your questions about your condition, the treatment he or she can offer, and possible outcomes. This type of physician will take a lengthy, detailed history in addition to asking you to fill out a comprehen-

sive questionnaire, which is very important in helping to make a complete diagnosis and to identify all of your health problems.

In addition, you should be given educational literature to help you learn about and understand your condition. Your environmental medicine physician should provide suggestions to improve the quality of your life, as well as referrals to any support groups that might be helpful to you. This type of physician will consider you to be a partner in your treatment, and you will be assuming equal responsibility in your health care. No one can offer a "magic pill," and it will take effort on your part to get well. However, with a caring and competent physician to help and encourage you, your health can be improved to levels you might not have thought possible!

The organizations listed in *Recommended Sources and Organizations,* p. 299, can help you locate a physician who will have a treatment philosophy similar to the one described in this book. These organizations can refer you to a physician in your area (if there is one) who can diagnose and treat food, chemical, and inhalant sensitivities. As with any organizations, these groups are made up of people with widely differing personality types, areas of interest, and skill.

The Allergic Person's Guide to Surgery

Surgery is a traumatic physical and psychological experience for everyone. Those with allergies must be concerned about many additional aspects of the surgical experience. Since sensitivities vary greatly in type and severity, the amount of preparation you need depends on your situation. Be sure to take an active part in your care, as successful surgery is a team effort.

Unless your surgery is an emergency, get a second opinion. This step may prevent unnecessary surgery, and will reduce your anxiety regarding its necessity.

SURVIVING THE HOSPITAL

If you are unfamiliar with the hospital where the surgery will be performed, you should make an inspection tour. During your visit, observe the following to help you determine your ability to tolerate the hospital:

- Is the building well maintained?
- Are the emergency exits, fire extinguishers, and smoke detectors clearly visible?
- Are the patient rooms clean and adequately furnished?
- Can windows be opened?
- Are the rooms air-conditioned?
- Is there a thermostat in each room?
- Are there fluorescent lights only in the room?
- Does each room have a private bathroom?
- Are there grab bars in the bathroom?
- Do the rooms and halls smell of perfume, room deodorizers, or human excrement?
- Can the call buttons be reached easily?
- Are fresh fruits and vegetables served?
- Will the kitchen accommodate special diets?
- Do the visiting hours seem reasonable?
- Does the staff seem friendly?
- Are there enough nurses, nurses' aides, and orderlies on duty?
- Is the staff cleanly and neatly dressed?

When you talk to hospital admissions personnel, ask for a "No Smoking" private room (if available and affordable). If you have to share a room with another person, you will be exposed to their personal care products as well as those of visitors. Obviously, you will have no control over the gifts, flowers, or books your roommate will receive. If you have to share a room, insist that your roommates be nonsmokers, and that

they not be allowed to use scented products. When you meet your roommates, either you or a family member should explain your problems tactfully so that they will understand and cooperate.

Make a list of your questions about the surgery, and make an appointment well in advance of the operation to talk with your environmental medicine physician, surgeon, anesthesiologist, admissions personnel, hospital dietitian, nurses, and hospital housekeeping staff.

Your environmental medicine physician may want to test you for sensitivity to surgical scrub, tape, suture materials, and local and general anesthetic, if you do not already know to which of those materials you are sensitive. You also need to find out which vitamin and mineral supplements you should take or increase.

After you have discussed your sensitivities with your environmental medicine physician, you need to talk about the following items with your surgeon:

- Any other medical problems you have (such as asthma, diabetes).
- Any past severe allergic (anaphylactic) reactions you have experienced.
- Your specific chemical, food, or inhalant allergies and their symptoms.
- Your medication sensitivities.
- Your IV intolerance (lactose IV's are milk-based. D5W and dextrose IV's are corn-based).
- Your allergies to surgical scrub (Betadine), tape (paper tape is usually tolerated), or suture materials (nylon or silk are generally used).
- Present medication that you need to continue during your hospital stay, including your allergy extracts. (You will need your surgeon to write the order for you to be able to

take these while you are in the hospital.)

- Vitamin/mineral supplements you need to take during your hospital stay. (You will need your surgeon to write the order for you to be able to take these while you are in the hospital.)

- The possibility of the need for a blood transfusion and your desire to donate your own blood for that purpose.

- The availability of oxygen in your room for treatment of your allergy symptoms (wheezing, chest tightness). Oxygen will aid in clearing almost all allergic reactions. You will need your surgeon to write an order stating that you may use the oxygen to clear a reaction. You may also need to take your own ceramic mask if you have difficulty tolerating plastic oxygen masks.

It is also very important that you talk to your anesthesiologist well before your surgery. Several anesthesia medications cause allergic reactions and the anesthesiologist needs to be aware of your allergies. Be certain to speak to the person who will be administering your anesthesia. Discuss the following things, if applicable:

- Any history or present condition of asthma or throat swelling.

- Your medication allergies.

- Your specific chemical, food, or inhalant allergies and their symptoms.

- Your present medications.

The formula for anesthesia that usually works well for the allergic person is 100 percent oxygen for five minutes followed by a bolus of Pentothal or Brevital to induce anesthesia. Anectine or Curare can be administered to paralyze during the surgery. Sublimaze can be used to obliterate memory, and Innovar or Demerol are usually well tolerated. Of course, known allergies to any of these medications would prevent their use.

Acupuncture has been used for centuries in other countries to aid in the control of pain caused during surgery. It is sometimes used alone, and at other times it is used in conjunction with more standard anesthesia. If your surgeon and anesthesiologist are willing, and if there is a competent and cooperative acupuncturist in your area, you may want to investigate the possibility of using a combination of acupuncture and anesthesia for your surgery. This could lessen your exposure to the volume of pharmacologicals necessary to perform your surgery.

Hypnosis can be helpful in preparing the patient for more extensive surgery. In some cases of repair or removal of skin lesions, local anesthetic may not be required when hypnosis is used. A combination of acupuncture and hypnosis may also be helpful in many surgical cases.

Discuss your major food allergies, if any, with the hospital dietitian, keeping this list as brief as possible. Do not give the dietitian a list of 50 foods to which you are sensitive if only six cause significant reactions; you do not want to cause confusion and disbelief. Ask only that the major foods to which you are allergic be omitted. It may be necessary to educate the dietitian about the contents of prepackaged foods and about reading labels. Suggest that whole, unprocessed foods be served, and inspect each meal tray to be sure that the foods you want to avoid have not inadvertently been served.

Before your surgery, you should also inform hospital housekeeping personnel about your chemical allergies, if any. Ask that room deodorizers, disinfectants, detergents, soaps, or bleaches not be used in your room during your stay. Suggest that clear, hot water or baking soda be used instead, or you may want to bring a "safe" cleaner with you for use in your room.

If you plan to take an air cleaner with you, ask if someone on the staff needs to see it first. Some hospitals require that the wiring and plug type be inspected ahead of time. If you need to take your own bedding, you must also notify the housekeeping staff.

Preparing for Surgery

For as long as possible before your surgery, reduce your total allergic load. Strictly avoid all exposure to the foods, chemicals, and inhalants to which you are allergic so that your immune system can be as strong as possible before the stress of surgery. Also increase your intake of vitamin C, as it strengthens your immune system, promotes wound healing, lessens post-surgical pain, and detoxifies your body of medications and anesthesia—but do not take it the night before surgery because it reduces the effectiveness of the anesthetic. Vitamin C supplements can be resumed as soon as you can tolerate something by mouth, if approved by your surgeon.

Vitamin E should be stopped two days prior to surgery and should not be resumed until five to six days afterwards, because it increases fragility of blood vessels and can result in excessive bleeding during and after surgery. Begin taking coenzyme Q_{10} if you are not already doing so. Both it and GeOxy 132 act as buffers against the effects of hypoxia (oxygen deficiency in body tissues) during surgery and combats the free radicals produced by damaged tissue.

Make a list of special items you need to take to the hospital, such as soap, shampoo, vitamins, allergy extracts, charcoal mask, air cleaner, bottled water, bedding, bathrobe, and pajamas or nightgown that are "safe" for you.

Once you have been admitted to the hospital—and before surgery—talk to the nurses at your station. They need to know if you have allergies to flowers, plants, or molds so that live plants will not be placed in your room. You must also inform them of your medication allergies, to prevent accidental administration of a medication that could cause a serious reaction when your immune system is already weakened by surgery. Some extremely sensitive people may also need to ask the nurses and aides not to wear perfumes, scented hand lotion, or scented hair spray.

Support from your family and friends during this time is especially important. They can watch for and prevent exposures that might cause a reaction when you are unable to be vigilant. You may want to have someone sit with you during the first two days and nights after your surgery; be sure they are aware of the foods and other substances you need to avoid.

Following Surgery

After the surgery, you can do several things to speed your recovery. Move around as soon as possible, within the limits set by your surgeon. This prevents fluid from collecting in your lungs, causing further complications, such as pneumonia. Muscles, nerves, and many body functions begin to suffer from just a few days of inactivity, so you should exercise as soon as your condition permits. Begin your exercise program slowly and increase as tolerated; walking is a good starting point. Do only what is permitted by your surgeon and what feels comfortable to you.

Exercise, increased water intake, vitamin C, germanium (Geo Oxy 132), and coenzyme Q_{10} help to detoxify the medications and anesthesia in your body. Increase your vitamin C intake until you reach your bowel tolerance level, and then take a maintenance dosage just slightly below that amount. These nutrients promote healing of your surgical wound, help reduce pain, and increase your sense of well-being.

Your food is another important factor in your recovery. Once you are at home you can avoid allergenic foods easily. Stay away from high-sugar and "empty calorie" foods; focus on fruits, vegetables, meats, and fish.

Finally, allow yourself to get plenty of rest and do not push yourself to recover too quickly. Everyone's body recovers at its own rate. Give your body and immune system the time it needs to rebuild after the stress of surgery.

While these suggestions are a good starting point, there may be additional problems or situations for you to consider. With careful planning and patience, you can do well, even with allergies, in a hospital setting.

Dental Care for Allergic People

Our teeth are living structures—even their enamel, which most of us think of as a white, hard, inanimate casing, is alive. Our teeth are intended to last us for a lifetime. If we do not care for them properly, they can become a source of pain, and can adversely affect our general health. Diseased teeth can become a focus of infection; improper grinding surfaces can result in poor digestion, which can lead to food sensitivity. Materials used in teeth restoration can be toxic. Regular dental care and personal dental hygiene are imperative for good health.

Choosing a Dentist

Choosing a health care professional is often difficult, and when allergies and chemical sensitivities must be considered, it becomes even more difficult. Most medical and dental offices are loaded with chemical exposures, and many health professionals and their staff have mini-

mal or no understanding of allergies.

If you do not have a dentist, perhaps the best person to ask for a recommendation is the physician treating your sensitivities. You may also check with friends and acquaintances who have similar problems; their dentists may be suitable for you.

When you are considering a dentist, go to the office rather than calling to make your appointment. Observation will help you determine whether the office is safe for you.

- Does the office appear to be clean and well maintained?
- Can you detect chemical odors, strong perfumes or tobacco smoke?
- Does the staff seem interested in what you have to say, and do they appear to be cooperative after you explain your limitations?
- Is the staff wearing scented personal care products?
- Does the dentist appear to be on schedule, or is the waiting room full of people?
- How many treatment rooms does the dentist use? Generally, you will spend less time in an office with fewer rooms.
- Is the atmosphere one of disorganization and stress, or of calm, efficient functioning?

Introduce yourself to the receptionist, ask for an appointment for an examination/consultation. Explain that you have chemical sensitivities and may need some special help, but do not go into extreme detail. The receptionist may not know about chemical sensitivities, and you do not want to seem antagonistic so that the office staff will be unwilling to help you. Simply say that because of your chemical sensitivities, some common materials and exposures can make you ill.

Make it clear that your physician has recommended that you receive your dental treatment:

- In the absence of aftershave; perfume; fabric softener; scented hair sprays, hand lotions, and deodorants; and tobacco smell on the dentist and assistants.
- With a minimum of chemical exposures within the office.
- After the dentist has talked with your physician. (A simple letter from your physician may be helpful.)

If the staff's initial response seems favorable, make an appointment for the examination/consultation. The first appointment on a Monday may be best for you, since the office will have aired out over the weekend.

If, after you leave the office, you can tell that the exposures are too great, or that you will not receive the cooperation you need, cancel your appointment. It might be wise to wait a day or two to be sure of your decision.

During your first examination appointment you can discuss your specific problems with the dentist, as well as the proposed treatment plan. If it seems that there are too many exposures, or that the dentist is not cooperative, you will need to look for another dentist. If everything seems to be acceptable, and you make more appointments, space your visits far enough apart to give you recovery time from the exposures you do encounter.

During your discussion with the dentist, explain the type of symptoms you generally experience, and indicate that your physician is willing to answer any questions. While you want your dentist to understand your problems, you do not want him or her to be afraid to treat you.

Chemical Exposures in Dental Offices

There are five chemicals indigenous to most dental offices: formaldehyde; acrylic; nitrous oxide; phenol; and mercury. Mercury is the most toxic of these substances.

In addition to general office exposures, you will have to consider the exposure to dental materials used in your mouth. There are literally thousands of materials a dentist may use. Some people tolerate the majority of these, while more severely ill people may have difficulty with many of them.

The dentist will examine your teeth and will probably need to take X-rays. A lead apron should be provided to cover your vital organs as a precaution, although today's X-ray equipment is relatively safe. The X-ray film is wrapped in vinyl, which may be a problem for severely sensitive people. X-ray film wrapped in paper is available.

Professional "cleaning" (prophylaxis) by the dentist or hygienist is an important part of dental care. Plaque which has hardened to calculus is impossible for you to remove with home dental care. The final step in prophylaxis is polishing the teeth with a paste made of pumice, water, flavorings, and colorings. An alternative material is flower of pumice moistened with water.

If study models are necessary, the dentist must make an impression of your teeth. The impression material usually used contains alginate, flavorings, and colorings. There are no problem-free alternatives, so it is best to avoid study models unless they are necessary for making crowns and partial plates.

Local anesthetics used during dental procedures are frequently a problem for people with chemical sensitivites. If testing is available, it would be wise to have local anesthetics screened for tolerance before dental work is begun. Hypnosis and acupuncture can be alternatives to local anesthetic. (See "The Allergic Person's Guide to Surgery," p. 272.)

PROBLEMS WITH AMALGAM FILLINGS

Amalgam fillings (silver fillings) contain approximately 50 percent mercury and 20–30 percent silver, with zinc, copper, and tin making up the balance. Amalgams release mercury in minute amounts, especially during chewing. Mercury is also released when amalgams are polished as the final step in a prophylaxis. The mercury itself may cause problems for many people, or may contribute to an overload phenomenon. For a person with numerous sensitivities, those fillings should be removed and replaced with a tolerated alternative.

While the American Dental Association and most dentists believe that amalgam fillings are safe, debate over the fillings and their mercury content has flourished since the 1930s. Recent amalgam studies done on sheep at the University of Calgary's Faculty of Medicine show that labelled mercury from amalgam fillings appeared in organs and tissues within 29 days after the fillings were placed in the mouths of the sheep. Whole-body scanning revealed three absorption sites; the lungs, the gastrointestinal tract, and the jaw tissue. Once absorbed, high concentrations of mercury from the dental amalgams were found in the kidneys and liver of the sheep.

According to Dr. Anne O. Summers of Dallas, Texas, the release of mercury from dental fillings increases the mercury resistance and the antibiotic resistance of common mouth and intestinal bacteria. In this study done on monkeys, the mercury-resistant bacteria were also resistant to such antibiotics as Ampicillin, Erythromycin, Streptomycin, Kanamycin, Chloamphenicol, and Tetracycline.

Other studies have demonstrated that mercury does leach out of amalgam fillings. The American Dental Association admits this fact, but maintains that the mercury levels are too low to be harmful. However, mercury is considered a hazardous material before it is put into the mouth. When amalgams are removed, they must be disposed of by the dentist as hazardous waste.

Some dentists will remove and replace amalgam with safer materials. However, the amalgam fillings must be removed in the proper order because of the "charges" that build up on them. The "charges" are the result of the "battery effect" of dissimilar metals in the mouth in the presence of saliva. Continuous exposure to small currents, such as these on the amalgams, stresses the endocrine glands, decreasing immune system activity.

Other precautions should also be taken when amalgam fillings are removed. Using a rubber dam in the mouth and maintaining an oxygen supply during amalgam removal reduces the absorption of mercury released as the filling is drilled out. Vitamin C should not be taken for 24 hours before your appointment as it reduces the effectiveness of the anesthesia.

It takes several months—perhaps up to a year—for the body to completely detoxify from the mercury after amalgam fillings have been removed and replaced. Vitamin C; vitamin B_1; vitamin B_2; vitamin E; glutathione, cysteine, or methionine; selenium; zinc; beta-carotene; manganese; and magnesium all aid in detoxification. Taking detoxification baths or dry sauna treatments will speed the detoxification process. (See *Detoxification*, p. 250.) Many people improve dramatically after having their amalgams removed; others see little or no improvement.

ALTERNATIVE FILLING MATERIALS

Restorations or fillings should be carefully considered since they become a permanent part of your teeth. To be considered an acceptable restoration material, a substance must be:

• Durable.
• Biologically inert.
• Soft enough to fit into the cavity preparation, and then harden.
• Stable, able to withstand chewing forces.
• Able to expand and contract similarly to the tooth.
• A poor heat conductor, so as not to damage the tooth pulp.
• Able to seal the cavity preparation to prevent decay.

Amalgam fillings are the most commonly used restoration material for back teeth. These fillings contain silver, tin, copper, zinc, and mercury. Composite fillings and gold restorations are alternatives.

Silicate fillings are used in front teeth and contain silver, alumina, calcium or sodium phosphate, calcium fluoride, sodium aluminum fluoride, phosphoric acid, and aluminum and zinc phosphate. Composite fillings are an alternative to silicate fillings.

Composite fillings may be used for both front and back teeth. They bond well with enamel and make the tooth more resistant to decay at the margin between the tooth and the filling. Composites are basically ground glass powder with quartz fillers in a plastic binder. Other ingredients may include methylmethacrylate or aromatic dimethacrylates with additives of urethane, diacrylate, vinyl silane, benzoyl peroxide, and benzophenone ether. Composites may be either light cured or chemically cured, depending on their formulation. Sensitive persons tolerate the light-cured form better than the chemically-cured form.

Gold alloyed with palladium, silver, and trace amounts of copper, iron, indium, tin, and zinc is used in cast restorations. Crowns, inlays, and bridgework are all cast restorations. Non-precious metal crowns and bridges are an alternative, but nickel should not be used—it has both toxic and allergenic properties. The cement used to put cast restorations in place can be a problem for the sensitive person.

Porcelain, composed of minerals in a glass matrix, may be used for crowns. Gold restorations are an alternative.

Temporary fillings are used while crowns and bridgework are being prepared. They contain zinc oxide, eugenol, and trace amounts of alcohol, acetic acid, and silica. There are no substitutes with less toxic properties.

OTHER DENTAL PROCEDURES

Many dentists now use fluoride treatment for both children and adults. This is a controversial measure. Some authorities feel it has no benefit after age 11, while others feel it is beneficial for all ages. Still others regard fluoride treatment as administering a poison because of its toxicity.

Those sensitive to fluoride should avoid this treatment. Solutions commonly used all contain a flavoring agent to mask the taste of the fluoride compound, and some also have a coloring agent. In addition to the toxicity of the fluoride itself, the flavoring and coloring agents may also cause reactions in sensitive people.

Recent evidence points to the possibility that root canals may also be a problem for some people. Bacteria remaining in the tubules of the tooth are anaerobic (can survive without oxygen) and produce toxins. If these toxins seep out of the tooth and into the body, they can overload the immune system. A variety of symptoms and seemingly unrelated problems can be produced by these toxins.

Good dental hygiene is important and should include brushing and flossing after each meal and at bedtime. Chemically sensitive people should use a natural bristle toothbrush with a bone handle. Baking soda is a good substitute for toothpaste, although there are a few health store toothpastes that are acceptable (most commercial toothpastes contain glycerine and corn syrup). A good mouthwash is a capful of three percent hydrogen peroxide, several pinches of baking soda, and a little bit of water. Vitamin C (ascorbic acid) dissolved in water also makes an effective mouthwash; use three times per day. Follow with a water rinse to prevent damage to the tooth enamel.

Taking proper care of your teeth is important, not only for your general health, but in order to avoid the exposure of restoration materials used in fillings, crowns, bridges, and dentures. Good dental hygiene will help protect your teeth. Proper nutrition also will contribute to your health and aid in maintaining gum and tooth quality. Vitamin C, germanium (GeOxy 132), and coenzyme Q10 are important in restoring and preserving gum integrity. Calcium and magnesium are also essential for healthy tooth enamel and strong root and bone structure.

Trouble-Free Travel

Travelling, whether for short or long distances, can be a challenge for a person with allergies. However, you *can* travel safely and enjoyably when certain measures are taken.

Our usual mode of travel is by car, whether we are going to the local grocery store or across the country. Because new cars abound with chemical exposures from their interior materials, the chemically sensitive should purchase a well-outgased, used car that previously belonged to a non-smoker. Ideally, the car should be at least two years old, and have outside air vents that can be closed against traffic fumes.

Carefully examine a car before purchasing it. Test-driving the car for a few blocks may help identify major incompatibilities, but for more subtle problems, a drive in traffic, as well as an hour or two on the highway, is essential.

Your tolerance to upholstery fabrics and padding will have to be determined. Leather interiors may be a safe alternative to cloth or vinyl for some sensitive people. If the trunk lining causes a problem because of strong odors, leaking in around the back seat, the area between the back seat and the trunk may have to be sealed.

The car's exhaust and fuel systems should be maintained in top condition as leaks from both systems can find their way to the passenger area, especially in an older car. Leaks of engine oil, transmission fluid, antifreeze, and power brake fluid can also cause troublesome chemical exposures if they come in contact with a hot manifold or exhaust pipe.

When travelling in the city, keep the windows closed to avoid traffic fumes and operate the air conditioner on its maximum setting to recirculate inside air. Passengers in the front seat are usually exposed to fewer exhaust fumes than passengers in the back. Try to take less travelled, open air routes. When stopping in traffic, try to stay two to four car lengths from the vehicle in front of you. Using an automobile model air cleaner filters out chemicals, and wearing a charcoal mask while travelling is also helpful. Using oxygen while in your car will help some sensitive people prevent exposure to circulating allergens and clear reactions.

When travelling for long distances, it is usually necessary to find safe lodgings. Bed and breakfast establishments are a possibility if you can call ahead and inquire about smoking, cleaning products, clothes washing products, room deodorizers, and heating and cooling systems.

It is possible to minimize allergic reactions when staying in a motel or hotel if you ask for the following when you call for reservations:
• A nonsmoking room.
• A room without a deodorizer.
• A room not recently treated with pesticides or redecorated.
• A room cleaned with only baking soda in water (if possible).
• Airing of the room prior to your arrival.
• A room away from the pool, laundry area, and heating plant.
• A room in which windows can be opened.

You may have to take your own linens (sheets, pillowcases, and towels). Air cleaners are essential; you may need to open a window and run the air cleaner as well. Upon your arrival at the hotel or motel, it is wise to call the housekeeping personnel and reiterate cleaning instructions. If you are using your own linens, you will want to advise them about this. If you use their linens, request no linen changes during your stay to reduce your exposure to detergent, fabric softener, or gas dryer residue.

Water is often a concern when travelling. You can take your own, buy water after you arrive, carry a water purifying thermos or pitcher (available at health stores), or set water aside to outgas chlorine after you arrive.

Those with severe food allergies may need to take their own food to ensure an adequate supply of safe food. Alternatives include contacting the chef either before or just after you arrive to make specific arrangements for your meals. (We have found the majority of chefs to be very helpful and cooperative.) Purchasing food at a natural food store after you arrive is another option.

Airplane travel presents many challenges. Airports frequently are difficult to endure if smoking is allowed and ventilation is poor. Jet fuel exhaust is always present, as are the odors of the personal care products of your fellow passengers. Wearing a charcoal mask is helpful. Being prepared with chemical extracts to gas and diesel, smog, perfume mix, fabric softener, ethanol, phenol, formaldehyde, and cigarette smoke will reduce your allergic load. If the flight is an international one, the plane may be sprayed with pesticide before passengers are allowed to disembark. In some cases, arrangements can be made to deplane before the pesticide is applied.

A comfortable way to travel is with a travel trailer. Your safe bedroom goes with you, and you have a clean kitchen facility in which to prepare meals, and there can also be a safe bath and shower. Motor homes are not recommended, however, since engine odors can easily enter the vehicle's interior.

CHAPTER 19

The Emotional and Psychological Impact of Environmental Illness

All illness has an emotional and psychological impact. Perhaps more than any other illness, environmental sensitivity illustrates our mind/body interrelationship very graphically. Environmental illness can masquerade as virtually any type of physical or psychological disorder. The healing process draws attention to the subtle, complex interplay between our mind (psychological) and our body (physiological). The more severe the environmental illness, the more important this relationship becomes.

Basis for Emotional and Psychological Impact

Chemical Changes

Chemical changes, which occur in our body when we experience an adverse reaction to something in our environment, are one cause of the emotional and psychological dimensions of environmental illness. During a reaction, histamine, endorphins, neurotransmitters, hormones, leukotrienes, or enkephalins (all chemicals produced by the body) are either released in excess, suppressed, or altered, and they affect normal brain functions. These changes in the brain cause symptoms, including alterations in thought, feelings, behavior, mood, and personality. Symptoms vary from one person to the next depending on the severity of the sensitivity and the degree of allergen exposure. Those mildly affected may feel only anger or depression, while more severely ill people may experience the entire range of symptoms.

A considerable number of clinical ecologists have demonstrated conclusively that behavioral and emotional disturbances can result from adverse reactions to toxic and nontoxic substances found in our everyday environment. Symptoms may include depression, anxiety, cognitive malfunctions, perceptual disorders, suicidal feelings, hyperactivity, and lethargy.

This same range of symptoms can occur with illnesses such as Epstein-Barr virus, *Candida albicans*, parasitic or bacterial infections, and Chronic Fatigue Syndrome. One may react to the organism itself, to the toxins released by the organism, to debris left by the dead organism, or to one's own immune response to the organism. The presence of these organisms in an environmentally sensitive person can complicate diagnosis.

Affected people suffer a great amount of emotional and psychological stress as they react to nontoxic, common substances that a healthy person can tolerate. The environment suddenly becomes painfully different and threatening.

Effects of Diagnosis and Treatment

The second cause of emotional and psychological problems for the environmentally ill is directly related to the diagnosis and treatment of the illness.

One's health history often reveals a prolonged, gradually deteriorating picture before an accurate diagnosis of environmental illness is made. Usually, a variety of medical specialists have been consulted, resulting in thick medical files and high costs. Often the person is labelled a hypochondriac, and other people become weary of hearing the various incessant complaints. The severely ill person becomes exhausted, financially depleted, dependent on society, worried that perhaps there is no explanation or treatment, or frightened that this disease will prove totally disabling or fatal. All of these factors place an enormous stress load on an already burdened psyche.

When the diagnosis is made, your response may be one of relief that the problem is not "all in your mind." This may be mixed with feelings of anger that it took so long to arrive at a diagnosis. You may feel angry toward the physician making the diagnosis—a type of "kill the messenger" phenomenon.

The diagnosis of severe environmental illness often precipitates a major life crisis. Harsh realities must be faced regarding lifestyle changes, changes in workplace, disruption of employment, financial burdens, and pressure caused by lengthy, often complicated allergy treatment. Even treatment of mild sensitivities necessitates some changes.

Often, friends and family are critical of the sufferer's need for change, and even small changes can upset others. The person may feel guilty for causing these problems, and also feel unsupported or, at times, even like a social outcast.

Sources of Stress

Additional sources of emotional and psychological stress are imposed on people with environmental illness. These stresses are similar to those imposed by any chronic illness.

Frustration

Frustrations mount from the process of the illness itself. Everything appears, at first, to be "off limits." For a long while, it may seem that every step forward necessitates giving up something familiar and important. It is frustrating being unable to count on your own ability to think, make decisions, or perform physically or sexually. You no longer feel in control of your life. Every hour of the day can be filled with changing symptoms, depending on various exposures.

You will encounter frustration as you and your clinician try to determine causes in the complex puzzle of this illness. There are additional frustrations as you temporarily become more ill when offending substances are withdrawn, or when invading organisms are eliminated (withdrawal syndrome). Responses of anxiety, depression, anger, or fear are understandable in the face of such an array of frustrations.

All environmentally ill people are temporarily overwhelmed by the need for dietary and environmental changes. You may experience feelings of rebellion, disbelief, and denial that such a problem really exists. Some reject, for a time, the measures that must be followed to attain good health. Added frustration ensues when an overnight cure cannot be offered. You may strongly resent that your lifestyle has been so rudely interrupted with health problems.

The steps that follow diagnosis also place a load on emotional stability.

RESPONSIBILITY

Responsibility for much of the treatment for environmental illness falls to the patient. This approach seems foreign to most people in an age where responsibility for disease control is placed on the health practitioner. A mental struggle often ensues between a desire for improved health and an aversion to so much responsibility. This is complicated by the fact that the sufferer is already exhausted and severely stressed. At this point, it may take time for the sufferer and the family to accept the realities of this illness.

If you are unable to accept responsibility for your own health improvement, an unfortunate state of dependency may result, carrying a large, psychological impact. You may become unnaturally dependent on society, spouse, friends, or health practitioners, and be "stuck" in a mode of recounting symptoms, laying blame on others, and making unrealistic and unnecessary demands on those people involved with your care. You may give up trying to help yourself, and may become rebellious, withdraw into despair and isolation, or reject treatment.

SELF-EDUCATION

Self-education is the next stage toward controlling environmental illness. Well-thought-out decisions need to be made to make the environment as safe as possible and conducive to healing. Practitioners in environmental medicine can provide a wealth of information so you can make choices. Your choices should be acceptable to family and employers, involve the least risk, require the least financial commitment, and provide the greatest health benefit. This major life reorientation will require a great deal of attention and constitutes an enormous stress.

IDENTITY CRISIS

An identity crisis may also surface at some time during recovery. Having to change your self-image from a productive, functioning person to a chronically ill person can be devastating to the ego. This problem has to be faced by anyone experiencing a chronic or debilitating illness. Fear of doing "irreversible damage" to your body accompanies this change in self-concept. Losing your ability to cope with the everyday environment can also damage your self-worth.

In our society, a person's identity is strongly associated with career. When your career is terminated or changed because of environmental illness, self-pride and identity are assaulted. As your self-awareness increases, the patterns that have contributed to a state of overload become apparent. Many of us are forced to re-examine fundamental beliefs and goals, to reconsider our life values, and to reassess our talents and skills.

DILEMMA

When treatment begins, you may find it baffling that progress toward recovery is not always upward. One day you feel quite well and see improvement from treatment. Another day, you react severely to an allergen exposure and fear once again that you will never be well. Another hour or day passes, the allergen is removed, the reaction clears, and improvement begins again. This "bouncing" toward recovery is a continuing stress, and others around you are confused by these shifts in health and mood. Others' reactions may range from sympathetic curiosity to disbelief, from sincere offers of help to anxious avoidance, and from warm acceptance to personal blame. In order to test the validity of your illness, others may even deliberately initiate exposures that can cause debilitating reactions.

RELATIONSHIPS

The environmentally ill person needs stable, constructive, unconditional support. Often that personal network of support is lost when family and friends fail to understand the sufferer's fluctuations in personality and health.

The stress of changes in interpersonal relationships creates another burden on your psyche at a time when you most need nurturing, acceptance, and understanding. Expectations of permanence and predictability in relationships are sometimes shattered.

SELF-PITY

A feeling of entrapment can affect your approach to life, if you succumb to the idea that you are a "victim" rather than a "victor." You may be tempted to blame the environment, the government, physicians and staff, family, friends, time of day or night, world affairs, or the weather. If this outlook continues, progress toward health will be impeded. The "poor me" approach includes:

- Repeatedly reviewing symptoms and past history.
- Indulging in negative thinking and wallowing in self-pity.
- Projecting anger and blame onto other people or circumstances.
- Bemoaning your fate.
- Creating internal stress with dispirited or hopeless thoughts and self-defeating beliefs or fears.
- Searching for "miracle" cures.
- Isolating and insulating yourself from every perceived threat.

You can see the world differently by changing your mind about what you want to see. See yourself as happy and healthy!

In the *Chronic Fatigue Syndrome*, Dr. Jesse Stoff claims that "if you argue for your disease and its limitations—they are yours." A "poor me" attitude can indeed make the disease yours forever, unless you take charge and reclaim your life and health.

SHAME

Some people are deeply ashamed when they cannot solve their own problems or direct the course of their lives. Shame also occurs for some when they become preoccupied with themselves as a result of environmental illness. In response to this temporary awkward feeling, they will hide their emotions, only to have them surface later in anxiety and confusion. As true awareness is gained, illusions and assumptions about oneself and one's weaknesses also become apparent, and there may be a temporary loss of self-esteem.

GIVING UP

Dr. Hans Selye concluded, after 50 years of research, that the factors that cause stress are not as important as the way we react to the stress. Fortunately, only a few people view their illnesses as hopeless. They believe that neither they nor anyone else can do anything about their problem. They respond with negativity to any suggested form of therapy:

"I tried that and it didn't work."

"My body tells me that I can't stand this treatment."

"I tried the diet for a week and it didn't do anything."

"It is impossible for me to give that up because...."

These people may try a form of treatment but stop it within a few days because "they are reacting to the treatment." This is not a valid assessment; in almost all cases, reactivity symptoms are those the sufferer had before treatment began.

With such a negative attitude, this person will withdraw further from other people and will eventually retreat into a shell. This mechanism, known as conservation/withdrawal, is a maladaptive emergency coping system used when adverse stimuli are too great.

NEEDING TO BE ILL

Another trap that sometimes develops is learning that others can be manipulated through chronic illness. This can occur when there are unresolved psychosocial problems. Illness can be an attention-getting or controlling device, a way to cope with rejection, or a method of extracting love from another. Some use their illness to escape from unpleasant circumstances with which they can no longer cope.

ANXIETY OR FEAR

The unknown or the future have always been sources of apprehension for many of us. During illness, this tendency easily becomes accentuated because coping skills are compromised.

You may feel fearful of the consequences of changes in lifestyle, occupation, living accommodations, or financial status. These unknowns create severe stress if they are not addressed. If you dwell on negative possibilities, they multiply, insidiously, into energy blocks that can lead to worsening of physical and emotional symptoms.

Stages of Loss

Interwoven with the emotional and psychological impacts of environmental illness is an added burden of loss—the loss of health and well-being. This loss makes us aware of our human frailty, and causes changes in us and in the course of our lives.

Dealing with the loss of health is similar to coping with loss of a loved one. There is a series of stages, outlined by Dr. Elizabeth Kubler-Ross in her book, *On Death and Dying*, which a person must experience to properly address the grief associated with a loss. The following process has been paraphrased to describe the loss of health in environmental illness.

The grieving process is very complex—there is no strict sequence for these stages. You may experience fluctuations between the stages, and one can occur before another. Each stage must be accepted and experienced to progress toward improved health. If movement from one phase to another does not occur, you may become "stuck," and the process of recovery may be delayed.

SHOCK

Even though you are aware of all of your symptoms, the shock of knowing that they are part of a larger, more complex picture can be temporarily overwhelming. A period of numbness may set in, where you cannot act on the information you have received about this type of illness and treatment.

Denial and Isolation

Since the course of environmental illness varies from day to day, depending on exposures to allergens or on the overload phenomenon, it is very easy to deny the existence of a long-term problem. Denial is readily reinforced by both popular and medical opinions, since treatment for environmental illness is unorthodox, unfamiliar, and often misunderstood. You are confronted with making a decision to accept treatment involving lifestyle changes and unconventional therapy at a time when decision-making is difficult and stressful.

The easier road is to deny the existence of a health problem or to search for another type of therapy. Some people remain in the denial stage by isolating themselves in remote areas in order to avoid exposures. They hope that the problem will magically disappear, rather than pursuing the causes of the illness and subsequent treatment. Others maintain denial by hiding under a canopy of psychotherapy, concluding that they would rather accept a diagnosis of mental illness than one of environmental illness.

Anger

It is not difficult to understand an angry response to ecological illness. Sometimes the anger is suppressed or mixed with liberal doses of self-pity. At other times, anger is expressed as blame against those who have tried to help, or as rejection of those who have expressed love or support.

The person affected by environmental sensitivities must fully experience this stage of anger before more progress can be made. Anger must be acknowledged, not suppressed, even if it is upsetting and volatile. You need assurance that this phase is inevitable, expected, and acceptable in the process of grief. You have real cause to be angry, hostile, and resentful. You may also express anger by being envious of people who enjoy good health. Ineffectual and unexpressed anger is damaging to your body's homeostasis.

Bargaining

This stage involves making secret deals with fate, with God, with a higher being, or with yourself. When indulging in a known allergen, you may promise that if you can be free of reaction from the offending substance, you will "be good" for a week or a month. If your allergic load is light enough at the time of the indulgence, you may not experience a reaction, and the bargaining may appear to have worked. This reinforces your actions and you will be apt to try this behavior again until the cumulative effect becomes overwhelming.

Another form of bargaining occurs when you fantasize that your physician can magically dispense good health in exchange for cooperative behavior. How marvelous it would be if this were true. The fantasy is dispelled, however, when you finally realize that this type of thinking is erroneous and manipulative, and that the final responsibility for good health lies with you.

Depression

Depression can be a primary physical reaction to an allergenic substance. It can also be a psychological response to the complexities of environmental illness. Your coping skills will be tested to the limit at this stage. Discouragement and often despair result whenever there is a setback. The question "Will I ever be well?" is followed by "Can I accept the limitations imposed by this illness?" This stage will weave throughout every other stage of grief, haunting the ill person with unresolved questions. Responses may vary from sadness to despair, crying to numbness, slowed responses to weakness, withdrawal to apathy, loneliness to self-imposed isolation, and from forgetfulness to feeling out of touch with reality. Again, this phase will pass if it is accepted and dealt with properly. This is a time when quality help and support from your physician, friends, and relatives should be accepted.

GUILT

Guilt is always lurking in the background for the environmentally sensitive person. "If only I had…" becomes a frequent indulgence. Guilt can become a special psychological burden, and self-forgiveness is imperative. It is easier to forgive others than to forgive yourself for real or imagined offences. You may feel that if you had done more, felt more, and been more of everything that this illness would not have occurred.

LONELINESS

Loneliness can develop when severely sensitive people change their lifestyle by giving up or changing employment or residence; when they are rejected by family or friends because of their "different" lifestyle; or when they isolate themselves from others to prevent reactions to normal, everyday substances.

ANXIETY AND PANIC

Anxiety is understandable when you must face the possibility of lifestyle changes. These changes not only affect you, but also others in close personal relationships. In addition, the stress of these stages of grief places a great demand on your adrenal glands. Continued stress will temporarily exhaust the adrenal system and a physical state of anxiety can result.

Another factor that can provoke temporary anxiety occurs when an environmentally ill person becomes acutely aware of situations or substances that cause reactions. Until you learn that steps can be taken to avoid or relieve reactions, you will probably feel threatened and anxious. If this anxiety is not alleviated, it can become a conditioned response.

ACCEPTANCE

Acceptance is not a one-time commitment leading to perfect health, but rather is a daily—sometimes hourly—dedication to working toward better health. The battle is not only with the physiology of your body but also with your psyche. Acceptance involves recognizing the limitations of your illness as well as the expansion to a new self with different coping skills. At some stage in every illness, we have to assume a degree of responsibility for ourselves, whether it involves completely revamping our lifestyles, changing our diets, or remembering to take supplements and extracts. Understanding the underlying concepts of the disease process and the preventive measures that can help alleviate our distress is essential. This open attitude and acceptance will help you progress to the final stage of hope.

THE FOCUS OF HOPE

There are many health-supporting mechanisms that can be used to change one's perception of environmental illness. Norman Vincent Peale proved that there is power in positive thinking. Norman Cousins' recovery from illness was a prime example of the curative powers of personal belief. He asks in his book, *Anatomy of an Illness*: "If negative emotions produce negative chemical changes in the body, wouldn't the positive emotions produce positive chemical changes? Is it possible that love, hope, faith, laughter, confidence, and will to live have therapeutic value?"

An environmentally sensitive person does not have to get stuck in depression or grief. We have been given the gift of an innate ability to maintain hope. Positive, constructive, enervating thoughts can aid recovery, and should be applied on a daily or hourly basis along with the other aspects of your therapy. In *Love, Medicine, and Miracles*, Dr. Bernie Siegel states that healing is a creative art, calling for all the hard work and dedication needed for other forms of creativity.

Taking Steps to Wellness

- Reduce stress in those areas over which you have control.
- Simplify your lifestyle.
- Determine your limits by "testing the waters." Reconcile what you want from life with what you can do.
- "Whatever you do, do it with a sense of joy, enthusiasm, and a purpose. This will gradually help with extending your powers of concentration, and strengthening your ability to make decisions." (Dr. Jesse Stoff, *Chronic Fatigue Syndrome*)
- Habits are hard to break; repetition is essential. Follow the adage, "Fake it until you make it."
- Take off the mask of adulthood and become a child again. The child in us loves to laugh. Aristotle described laughter as a "bodily exercise precious to health."

- Use visual imagery—see yourself as a healthy person.
- Start each day by concentrating on a beautiful music or a scene, poem, or affirmation. An affirmation can be as simple as one word: determination, energy, strength, hope, courage. Be inventive and design a new affirmation each week.
- Adopt a positive, hopeful attitude toward recovery from your illness. Concentrate on the present, not the past.
- Forgive yourself and others for any wrong-doing.
- Seek a personal sense of purpose and meaning by looking at new dimensions and definitions for your life. As Siegel said, "You can create your own opportunities out of the same raw materials from which other people create their defeats."
- Gain self-confidence in your coping ability.
- Adopt a spirit of thankfulness for the inherent gifts, talents, and abilities you possess. Give yourself a positive message.
- Improve your self-esteem. Hold on to your identity.
- Focus on wellness rather than on illness.
- Nurture a sense of humor—read comedies, cartoons. Let laughter be your best medicine.
- Focus on changes rather than on problems. Remember that you are in control.
- Seek spiritual support and comfort through meditation and prayer.
- Strengthen your interpersonal relationships.
- Work on a hobby that is compatible with your illness. When a negative thought occurs, replace it with positive, constructive work that will absorb you and stop the negative pattern from becoming a habit. Dr. Jesse Stoff writes: "Transforming negative thoughts is not merely saying 'no' to the negative thought. It

is a creative process of generating positive feelings from within."

- Recognize emotions and allow yourself to feel joy, hope, life, peace, love, and even anger, fear, and pain.
- Look for new beginnings in your lifestyle or occupation.
- Release feelings of anger, fear, guilt, or pain. Our emotions do not just happen to us—we choose them.
- Extend your talents and personality into the community around you. That community may consist of other environmentally ill people elsewhere in the country. Network with others.
- Learn to benefit each day from your experiences.
- Gradually restructure your faulty psychological defenses.
- Remember that you have choices and options as you learn how to live.
- Live life to the fullest each day even though you may experience some limitations. Stretch yourself a bit further in your endeavors each day.

In *Love, Medicine, and Miracles*, Dr. Siegel tells of a quotation found on a wall in a bombed-out basement in Germany, after the close of World War II. "I believe in the sun—even when it does not shine. I believe in God—even when I do not hear him speak." As you begin taking a positive approach to your life, this attitude may last only for a fleeting moment each day. However, your approach will expand and become a large part of your recovery from environmental illness. Set realistic goals by taking into consideration your strengths and weaknesses. Do not pass the point of exhaustion; these exercises of faith can be just as tiring as physical activity. It may be wise to set aside a few minutes each day to practice these positive concepts. By taking short breaks away from depressing thoughts, even physical symptoms of depression will begin to lift.

You have the innate ability—and the responsibility—to do something about your health. Working on a positive program to improve your health will give you an increased sense of well-being. Take one small step at a time that will lead to conscious control of your illness. Dr. Siegel describes a person who exercises hope and control as "an exceptional patient." These people learn to take charge of their lives, and they work hard to achieve health and peace of mind.

Seek out every avenue of help and support from traditional medicine as well as from alternative forms of healing. Use your symptoms as signposts for discovering treatments that are most effective, rather than as indicators of doom. Use your inner strength to overcome what may seem to be impossible; allow the innate restorative powers of your body to work their miracles.

GLOSSARY OF TERMS

Absorption: The process by which nutrients are taken up through the intestinal wall and passed into the bloodstream.

Acetaldehyde: An aldehyde found in cigarette smoke, vehicle exhaust, and smog. It is a metabolic product of *Candida albicans* and is synthesized from alcohol in the liver.

Acetylcholine: A neurotransmitter manufactured in the brain, used for memory and control of sensory input and muscular output signals.

Acid: Any compound capable of releasing a hydrogen ion; it will have a pH of less than 7.

Acute: Extremely sharp or severe, as in pain; can also refer to an illness or reaction that is sudden and intense.

Adaptation: Ability of an organism to integrate new elements into its environment.

Addiction: A dependent state characterized by cravings for a particular substance if that substance is withdrawn.

Additive: A substance added in small amounts to foods to alter the food in some way.

Adrenalin: Trade mark for preparations of epinephrine, which is a hormone secreted by the adrenal gland. It is used sublingually and by injection to stop allergic reactions.

Aerobic: Organisms or metabolic processes that require oxygen.

Aldehydes: A class of organic compounds obtained by oxidation of alcohols. Formalde-hyde and acetaldehyde are members of this class of compounds.

Alkaline: Basic, or any substance that accepts a hydrogen ion; its pH will be greater than 7.

Allergenic: Causing or producing an allergic reaction.

Allergens: Substances that cause adverse symptoms, such as pollens; molds; animal danders; food and drink (often those most liked or disliked); or chemicals found in air, water, or food.

Allergic reaction: Adverse, varied symptoms or a group of symptoms, unique to each person, resulting from the body's response to exposure to allergens.

Allergic shiners: Dark circles under the eyes, usually indicative of allergies.

Allergy: Attacks by the immune system on harmless or even useful things entering the body. Abnormal responses to substances usually well-tolerated by most people.

Amino acid: An organic acid that contains an amino (ammonia-like) chemical group; the building blocks that make up all proteins.

Anabolism: Metabolic process by which simple substances are synthesized into complex substances; shifts the body pH toward alkalinity. It involves the production of energy.

Anaerobic: Organisms or metabolic processes that do not require oxygen.

Anaphylactic shock: An infrequent, extreme, and immediate allergic reaction that can cause difficulty in breathing or even death.

Antibody: A protein molecule produced to protect the body. It is made by B-lymphocytes or plasma cells in response to a perceived foreign or abnormal substance or organism.

Antigen: Any substance recognized by the immune system that causes the body to produce antibodies; also refers to a concentrated solution of an allergen.

Antihistamine: A chemical that blocks the action of histamine that is released by the mast cells and basophils during an allergic reaction.

Antioxidant: A substance that slows oxidation. In nutrition, a substance that prevents damage from free radicals and results in oxygen sparing.

Artificial: Manmade in imitation of something natural.

Assimilate: To incorporate into a system of the body; to transform nutrients into living tissue.

Autoimmune: A condition resulting when the body makes antibodies against its own tissues or fluid. The immune system attacks the body it inhabits, which causes damage or alteration of cell function.

Basal temperature: A "resting" temperature used to determine hypothyroidism. Also used as a marker to follow effects of treatment for hypothyroidism.

Basophils: A type of white blood cell that mediates inflammatory reactions. They are functionally similar to mast cells and are found in mucous membranes, skin, and bronchial tubes.

B-cell: A white blood cell. It produces antibodies as directed by the T-cells.

Binder: A substance added to tablets to help hold them together.

Binding: The uniting of two substances, such as a mineral binding to an enzyme, or a neurotransmitter to a receptor site.

Bioaccumulation: Buildup of chemicals or substances in cells and tissues.

Biochemical individuality: A distinct cellular makeup that is basic and unique to each person. This determines cellular needs, responses, and metabolism.

Blood brain barrier: A cellular barrier that prevents certain chemicals from passing from the blood to the brain.

Buffer: A substance that minimizes changes in pH (acidity or alkalinity).

Candida albicans: A genus of yeastlike fungi normally found in the body. It can multiply and cause infections, allergic responses, or toxicity.

Candidiasis: An overgrowth of Candida organisms, which are part of the normal flora of the mouth, skin, intestines, and vagina.

Carbohydrate, complex: A large molecule consisting of simple sugars linked together, found in whole grains, vegetables, and fruits. Metabolizes more slowly to glucose (a body nutrient) than refined carbohydrates.

Carbohydrate, refined: A molecule of sugar that metabolizes quickly to glucose (a nutrient), for example, white flour, sugar, and white rice.

Cascade: A succession of metabolic events that accelerate an allergic reaction or immune response.

Catabolism: Metabolic process in which complex substances are broken down into simpler substances; shifts the body pH toward acidity. It involves the release of energy.

Catalyst: A chemical that speeds up a chemical reaction without being consumed or permanently affected in the process.

Cerebral allergy: Mental dysfunction caused by

sensitivity to foods, chemicals, inhalants, or toxins in the environment.

Cerebral symptoms: Symptoms that affect the brain, cognitive functions, and emotions.

Chelation: A process whereby an amino acid is combined with another substance to increase its absorption and ease its assimilation into the body.

Chronic: Of long duration; refers to constant pain, condition, or illness that has been present for a long time.

Clinical ecology: A branch of medicine that treats allergies and sensitivities through diet, environmental control, and immunotherapy techniques.

Coenzyme: Organic molecules that enhance or are necessary for enzyme function. Vitamins are among compounds that serve as coenzymes.

Cofactor: In nutrition, a substance necessary to cause a given process to take place. Minerals serve as cofactors.

Cumulative reaction: A type of reaction caused by an accumulation of allergens in the body.

Cyclic allergy: A type of allergy which, with abstinence and/or non-exposure, will disappear and will not reappear unless there is over-exposure to the substance.

Cytokine: A chemical produced by the T-cells during an infection as our immune system's second line of defense. Examples of cytokines are interleukin 2 and gamma interferon.

Desensitization: The process of building up body tolerance to allergens by the use of extracts of the allergenic substance.

Detoxification: A variety of methods used to reduce toxic materials accumulated in body tissues.

Die-off: Uncomfortable symptoms caused when cells of organisms rupture and release toxic metabolic products in the body.

Digestive tract: Includes the mouth, esophagus, stomach, small and large intestines, salivary glands, and portions of the liver and pancreas. Its function is to digest food and transfer nutrients and water from the external environment to the body's internal environment.

Disorder: A disturbance of regular or normal functions.

Eczema: Dry, itchy, noncontagious skin rash frequently caused by allergy.

Edema: Excess fluid accumulation in tissue spaces. May be local or generalized.

Electromagnetic: Refers to emissions and interactions of both electric and magnetic components. Magnetism arising from electric charge in motion. Has a definite amount of energy.

Elimination diet: A diet in which common allergenic foods and those suspected of causing allergic symptoms have been temporarily eliminated.

Endocrine: Refers to ductless glands that manufacture and secrete hormones into the bloodstream or extracellular fluids.

Endocrine system: Thyroid, parathyroid, pituitary, hypothalamus, adrenal glands, pineal glands, and the gonads. The intestinal tract, kidneys, liver, and placenta may also be included.

Endogenous: Originating from or due to internal causes.

Endpoint: The treatment dose as determined by serial dilution titration.

Environment: A total of circumstances and/or surroundings in which an organism exists. May be a combination of internal or external influences that can affect an individual.

Environmental illness: A complex set of symptoms caused by adverse reactions of the body to external and internal environments.

Environmental medicine physician: A physician who specializes in the diagnosis, management, and prevention of the disruption of body homeostasis that results from environmental exposures (foods, inhalants, and chemicals). Treatment may include a combination of environmental control, immunotherapy, nutritional supplements, and rotation diet, with minimal use of drugs.

Enzyme: A substance, usually protein in nature and formed in living cells, which starts or stops biochemical reactions.

Eosinophil: A type of white blood cell. Eosinophil levels may be high in some cases of allergy or parasitic infection.

Erythrocyte: Red blood cell.

Excipient: An inert substance added to a prescription or vitamin to give a certain consistency or form to the preparation.

Exocrine: Refers to substances released through ducts that lead to a body compartment or surface.

Exogenous: Originating from or due to external causes.

Extracellular: Situated or occurring outside a cell or cells.

Extract: Treatment dilution of an antigen (allergen) used in immunotherapy, such as a food, chemical, or pollen extract.

"Fight or flight": The activation of the sympathetic branch of the autonomic nervous system, preparing the body to meet a threat or challenge.

Fixed allergy: See *Permanent allergy*.

Food addiction: Similar to drug addiction; the person becomes "hooked" on a particular allergenic food and must keep eating it regularly in order to prevent withdrawal symptoms.

Food family: A grouping of foods according to their botanical or biological characteristics.

Free radical: A substance with unpaired electrons, which is attracted to cell membranes and enzymes where it binds and causes damage.

Gastrointestinal: Relating both to stomach and intestines.

Heparin: A substance released during allergic reactions. Preparations of heparin, in the proper concentrations and administered sublingually, have an anti-inflammatory action.

Histamine: A body substance released by mast cells and basophils during allergic reactions, which precipitates allergic symptoms.

Holistic: Refers to the view that health and wellness depend on a balance between mind, body, emotions, and spirit.

Homeopathic: Refers to giving minute amounts of remedies that in massive doses would produce effects similar to the condition being treated.

Homeostasis: The balance of functions and chemical composition within an organism that results from the actions of regulatory systems.

Hormone: A chemical substance that is produced in the body, secreted into body fluids, and is transported to other organs, where it produces a specific effect on metabolism.

Hydrocarbon: A chemical compound that contains only hydrogen and carbon.

Hypersensitivity: An acquired reactivity to an antigen that can result in bodily damage upon subsequent exposure to that particular antigen.

Hyperthyroidism: A condition resulting from over-function of the thyroid gland.

Hypoallergenic: Refers to products formulated to contain the fewest possible allergens. Such products are not necessarily safe for everyone.

Hypothyroidism: A condition resulting from under-function of the thyroid gland.

IgA: Immunoglobulin A, an antibody found in secretions associated with mucous membranes.

IgD: Immunoglobulin D, an antibody found on the surface of B-cells.

IgE: Immunoglobulin E, an antibody responsible for immediate hypersensitivity and skin whealing.

IgG: Immunoglobulin G (known as gammaglobulin), the major antibody in the blood that protects against bacteria and viruses.

IgM: Immunoglobulin M, the first antibody to appear during an immune response.

Immune system: The body's defense system, composed of specialized cells, organs, and body fluids. It has the ability to locate, neutralize, metabolize, and eliminate unwanted or foreign substances.

Immunocompromised: A person whose immune system has been damaged or stressed and is not functioning properly. May or may not be reversible, depending on the extent of the damage.

Immunity: Inherited, acquired, or induced state of being able to resist a particular antigen by producing antibodies to counteract it; mechanisms that maintain the uniqueness of self.

Immunoglobulin: A specific antibody.

Immunotherapy: Treatment with allergy extracts over a period of time, with doses of the extract based on individual test results.

Incitant: See *Allergen*.

Inflammation: The reaction of tissues to injury from trauma, infection, or irritating substances. Affected tissue can be hot, reddened, swollen, and/or tender. Oxygen availability may be reduced in these tissues.

Inhalant: Any airborne substance small enough to be inhaled into the lungs; e.g., pollen, dust, mold, and animal danders.

Intolerance: Inability of an organism to endure a substance.

Intracellular: Situated or occuring within a cell or cells.

Intradermal: Method of testing in which a measured amount of antigen is injected between the top layers of the skin.

Ion: An atom that has lost or gained an electron and thus carries an electrical charge.

Kinins: Peptides split from protein in inflamed areas. They affect specific target tissues and facilitate vascular changes in inflammation.

Latent: Concealed or inactive.

Leukocytes: White blood cells.

Lipids: Fats and oils that are insoluble in water. Oils are liquid at room temperature and fats are solid.

Lymph: A clear, watery, alkaline body fluid found in the lymph vessels and tissue spaces. Contains predominantly white blood cells.

Lymphocyte: A type of white blood cell, usually classified as T- or B-cells. There are many subsets.

Macrophage: A white blood cell that kills and ingests microorganisms and other body cells.

Maladaption: An alternative term used to describe sensitivity.

Masking: Suppression of symptoms due to frequent exposure to a substance to which a person is sensitive.

Mast cells: Large cells containing histamine, found in mucous membranes and skin cells. The histamine in these cells is released during certain allergic reactions.

Mediated: Serving as the vehicle to bring about a phenomenon. An IgE-mediated reaction is one in which IgE changes cause - the symptoms and the reaction to proceed.

Membrane: A thin sheet or layer of pliable tissue that lines a cavity, connects two structures, or provides a structural, selective barrier (e.g., cell membranes).

Metabolism: Complex chemical and electrical processes in living cells by which energy is produced and life is maintained. New material is assimilated for growth, repair, and replacement of tissues; waste products are excreted.

Metabolite: Any product of metabolism.

Migraine: A condition marked by recurrent severe headaches on one side of the head, often accompanied by nausea, vomiting, and light aura. These headaches are frequently attributed to food allergy.

Mineral: An inorganic substance. The major minerals in the body are calcium, phosphorus, potassium, sulfur, sodium, chloride, and magnesium.

Modulator: A molecule attached to a protein, which adapts the properties of other binding sites and regulates the functional activity of the protein.

Monocyte: A type of white blood cell.

Mucous membranes: Moist tissues forming the lining of body cavities that have an external opening, such as the respiratory, digestive, and urinary tracts.

Nervous system: A network made up of nerve cells, the brain, and the spinal cord, which regulates and coordinates body activities.

Neurotransmitter: A molecule that transmits electrical and/or chemical messages from nerve cell to nerve cell (neuron) or from nerve cells to muscle, secretory, or organ cells.

Neutralize: To render an allergic reaction inactive. In chemistry, rendering a substance neither acidic nor alkaline.

Neutralizing dose: The dilution of a particular antigen that gives relief from or prevents allergic symptoms. This treatment dose is determined by provocative-neutralization testing.

Nutrients: Vitamins, minerals, amino acids, fatty acids, and glucose, which are the raw materials needed by the body to provide energy, effect repairs, and maintain functions.

Optimal dose: Dose that gives the most complete relief for the longest period of time.

Organic foods: Foods grown in soil free of chemical fertilizers, and without pesticides, fungicides, or herbicides.

Orthomolecular: Pertaining to the "right" molecule; treating disease by supplying the proper balance and concentration of substances found in the body, such as vitamins, minerals, trace elements, amino acids, enzymes, and hormones.

Outgasing: The releasing of volatile chemicals that evaporate slowly and constantly from seemingly stable materials such as plastics, synthetic fibers, or building materials.

Overload: The overpowering of the immune system due either to massive, concurrent exposure or to low-level continuous exposure caused by many stresses, including allergens.

Oxidation: The chemical process by which a substance combines with oxygen and changes to another form. In chemistry, refers to that portion of a chemical reaction in which an electron is lost by an atom or group of atoms.

Parasite: An organism that depends on another organism (host) for food and shelter, contributing nothing to the survival of the host.

Pathogenic: Capable of causing disease.

Pathology: The scientific study of disease; its cause, processes, structural or functional changes, developments and consequences.

Pathway: The metabolic route used by body systems to facilitate biochemical functions.

Permanent allergy: An allergy to a substance that always provokes symptoms, even after prolonged abstinence.

Petrochemical: A chemical derived from petroleum or natural gas.

pH: A scale from 1 to 14 used to measure acidity and alkalinity of solutions. A pH of 1–6 is acidic; a pH of 7 is neutral; a pH of 8–14 is alkaline or basic.

Phagocyte: White blood cells possessing the ability to ingest bacteria, foreign particles, and other cells.

Phagocytosis: The process of ingestion and digestion by cells (for example, lymphocytes ingest bacteria).

Postnasal drip: The leakage of nasal fluids and mucus down into the back of the throat.

Precursor: Anything that precedes another thing or event, such as a physiologically inactive substance that is converted into an active enzyme, vitamin, or hormone.

Prostaglandins: A group of unsaturated, modified fatty acids with a regulatory function.

Provocative-neutralization: An allergy test that uses an antigen to provoke a reaction and then neutralizes the reaction with a lower or higher dose of the same antigen.

Radiation: The process of emission, transmission, and absorption of any type of waves or particles of energy, such as light, radio, ultraviolet, or X-rays.

Receptor: Special protein structures on cells where hormones, neurotransmitters, and enzymes attach to the cell surface.

Respiratory system: The system that begins with the nostrils and extends through the nose to the back of the throat and into the larynx and lungs.

Rotation diet: A diet in which a particular food and other foods in the same "family" are eaten only once every four to seven days.

Sensitivity: An adaptive state in which a person develops a group of adverse symptoms to the environment, either internal or external. Generally refers to non-IgE "allergic" reactions.

Sensitization: The process that leads to the development of allergic symptoms in persons intolerant to a specific substance.

Serotonin: A constituent of blood platelets and other organs that is released during allergic reactions. It also functions as a neurotransmitter in the body.

Steroid: A subclass of naturally occurring lipid molecules such as hormones, bile acids, precursors for vitamins, and certain natural drugs; in pharmacology, a synthetic compound used to suppress the action of the immune system.

Stress: Anything that places undue strain upon normal body functions. Stress may be internal in origin (disease, malnutrition, dysfunction of a system, or allergic reaction) or external (environmental factors or interpersonal relations).

Sublingual: Under the tongue; method of testing or treatment in which a measured amount of an antigen or extract is administered under the tongue, behind the teeth. Absorption of material is rapid.

Supplement: Nutrient material taken in addition to food in order to satisfy extra demands, effect repair, and prevent degeneration of body systems.

Susceptibility: An alternative term used to describe sensitivity.

Symptoms: A recognizable change in a person's physical or mental state, that is a departure from normal function, sensation, or appearance and may indicate a disorder or disease.

Synapse: A specialized junction between two nerve cells where the electrical and chemical activity in one cell affects the action of the second.

Syndrome: A group of symptoms or signs that, occurring together, produce a pattern typical of a particular disorder.

Synthesis: Combining of separate elements and substances to make a new, coherent whole.

Synthetic: Made in a laboratory; not normally produced in nature, or may be a copy of a substance made in nature.

Systemic: Affecting the entire body.

Target organ: The particular organ or system in an individual that will be affected most often by allergic reactions to varying substances.

T-cell: A white blood cell that instructs B-cells to produce antibodies in an allergic or immune reaction.

Tolerance: The capacity of the body to withstand repeated exposures without symptoms.

Tolerance threshold: The maximum amount of allergens, stress, and exposures that an individual can tolerate without having symptoms.

Toxicity: A poisonous, irritating, or injurious effect resulting when a person ingests or produces a substance in excess of his or her tolerance threshold.

Toxin: Poisonous, irritating, or injurious substance.

Trace mineral: An inorganic substance found in minute quantities in the body. The major trace minerals are chromium, cobalt, copper, iodine, iron, zinc, manganese, molybdenum, selenium, and vanadium.

Transmission: The conveyance or spread of an infectious disease from one person to another.

Universal reactor: A person who is allergic to or has symptoms from numerous materials.

Urticaria: Allergic hives or welts.

Vascular: Pertaining to blood vessels.

Vitamin: A complex organic molecule that must be present in trace amounts to maintain normal metabolic processes. Insufficient amounts result in deficiency states. Occurs naturally in plants and animals.

Wheal: A raised bump on the skin surface caused by injection of an antigen between the top layers of skin.

Withdrawal: Short-term, adverse symptoms experienced when a person avoids a substance to which he or she is allergic or addicted.

Xenobiotic: A substance that is foreign to the body, such as drugs, chemicals, fertilizers, insecticides, herbicides, or fungicides.

RECOMMENDED SOURCES
AND ORGANIZATIONS

Sources for Personal Use

For information on detoxification centers and testing, see "Sources for Professional Use."

CELLOPHANE BAGS

Erlander's Natural Products
P.O. Box 106, Dept. NN
Altadena, CA   91001
(818) 797-7004

CERAMIC OXYGEN MASKS
AND STAINLESS STEEL TUBING

Environmental Purification Systems
P.O. Box 191
Concord, CA   94522
(415) 682-7231

CERAMIC OXYGEN MASKS
AND TYGON TUBING

American Environmental Health
  Foundation
8345 Walnut Hill Lane
Dallas, TX   75231-4262
(214) 361-9515

COTTON CLOTHING
(FORMALDEHYDE FREE)

Canary Clothes
1173A Second Ave., Suite 320
New York, NY   10021

COTTON/SILK CHARCOAL MASKS

Diane Anderson
(cotton surgical-style flat masks)
52204 Avenida Juarez
La Quinta, CA   92253
(619) 564-1709

Sandra DenBrader, RN
(cotton and silk fitted masks)
114 Ray Street
Arlington, TX   76010
(817) 860-9299

ENVIRONMENTAL DESIGNER

Donna Shrier
825 Northlake
Richardson, TX   75080
(214) 235-0485

FURNITURE POLISH (PURE LEMON OIL)

Vermont Country Store
P.O. Box 3000
Manchester Center, VT   05255-3000
(802) 362-2400

Karen's Non-Toxic Products
P.O. Box 15
Malaga, NJ   08328
(800) 527-3674

Housing Consultants

Wayne Baltz
829 Gallup Road
Ft. Collins, CO   80521
(303) 493-6593

John Bower
Ecology Safe Homes
7471 North Shiloh Road
Unionville, IN   47468
(812) 332-5073

Masters Corporation
P.O. Box 514
New Canaan, CT   06840
(203) 966-3541

Mary Oetzel
Environmental Health Services
3202 W. Anderson Lane, #208-249
Austin, TX   78767
(512) 288-2369

David Rousseau
ArcRemy Consulting Ltd.
3683 West 4th Avenue
Vancouver, B.C.   V6R 1P2
Canada
(604) 737-8068

Bruce Small and Associates
Sunnyhill Research Centre
RR #1
Goodwood, ON   L0C 1A0
Canada
(416) 294-3531

Impregnated Fiber Charcoal Face Masks

E.L. Foust Co., Inc.
P.O. Box 105
Elmhurst, IL   60126
(800) 225-9549

Magnets

Enviro-Tech Products
17167 S.E. 29th Street
Choctaw, OK   73020
(405) 390-3009

Mold Test

Mold Survey Service
Dr. Sherry A. Rogers
2800 W. Genesee Street
Syracuse, NY   13219
(315) 488-2856

Nutritional, Antiparasitic and Antiviral Materials

Biological Homeopathic Industries, Inc.
   (BHI)
11600 Cochiti S.E.
Albuquerque, NM   87123
(800) 621-7644
(homeopathic remedies)

Cardiovascular Research/Arteria
1061-B Shary Circle
Concord, CA   94518
(800) 351-9429
(tapioca and sago palm vitamin C, Tri-Salts,
antiparasitic and antiviral preparations, and
other nutritional materials)

L. and C. Associates
5581 Woodsong Drive
Atlanta, GA   30338
(404) 396-8675
(carrot, potato, and sago palm vitamin C,
and other nutritional materials)

Miles Consumer Healthcare Division
1127 Myrtle Street
Ellehart, IN   46515
(219) 264-8111
(Alka Seltzer Gold)

Nutricology, Inc./
   Allergy Research Group
400 Preda Street
San Leandro, CA   94577
(800) 545-9960
(sago palm vitamin C, antiparasitic
preparations, and other nutritional materials)

Thorne Research
P.O. Box 3200
Sandpoint, Idaho   83864
(208) 263-1337
(Mycocidin)

Vital Life (Klaire Laboratories)
1573 W. Seminole
San Marcos, CA   92069
(619) 744-9680
(Bi-Carb Formula, powdered ascorbic acid,
and other nutritional materials)

SHOWER FILTERS

American Environmental Health
   Foundation
8345 Walnut Hill Lane
Dallas, TX   75231-4262
(214) 361-9515

Environmental Purification Systems
P.O. Box 191
Concord, CA   94522
(415) 284-2129

Purebasics
1903 Blake Drive
Richardson, TX   75081
(214) 231-2555

Sources for Professional Use

CAFFEINE METABOLISM TEST
FOR LIVER FUNCTION

Diagnos-Techs, Inc.
6620 S. 192nd Place, Suite J-104
Kent, WA   98032
(206) 251-0596

CHLORDANE TESTING

AccuChem Labs
990 N. Bowser Road, Suite 800
Richardson, TX   75081
(214) 234-5577

COMPREHENSIVE STOOL
AND DIGESTIVE ANALYSIS

Meridian Valley Clinical Laboratory
24030 132nd Avenue, S.E.
Kent, WA   98042
(206) 631-8922

Great Smokies Diagnostic Labs
18A Regent Park Blvd.
Ashville, NC   28806
(800) 522-4762

Detoxification Centers

Center for Environmental Medicine
7510 Northforest Drive
N. Charleston, SC   29418
(803) 572-1600

Environmental Health Center
8345 Walnut Hill Lane, Suite 205
Dallas, TX   75231
(214) 368-4132

Health Med
#1 Scripps Drive, Suite 201
Sacramento, CA   95826
(916) 924-8060

For information about detoxification in
Canada, contact:
Dr. Jozef Krop
RR #6
6901 Second Line West
Mississauga, ON   L5M 2B5
Canada

Dust/Dust Mite Collector

ALK Laboratories, Inc.
Indoor Allergen Analysis Laboratory
132 Research Drive
Milford, CT   06460
(800) 325-7354

Formaldehyde Test Kit

Occupational Health and
3M Safety Products Division
220-7W 3M Center
St. Paul, MN   55144-1000
(612) 733-8029

Heidelberg Gastrogram pH System

Heidelberg International, Inc.
6669 Peachtree Ind. Blvd., Suite K
Atlanta (Norcross), GA   30092
(404) 449-4888

Immunoglobulin E Test Kit

MAST Immunosystems Technical Service
630 Clyde Court
Mountain View, CA   94043
(800) 233-6273

Liver Function Test Kits for D-Glucaric Acid and Mercapturic Acid

Doctor's Data, Inc.
30 W 101 Roosevelt Road
West Chicago, IL   60185
(800) 323-2784

Parasite Test Kits for Mucosal Swabbing

Great Smokies Diagnostic Labs
18A Regent Park Blvd.
Ashville, NC   28806
(800) 522-4762

Sodium Thiosulfate Nose Drops

Idaho Falls Chem Lab
Judy Storms, Director
Homer Wolf, Pharmacist
862 10th Street
Idaho Falls, ID   83404
(208) 522-3246

Specimen Testing for Pesticides, Solvents, Herbicides, and Heavy Metals

AccuChem Labs
990 North Bowser, Suite 800
Richardson, TX   75081
(214) 234-5577

Vacuum Fume Extractor

Larry Ward
25885 Trabuco Road, #119
El Toro, CA   92630
(714) 770-9616

Organizations

Patient and Volunteer Organizations

H.E.A.L. (Human Ecology Action League)
P.O. Box 49126
Atlanta, GA   30359
(404) 248-1898

Human Ecology Foundation of Canada
46 Highway #8
Dundas, ON   L9H 4V3
Canada
(416) 628-8241

Professional Organizations

Contact for physician referrals.

Allergy Information Association
65 Tromley Dr., Suite 10
Etobicoke, ON   M9B 5Y7
Canada

American Academy of
  Environmental Medicine
P.O. Box 16106
Denver, CO   80216
(303) 622-9755

American Academy of Otolaryngic Allergy
1101 Vermont Ave. N.W., Suite 302
Washington, DC   20005
(202) 682-0456

Canadian Schizophrenia Foundation
7375 Kingsway
Burnaby, B.C.   V3N 3B5
Canada
(604) 521-1728

Pan American Allergy Society
P.O. Box 947
Fredericksburg, TX   78624
(512) 997-7467

Society for the Study of
  Biochemical Intolerance
1675 N. Freedom Blvd., Suite 11E
Provo, UT   84604
(801) 373-8500

RECOMMENDED BOOKS

You may want to read some of these books to further your understanding of your total health picture. Most of them are available at health stores and book stores.

A Consumer's Dictionary of Cosmetic Ingredients, Ruth Winter. Crown Publishers, Inc., New York, 1976.

Excellent for unraveling the mystery of cosmetic labelling. The material is understandable for people with no scientific training.

A Consumer's Dictionary of Food Additives, Ruth Winter. Crown Publishers, Inc., New York, 1984.

Helps consumers to understand food labelling and to make informed food choices.

The Allergy Self-Help Book, Sharon Faelten and Editors of *Prevention Magazine*. Rodale Press, Emmaus, PA, 1983.

Presents many practical tips on recognizing and avoiding specific allergens, and on understanding the effects of these substances. A section of the book discusses various types of allergy testing and treatment.

An Alternative Approach to Allergies, Theron G. Randolph and Ralph W. Moss. Harper and Row, New York, 1980.

Describes a new approach to allergy and chronic illness. Dr. Randolph shows that many illnesses, both physical and mental, are caused

by our contaminated indoor and outdoor environments.

Are Your Dental Fillings Hurting You? Guy Fasciana. Health Challenge Press, Springfield, MA, 1986.

Discusses the relationship between chronic illness and mercury toxicity from amalgam dental fillings. Written for dentists, physicians, and patients, this book includes dental physiology, evidence of toxicity and its effect on the immune system, and considerations for alternative filling materials.

Back to Health, Dennis Remington and Barbara Higa. Vitality House International, Provo, UT, 1986.

A comprehensive, easy-to-read guide to Candidiasis, its problems, and its treatments. A new approach to treating obesity is also introduced.

Biomagnetic Handbook, William Philpott and Sharon Taplin. Envirotech Products, Choctaw, OK, 1980.

A guide to the use of magnetic energy in diagnosing and treating health problems.

Brain Allergies, William H. Philpott and Dwight Kallta. Keats Publishing, Inc., New Canaan, CT, 1980.

Presents an overview of depression, schizophrenia, and degenerative disease as they relate to food allergy/addiction and to other substances to which our body is exposed.

Dr. Wright's Book of Nutritional Therapy, Jonathan Wright. Rodale Press, Emmaus, PA, 1979.

Explores the underlying cause of many illnesses that can be alleviated with natural and nutritional therapies. He also discusses the importance of preventive health care. The many case histories make this book easy to follow.

Dr. Wright's Guide to Healing with Nutrition, Jonathan Wright. Rodale Press, Emmaus, PA, 1984.

Reviews case histories with suggestions for treatment with nutritional supplements and diet adjustments.

The Electromagnetic Man, Cyril Smith and Simon Best. St. Martin's Press, New York, 1989.

Presents the effect on biosystems of electrical impulses, ranging from large-scale electromagnetic phenomena to the low-frequency fields produced by man-made sources.

Feed Your Kids Right, Lendon Smith. Dell Publishing Company, Inc., New York, 1979.

Discusses health problems that can be prevented by a proper diet. Dr. Smith presents a nutritional program, including both diet and supplements, which will give children optimal physical and mental health from infancy through adolescence.

Food, Mind, and Mood, David Sheinkin, Michael Schachter, and Richard Hutton. Warner Books, New York, 1979.

Explores the effects of cerebral allergy in a concise format. Food and nutrient excesses, deficiencies, or sensitivities can play a major role in brain function, mood, and chronic disease.

Freedom from Allergy Cookbook, Dr. Ron Greenberg and Angela Nori. Blue Poppy Press, Vancouver, B.C., 1991. 3rd edition.

Contains over 200 healthy and delicious wheat-, yeast-, and dairy-free recipes organized clearly for people on rotation diets.

How to Control Your Allergies, Robert Foreman. Larchmont Books, New York, 1979.

Enables the reader to begin to identify and control problems of mind and body that are caused by food allergies and chemical susceptibility.

Human Ecology and Susceptibility to the Chemical Environment, Theron Randolph. Charles C. Thomas, Publisher, Springfield, IL, 1962.

A classic book on clinical ecology written by a pioneer in this emerging field of medicine. Dr. Randolph describes chemical susceptibility problems and a working model of the stages of allergy/addiction.

If It's Tuesday, It Must Be Chicken, Natalie Golos and Frances Goldbitz. Keats Publishing, Inc., New Canaan, CT, 1983.

A practical guide to help incorporate the rotation diet concept into everyday menu planning.

Is This Your Child? Doris Rapp. William Morrow and Co., Inc., New York, 1991.

An excellent guide for identifying allergies related to health problems in children. All aspects of treatment are presented, and practical advice on diet and home environment is provided.

Mental and Elemental Nutrients, Carl Pfeiffer.

Keats Publishing, Inc., New Canaan, CT, 1975.

Approaches the subject of nutritional therapy from a psychiatrist's viewpoint. Dr. Pfeiffer discusses each nutrient, its effect in our body, the symptoms of deficiency, and its use in therapy.

The Nontoxic Home, Debra Lynn Dadd. Jeremy P. Tarcher, Inc., Los Angeles, 1986.

A complete guide to maintaining a nontoxic home and lifestyle, with an emphasis on safe products and alternatives.

Solved: The Riddle of Illness, Stephen E. Langer and James F. Scheer. Keats Publishing, Inc., New Canaan, CT, 1984.

Expands on the information about the thyroid gland first presented by Dr. Broda Barnes. The role of hypothyroidism in chronic fatigue and chronic illness is discussed.

Tired or Toxic? Sherry Rogers. Prestige Publishers, Syracuse, NY, 1990.

An informative book for laymen and physicians about the biochemical effects of the environment on individuals. It also includes methods of detoxifying our body and environment in order to return to healthful living.

Type I, Type II Allergy Relief Program, Alan Levin and Merla Zellerbach. Jeremy P. Tarcher, Inc., Los Angeles, 1983.

Describes varied syndromes presented by sensitive individuals to help identify the classic problems associated with allergy and the resulting breakdown of the immune system. Outlines self-help methods.

Victory Over Diabetes, William Philpott and Dwight Kalita. Keats Publishing, Inc., New Canaan, CT, 1983.

A comprehensive presentation of the effect of stress caused by allergic/addictive reactions, which can affect pancreatic function. Includes a detailed discussion of the rotation diet program and ways to enhance our body's resources for maintaining a healthy lifestyle.

Vitamin C Connection, Emanuel Cheraskin, W. Marshall Ringsdorf, and Emily L. Sisley. Harper & Row Publishers, New York, 1983.

A well-documented text on the beneficial effects of vitamin C on cell metabolism, immune function, and biochemical processes in our body. Contains valuable aids in determining individual use and dose of vitamin C.

The Yeast Syndrome, John Parks Trowbridge. Bantam Books, New York, 1986.

Explores the clinical symptoms, physiological effects, diagnostic techniques, and treatment procedures of chronic yeast infections. It offers hope to those who have suffered from these organisms.

Your Home, Your Health, and Well-Being, David Rousseau, William Rea, and Jean Enwright. Hartley and Marks, Inc./Ten Speed Press, Pt. Roberts, WA, 1988.

A detailed guide for creating a living and working space that is free from toxic chemicals. Indoor health hazards, building materials, air quality products, water and electrical systems, and heating and cooling systems are all reviewed in careful detail.

BIBLIOGRAPHY

Abrahamson, E. M., and Pezet, A. W. *Body, Mind, and Sugar*. New York: Avon, 1951.

Altman, Philip L., and Dittmar, Dorothy S. *Metabolism*. Bethesda, MD: Federation of American Societies for Experimental Biology, 1968.

American Cancer Society. "General Facts on Smoking and Health." November 1985.

American Cancer Society. "Women and Smoking." November 1985.

Asai, Kazukiko. *Miracle Cure: Organic Germanium*. Tokyo: Japan Publications, Inc., 1980.

Ashford, Nicholas, and Miller, Claudia. *Chemical Sensitivity, A Report to the New Jersey State Department of Health*. December 1989.

Baines, T. M.; Somes, J. H.; and Hellman, K. H. "Effects of Fuel Variables on Diesel Emissions." *Journal of the Air Pollution Control Association* 32(8):810–15 (1982).

Baines, T.; Somers, J. H.; and Hellman, K. H. "EPA Motor Vehicle Emissions Characterization Projects on Light and Heavy Duty Diesels." *Journal of the Air Pollution Control Association* 32(7):725–28 (1982).

Baker, Sidney, and Galland, Leo. "Case Presentations: Magnesium, Histamine, Allergic Reactions." Presented at Evaluating and Treating the Environmentally Sensitive/Complex Patient, San Diego, CA, January 18, 1987.

Barbul, A., and Seifter, E. "Wound Healing and Thymotropic Effects of Arginine: A Pituitary Mechanism of Action." *American Journal of Clinical Nutrition* 37:786 (1983).

Barnes, Broda O., and Galton, Lawrence. *Hypothyroidism: The Unsuspected Illness*. New York: Harper & Row, 1976.

Bartholmew, Mel. *Square Foot Gardening*. Emmaus, PA: Rodale Press, 1981.

Beaver, P. C.; Jung, Rodney C.; and Cupp, Eddie W. *Clinical Parasitology*. Philadelphia: Lea and Febiger, 1984.

Becker, Robert O. *Cross Currents*. Los Angeles: Jeremy P. Tarcher, Inc., 1990.

Becker, R. O., and Selden, G. *The Body Electric*. New York: William Morrow and Company, 1985.

Bell, Iris. *Clinical Ecology*. Bolinas, CA: Common Knowledge Press, 1982.

Bell, Iris. "Environmental Illness and Health: The Controversy and Challenge of Clinical Ecology for Mind–Body Health." *Advances* IV(3):45–55 (1987).

Bellanti, Joseph A. *Immunology III*. Philadelphia: W. B. Saunders Company, 1985.

Bender, Arnold E. *Dictionary of Nutrition and Food Technology*. Stoneham, MD: Butterworth, 1982.

Bionic Products. "Components of Sidestream Smoke." *Manual for Eleventh Clinical Ecology Instructional Course, Part I—Primary*. Aurora, CO: 15 (April 18–20, 1986).

Bland, Jeffrey. *Your Health Under Siege*. Brattleboro, VT: Stephen Greene Press, 1982.

Bland, Jeffrey. "Therapeutic Uses of Nutrition: Vitamins A to Zinc." Presented at Denver, CO, December 8–9, 1984.

Bland, Jeffrey. "Introductory Nutrition." Audio Training Series. Torrance, CA: 1985.

Bland, Jeffrey, ed. *The 1984–1985 Yearbook of Nutrition Medicine*. New Canaan, CT: Keats Publishing, Inc., 1985.

Bland, Jeffrey, ed. *Medical Applications of Clinical Nutrition*. New Canaan, CT: Keats Publishing, Inc., 1985.

Bliznakov, Emile, and Hunt, Gerald. *The Miracle Nutrient Coenzyme Q_{10}*. Toronto: Bantam Books, 1987.

Bradshaw, John. *Homecoming: Reclaiming and Championing Your Inner Child*. New York: Bantam Books, 1990.

Braverman, Eric R., with Pfeiffer, Carl. *The Healing Nutrients Within*. New Canaan, CT: Keats Publishing, Inc., 1987.

Breneman, James C. *Basics of Food Allergy*. Springfield, IL: Charles C. Thomas, 1984.

Bricklin, Mark, and Claessens, Sharon. *The Natural Healing Cookbook*. Emmaus, PA: Rodale Press, 1981.

Brodeur, Paul. *Currents of Death*. New York: Simon and Schuster, 1989.

Brody, Jane. *Jane Brody's Nutrition Book*. New York: W. W. Norton & Company, 1981.

Brostaff, Jonathan. "The Brain–Allergy Axis." *American Academy of Environmental Medicine Newsletter* 20(3):1 (Summer 1985).

Brostaff, Jonathan, and Challacombe, Stephen J. *Food Allergy and Intolerance*. London: Bailliere Tindall, 1987.

Brown, Norman. "10 Foods to Keep Your Immune System Fit." *Let's Live* (August 1986):32–34.

Bucholz, Ilene K.; Cook, Karen S.; and Randolph, Theron G. *An Alternative Measure*. Chicago: Human Ecology Research Foundation, 1982.

Budoff, Penny Wise. *No More Menstrual Cramps and Other Good News*. New York: Penguin Books, 1980.

Buist, Robert. *Food, Chemical Hypersensitivity*. Garden City Park, NY: Avery Publishing Group, Inc., 1988.

Buist, Robert. "New Light on Chronic Fatique Syndrome." *Journal of Orthomolecular Medicine* III(3):186–89 (1988).

Burks, A.; Mallory, S.; Williams, L.; and Shirrell, M. "Atopic Dermatitis: Clinical Rebalance of Food Hypersensitivity Reactions." *Journal of Pediatrics* 113(3):447–51 (1988).

Calabrese, Edward J., and Dorsey, Michael W. *Healthy Living in an Unhealthy World*. New York: Simon and Schuster, 1985.

Cameron, Evan, and Pauling, Linus. *Cancer and Vitamin C*. Palo Alto, CA: The Linus Pauling Institute, 1979.

Cardiovascular Research. "Clinical Uses of Coenzyme Q_{10}." Pamphlet, Cardiovascular Research, Ltd. Concord, CA: 1985.

Cathcart, Robert F. "The Method for Determining Proper Doses of Vitamin by Titrating to Bowel Tolerance." *Journal of Orthomolecular Psychiatry* X(2):125–32 (1981).

Cathcart, Robert F. "Vitamin C: The Nontoxic Nonratelimited, Antioxidant Free Radical Scavenger." *Medical Hypothesis* 18:61–77 (1985).

Cathcart, Robert F. "The Vitamin C Treatment of Allergy and the Normally Unprimed State of Antibodies." *Medical Hypothesis* 21(3):307–21 (1986).

Cernansky, Nicholas P. "Diesel Exhaust Odor and Irritants: A Review." *Journal of the Air Pollution Control Association* 33(2):97–104 (1983).

Chaitow, Leon. *Amino Acids in Therapy*. Rochester, VT: Healing Arts Press, 1988.

Challem, Jack Joseph. *Vitamin C Updated*. New Canaan, CT: Keats Publishing, Inc., 1983.

Challem, Jack Joseph, and Lewin, Renate. "Turn Off Your Allergies with Neutralization Therapy." *Let's Live* (March 1987):34–36.

Challem, Jack Joseph, and Lewin, Renate. "War in the Wards: A Guide for Surviving Surgery and the Hospital." *Let's Live* (May 1987):10–14.

Cheraskin, E.; Ringsdorf, M. W.; and Clark, J. W. *Diet and Disease*. New Canaan, CT: Keats Publishing, Inc., 1977.

Cheraskin, E.; Ringsdorf, W. M.; and Sisley, E. L. *The Vitamin C Connection*. New York: Harper & Row, 1983.

Choy, Ray; Monro, Jean; and Smith, Cyril. "Electrical Sensitivities in Allergy Patients." *Clinical Ecology* IV(3):93–101 (November 1986).

Clark, Linda. "More Help for Your Allergies, Part II." *Let's Live* (February 1981):89–99.

Clendening, Logan. *Source Book of Medical History*. New York: Dover Publications, Inc., 1942.

Colgan, Michael. *Your Personal Vitamin Profile*. New York: William Morrow and Company, Inc., 1982.

Colgrove, Melba; Bloomfield, Harold; and McWilliams, Peter A. *How to Survive the Loss of a Love*. New York: Bantam Books, 1976.

Cousins, Norman. *Healing Heart*. New York: Avon Books, 1984.

Cousins, Norman. *Head First, The Biology of Hope*. New York: E. P. Hutton, 1989.

Cousteau, Jacques-Yves. *The Cousteau Almanac*. New York: Doubleday and Company, 1981.

Crook, William G. *Tracking Down Hidden Food Allergy*. Jackson, TN: Professional Books, 1980.

Crook, William G. *The Yeast Connection*. Jackson, TN: Professional Books, 1983.

Dadd, Debra Lynn, and Levin, Alan S. *A Consumer Guide for the Chemically Sensitive*. San Francisco: Nontoxic Lifestyles, Inc., 1982.

Dadd, Debra Lynn. *Nontoxic and Natural*. Los Angeles: Jeremy P. Tarcher, Inc., 1984.

Dadd, Debra Lynn. *The Nontoxic Home*. Los Angeles: Jeremy P. Tarcher, Inc., 1986.

Davis, Roy, and Rawls, Walter. *Magnetism and Its Effect on the Living System*. Kansas City, MO: Acres USA, 1988.

Dickey, Lawrence D., ed. *Clinical Ecology*. Springfield, IL: Charles C. Thomas, 1976.

Dickey, Lawrence D., and Maclennan, John G. *Clinical Ecology Office Procedures Manual*, 6th ed. (1981).

Duncan, Bruce. "Chronic Fatigue Syndrome." Pre-publication manuscript. Palmerston, North New Zealand (1989).

Eagle, Robert. *Eating and Allergy*. Garden City, NY: Doubleday and Company, 1979.

Ecological Formulas. "Free Radical Quenchers." Pamphlet, Ecological Formulas. Concord, CA: n.d.

Editors of *Prevention Magazine*. *Everyday Health Hints*. Emmaus, PA: Rodale Press, 1985.

Eurman, Nina. "The Immunity Arsenal vs. the Attackers." *Let's Live* (August 1986):16–19.

Faelten, Sharon, and Editors of *Prevention Magazine*. *The Allergy Self-Help Book*. Emmaus, PA: Rodale Press, 1983.

Fasciana, Guy S. "The E.I. Dentist—Dental Materials Part I." *The Human Ecologist* (25):9–11 (Spring 1984).

Fasciana, Guy S. "The E.I. Dentist—Dental Materials Part II." *The Human Ecologist* (26):11–12 (Summer 1984).

Fasciana, Guy S. *Are Your Dental Fillings Hurting You?* Springfield, MA: Health Challenge Press, 1986.

Feingold, Ben F. *Why Your Child Is Hyperactive*. New York: Random House, 1975.

Finn, R., et al. "Hydrocarbon Exposure and Glomerulonephritis." *Clinical Nephrology* 14(4):173–75 (1980).

Foreman, Robert. *How to Control Your Allergies*. New York: Larchmont Books, 1979.

Fox, Arnold. "The B Complex." *Let's Live* (February 1984):18–22.

Fox, Arnold, and Fox, Barry. "Take Care of Your Immune System." *Let's Live* (August 1986):10–14.

Fox, Arnold, and Fox, Barry. "Super Foods and Your Immune System." *Let's Live* (October 1986):10–14.

Fox, Arnold, and Fox, Barry. "Supplementing Your Immune System." *Let's Live* (July 1987):14–18.

Fox, Arnold, and Fox, Barry. "Immunity." *Let's Live* (October 1987):10–17.

Franz, Marion. *Fast Food Facts*. Wayzato, MN: Diabetes Center, 1987.

Frazier, Claude. *Coping With Food Allergy*. New York: Quadrangle Press, 1974.

Frazier, Claude. *Coping and Living With Allergies*. Englewood Cliffs, NJ: Prentice-Hall, 1980.

Frazier, Claude, and Brown, F. K. *Insects and Allergy*. Norman, OK: University of Oklahoma Press, 1980.

Fuchs, Kathryn. *The Nutrition Detective*. New York: St. Martin's Press, 1985.

Gaby, Alan. *The Doctor's Guide to Vitamin B6*. Emmaus, PA: Rodale Press, 1984.

Galland, Leo, with Buchman, Dian Dincin. *Superimmunity for Kids*. New York: C. P. Dutton, 1988.

Garfinkle, Ellen. "The Role of Psychotherapy in the Treatment of Environmental Illness." Source unknown.

Garrison, Robert Jr. *Lysine, Tryptophan and Other Amino Acids*. New Canaan, CT: Keats Publishing, Inc., 1982.

Gaul, John W. "The Immune System." *Let's Live* (October 1981):117–21.

Golos, N.; Golbitz, F.; and Leighton, F. *Coping With Your Allergies*. New York: Simon and Schuster, 1979.

Golos, N., and Golbitz, F. *If This Is Tuesday, It Must Be Chicken*. New Canaan, CT: Keats Publishing, Inc., 1983.

Golos, Natalie; O'Shea, James F.; and Waickman, Francis J.; with Golbitz, Frances Golos. *Environmental Medicine*. New Canaan, CT: Keats Publishing, Inc., 1987.

Grant, Alexander, ed. "Aspartame Headache." *Healthwise* XI(6):1 (June 1988).

GY&N–Nutrient Pharmacology. "L-Carnitine." Pamphlet, GY&N–Nutrient Pharmacology. Carlsbad, CA: n.d.

Hagglund, Howard E., and Ferrier, Marsha. *Help! I Feel Awful!* Norman, OK: HEH Medical Publications, 1985.

Hahn, L. J.; Kloiber, R.; Viney, M. J.; Takahashi, Y.; and Lorscheider, F. L. "Dental Silver Tooth Fillings: A Source of Mercury Exposure Revealed by Wholebody Image Scan and Tissue Analysis." *The FASEB Journal* III:2641 (1989).

Hallenbeck, W. H., and Cummingham-Burns, K. M. *Pesticides and Human Health*. New York: Springer-Verlag, 1985.

Huggins, Hal A., and Huggins, Sharon A. *It's All In Your Head*. Colorado Springs, CO: Huggins, 1985.

Huggins, Hal A. "Root Canals." *Let's Live* (November 1990):71.

Hunter, Beatrice Trum. *Consumer Beware*. New York: Simon and Schuster, 1971.

Hunter, Beatrice Trum. *The Great Nutrition Robbery*. New York: Charles Scribner's Sons, 1978.

Hunter, Beatrice Trum. *The Additives Book*. New Canaan, CT: Keats Publishing, Inc., 1980.

Hunter, Beatrice Trum. *How Safe is the Food in Your Kitchen?* New York: Charles Scribner's Sons, 1981.

Hunter, Beatrice Trum. *The Sugar Trap*. Boston: Houghton Mifflin Co., 1982.

Hunter, Beatrice Trum. "Gluten Intolerance." *Clinical Ecology* IV(3):120–26 (Fall 1986).

Inlander, Charles B., and Weiner, Ed. *Take This Book to the Hospital With You*. Emmaus, PA: Rodale Press, 1985.

Jacobson, Michael F. *Eaters Digest: The Consumer's Factbook of Food Additives*. Garden City, NY: Anchor Books, 1972.

Jampolsky, Gerald. *Love is Letting Go Fear*. Millbrae, CA: Celestial Arts, 1979.

Jampolsky, Gerald. *Out of Darkness and into the Light*. New York: Bantam Books, 1989.

Jelks, Mary. *Allergy Plants That Cause Sneezing and Wheezing*. Tampa, FL: World Wide Printing, n.d.

Johns, Stephanie Bernardo. *The Allergy Guide to Brand-Name Foods and Food Additives*. New York: New American Library, 1988.

Joklik, Wolfgang K.; Willett, Hilda P.; Amos, Bernard D.; and Wilfert, Catherine M. *Zinsser Microbiology*. Norwalk, CT: Appleton and Lange, 1988.

Joneja, Janice Vickerstaff, and Bielory, Leonard. *Understanding Allergy, Sensitivity and Immunity*. New Brunswick and London: Rutgers University Press, 1990.

Jones, M. H. *The Allergy Self-Help Cookbook*. Emmaus, PA: Rodale Press, 1984.

Jones, M. H. "Amaranth and Quinoa." *Mastering Food Allergies* I(3):1–2, 4 (March 1986).

Jones, M. H. "Superfood #4-Teff." *Mastering Food Allergies* IV(7):1–2 (July–August 1989).

Justice, Blair. *Who Gets Sick: Thinking and Health*. Houston: Peak Press, 1987.

Kalsner, S., and Richards R. "Coronary Arteries of Cardiac Patients are Hyperreactive and Contain Stores of

Amines: A Mechanism for Coronary Vasospasm." *Science* 223:1435–37(1984).

Kebbekus, Barbara; Greenberg, Arthur; Horgan, Liam; Bozzelli, Joseph; Darack, Faye; and Eveleens, Carol. "Concentration of Selected Vapor and Particulate-Phase Substances in the Lincoln and Holland Tunnels." *Journal of the Air Pollution Control Association* 33(4):328–30 (1983).

Kellerman, R. W., and Graham, Richard C., Jr. "Kinins—Possible Physiologic and Pathologic Roles in Man." *New England Journal of Medicine* 279(16):859–64 (1968).

King, Jonathan. *Troubled Waters.* Emmaus, PA: Rodale Press, 1985.

Kirschman, John D. *Nutrition Almanac.* New York: McGraw-Hill Book Company, 1979.

Kordash, Terance R. "Environmental Control of Molds." *Allergy Forum* II(3):1–7 (November 1990).

Krassner, Michael B. "Brain Chemistry." *Chemical and Engineering News* 61(35):22–33. (August 29, 1983).

Kubler-Ross, E. *On Death and Dying.* New York, Macmillan, 1969.

Lafavore, Michael. *Radon: The Invisible Threat.* Emmaus, PA: Rodale Press, 1987.

Langer, S., and Scheer, J. *Solved: The Riddle of Illness.* New Canaan, CT: Keats Publishing, Inc., 1984.

Langone, John. "Emerging Viruses." *Discover* (December 1990):63–68.

Larson, June, and Nugent, Bonnie. *Very Basically Yours.* Chicago: The Board of the Human Ecology Study Group, 1967.

Lesser, Michael. *Nutrition and Vitamin Therapy.* New York: Bantam Books, 1981.

Levin, Alan, and Zellerbach, Merla. *The Type 1/Type 2 Allergy Relief Program.* Los Angeles: Jeremy P. Tarcher, Inc., 1983.

Levine, Stephen, and Reinhardt, Jeffrey H. "Biochemical Pathology Initiated by Free Radicals, Oxidant Chemicals and Therapeutic Drugs." *Journal of Orthomolecular Psychiatry* XII(3):166–83 (1983).

Levine, Stephen, and Kidd, Parris M. *Antioxidant Adaptation.* San Leandro, CA: Biocurrents Division, Allergy Research Group, 1986.

Lieberman, Allan D., and Kline, Ellis. "Microbiological Flora: An Antigenic Source of Ecological Illness." Presented at the 19th Advanced Seminar of the American Academy of Environmental Medicine, Phoenix, AZ, November 3, 1985.

Lifton, Bernice. *Bugbusters.* New York: McGraw-Hill Book Company, 1985.

Lippman, Morton, and Schlesinger, Richard B. *Chemical Contaminations in the Human Environment.* New York: Oxford University Press, 1979.

Lorenzani, Shirley S. *Candida: A Twentieth Century Disease.* New Canaan, CT: Keats Publishing, Inc., 1986.

Mabray, C.; Burdett, M.; Martin, T.; Jaynes, C.; and Hayes, J. "Treatment of Common Gynecologic Endocrinologic Symptoms by Allergy Management Procedures." *Obstetrics and Gynecology* 50(5):560–64 (1982).

McElroy, William D. *Cell Physiology and Biochemistry.* Englewood Cliffs, NJ: Prentice-Hall, Inc., 1971.

McGilvery, Robert W., and Goldstein, Gerald W. *Biochemistry—A Functional Approach.* Philadelphia: W. B. Saunders Company, 1983.

McGrath, Mike, ed. "Dust Mites: A Microscopic Monster You Can Tame." *Rodale's Allergy Relief* I(9):1, 3 (1986).

McGrath, Mike, ed. "Do In Your Dust Mites Now!" *Rodale's Allergy Relief* II(8):1, 4–5 (1987).

Mackarness, R. *Not All In the Mind.* London: Pan Books, 1976.

Mackarness, R. *Chemical Victims.* London: Pan Books, 1980.

Mackarness, R. *Living Safely in a Polluted World.* New York: Stein and Day, 1980.

McKelway, Ben, ed. *Guess What's Coming to Dinner?* Washington: CPSI, 1987.

Male, David. *Immunology.* St. Louis, MO: The C.V. Mosby Company, 1986.

Mandell, Marshall, and Scanlon, Lynne. *Dr. Mandell's 5-Day Allergy Relief System.* Denver: The Nutri-Books Corporation, 1979.

Miller, Claudia. "Chemical Susceptibilities' Many Guises." *The Human Ecologist* (3):3–8 (June 1979).

Miller, Dana. "Electromagnetic Bodies, Electromagnetic Pollution." *The Human Ecologist* 34:7–11 (Spring 1987).

Miller, Joseph B. *Food Allergy Provocative Testing and Injection Therapy.* Springfield, IL: Charles C. Thomas, Publisher, 1972.

Moore, Raymond, and Moore, Dorothy. *Home Made Health.* Waco, TX: World Books Publisher, 1986.

Morales, Betty Lee. "Immunity: What Is It?" *Let's Live* (August 1986):56–57.

Morgan, Joseph T. "The Water Problem." *The Human Ecologist* (June 1980):3–4.

Moser, Penny Ward. "All the Real Dirt on Dust." *Discover* (November 1986):106–115.

Myers, John A. "Biological Medicine." Presented at Tacoma, WA, January 1976.

Nelson, P. F. "Evaporative Hydrocarbon Emissions from a Large Vehicle Population." *Journal of the Air Pollution Control Association* 31(11):1191–93 (1981).

Nelson, Ray. *Pollen Guide for Allergy.* Spokane, WA: Hollister-Stier/Miles Laboratories, 1990.

Newbold, H. L. *Mega Nutrients for Your Nerves.* New York: Berkley Publishing Company, 1978.

Nugent, Nancy, and Editors of *Prevention Magazine. Food and Nutrition.* Emmaus, PA: Rodale Press, 1983.

Null, Gary, and Null, Steven. *How to Get Rid of the Poisons in Your Body.* New York: Arco Publishing Company, Inc., 1978.

Ogle, Irving. *The Healing Mind.* Berkeley, CA: Celestial Arts, 1974.

Okamoto, W. K.; Gorse, Robert A.; and Pierson, W. R. "Nitric Acid in Diesel Exhaust." *Journal of the Air Pollution Control Association* 33(11):1098–1100 (1983).

Oldstone, Michael B. A. "Viral Alteration of Cell Function." *Scientific American* (August 1989):42–48.

Ory, Robert L. *Anti-Nutrients and Natural Toxicants In Foods.* Westport, CT: Food and Nutritional Press, Inc., 1981.

Oski, Frank A. *Don't Drink Your Milk.* Syracuse, NY: Mollica Press, Ltd., 1983.

Packard, Vernal S. *Processed Foods and the Consumer: Additives, Labeling, Standards, and Nutrition.* Minneapolis: University of Minnesota Press, 1976.

Pangborn, J. B. "Functions of Important Amino Acids." Lisle, IL: Technical Memorandum #2, Bionostics, Inc., February 1983.

Passwater, Richard A. *Super Nutrition.* New York: Pocket Books, 1975.

Passwater, Richard A. *Supernutrition for Healthy Hearts.* New York: The Dial Press, 1977.

Pauling, Linus. *Vitamin C and the Common Cold.* San Francisco: W. H. Freeman and Company, 1976.

Pearson, Durk, and Shaw, Sandy. *Life Extension.* New York: Warner Books, 1982.

Pearson, Durk, and Shaw, Sandy. *The Life Extension Companion.* New York: Warner Books, 1984.

Pfeiffer, Carl C. *Mental and Elemental Nutrients.* New Canaan, CT: Keats Publishing, Inc., 1975.

Pfeiffer, Carl C., and Audette, Lianne. "Pyroluria—Zinc and B$_6$ Deficiency." *International Chemical Nutrition Review* VIII(3):107–110 (July 1988).

Philpott, William H., and Taplin, S. *Biomagnetic Handbook.* Chocktaw, OK: Envirotech Products, 1980.

Philpott, William H., and Kalita, Dwight K. *Brain Allergies.* New Canaan, CT: Keats Publishing, Inc., 1980.

Philpott, William H., and Kalita, Dwight K. *Victory Over Diabetes.* New Canaan, CT: Keats Publishing Inc., 1983.

Pike, Arnold. "Feeding Your Immune System." *Let's Live* (October 1987):34–38.

Randolph, Theron. *Human Ecology and Susceptibility to the Chemical Environment.* Springfield, IL: Charles C. Thomas, 1962.

Randolph, Theron G., and Moss, Ralph W. *An Alternative Approach to Allergies.* New York: Harper & Row, 1980.

Randolph, Theron G., and Moss, Ralph W. *Allergies, Your Hidden Enemy.* Wellingborough, England: Thorsons Publishers, Ltd., 1981.

Randolph, Theron. *Environmental Medicine—Beginnings and Biographies of Clinical Ecology.* Fort Collins, CO: Clinical Ecology Publications, 1987.

Randolph, Theron G., and Wisner, R. Michael. *Detoxification: Personal Survival in a Chemical World.* N.p., Heathmed, Inc., 1988.

Rapp, Doris J. *Allergies and the Hyperactive Child.* New York: Simon and Schuster, 1979.

Rapp, Doris J. *Allergies and Your Family.* New York: Sterling Publishing Co., Inc., 1984.

Rapp, Doris J., and Bamberg, Dorothy. *The Impossible Child.* Buffalo, NY: Practical Allergy Research Foundation, 1986.

Rapp, Doris J. *Is This Your Child?.* New York: William Morrow and Company, 1991.

Rea, W. "Inter-Relationships between the Environment and Premenstrual Syndrome." *Functional Disorders of the Menstrual Cycle,* edited by M. Brush and E. Goudsmit: 135–37. New York: John Wiley and Sons Ltd., 1988.

Remington, Dennis, and Higa, Barbara. *Back to Health.* Provo, UT: Vitality House International, 1986.

Remington, Dennis, and Higa, Barbara. *The Bitter Truth About Artificial Sweeteners.* Provo, UT: Vitality House International, 1987.

Rennie, John. "The Body Against Itself." *Scientific American* (December 1990):107–15.

Ringsdorf, M. W., and Cheraskin, E. "Nutritional Aspects of Urolithiasis." *Journal of Orthomolecular Psychiatry* XII(2):142–46 (1983).

Rinkel, H.; Randolph, T.; and Zeller, M. *Food Allergy.* Springfield, IL: Charles C. Thomas, 1951.

Rippon, John W. *Medical Mycology.* Philadelphia: W. B. Saunders Company, 1982.

Robinson, Trevor. *The Organic Constituents of Higher Plants.* North Amherst, MA: Cordus Press, 1983.

Rogers, Sherry A., and Rea, William. "Surgery and the E.I. Patient." *The Human Ecologist* (30):10–11 (Fall 1985).

Rogers, Sherry A. *The E.I. Syndrome, An Rx for Environmental Illness.* Syracuse, NY: Prestige Publishing, 1986.

Rogers, Sherry A. *Tired or Toxic?* Syracuse, NY: Prestige Publishing, 1990.

Roitt, Ivan; Brostoff, Jonathan; and Male, David. *Immunology.* St. Louis, MO: The C. V. Mosley Company, 1985.

Rothschild, Jonathan. "The Thymus—Your Master Gland of Immunity." *Let's Live* (April 1982):43–47.

Rousseau, David; Rea, W.J.; and Enwright, Jean. *Your Home, Your Health, and Well-Being.* Point Roberts, WA: Hartley and Marks, Inc./Ten Speed Press, 1987.

Rowe, A. "Chronic Ulcerative Colitis—An Allergic Disease." *Annals of Allergy* VII(6):727–819 (1949).

Saifer, Mark, and Saifer, Phyllis. "A Guide to Drinking

Water." *The Human Ecologist* IX (June 1980).

Saifer, Phyllis. "Universal Reactivity—Some Underlying Causes." *The Human Ecologist* (20):4–5 (Winter 1982–83).

Saifer, Phyllis, and Zellerbach, Merla. *Detox.* Los Angeles: Jeremy P. Tarcher, Inc., 1984.

Satir, Virginia. *Making Contact.* Berkeley, CA: Celestial Arts, 1976.

Schauss, Alexander. *Diet, Crime, and Delinquency.* Berkeley, CA: Parker House, 1987.

Schroeder, Henry A. *The Trace Elements and Man.* Old Greenwich, CT: The Devin-Adair Company, 1973.

Schultzle, Dennis, and Perez, Joseph M. "Factors Influencing the Emissions of Nitrated-Polynuclear Aromatic Hydrocarbons (Nitro-PAH) from Diesel Engines." *Journal of the Air Pollution Control Association* 33(8):751–53 (1983).

Schutte, Karl H., and Myers, John A. *Metabolic Aspects of Health—Nutritional Elements in Health and Disease.* Kentfield, CA: Discovery Press, 1979.

Selye, Hans. *Stress Without Distress.* New York: New American Library–Dutton, 1975.

Selye, Hans. *The Stress of Life.* New York: McGraw-Hill, 1978.

Sheinkin, D.; Schachter, M.; and Hutton, R. *Food, Mind and Mood.* New York: Warner Books, 1979.

Sherris, John C., ed. *Medical Microbiology.* New York: Elsevier Science Publishing Company, 1984.

Siegel, Bernie S. *Love, Medicine, and Miracles.* New York: Harper & Row, 1986.

Sigsby, John E.; Tejada, Silvestre; Ray, William; Lang, John; and Duncan, John. "Volatile Organic Compound Emissions from 46 In-Use Passenger Cars." *Environmental Service and Technology* XXI(5):466–75 (1987).

Simonton, Carl O. *Getting Well Again.* New York: Bantam Books, 1982.

Small, Bruce M. *The Susceptibility Report.* Longueuil, PQ, Canada: Deco Books, 1982.

Smith, Cyril, and Best, Simon. *Electromagnetic Man.* New York: St. Martin's Press, 1989.

Smith, Lendon. *Feed Your Kids Right.* New York: Dell Publishing Company, Inc., 1979.

Smith, Lendon. *Feed Yourself Right.* New York: McGraw-Hill, 1983.

Spohn, Richard B. *Clean Your Room: A Compendium On Indoor Pollution.* State of California: Department of Consumer Affairs, 1982.

Stanier, Roger Y.; Duodoroff, Michael; and Adelberg, Edward A. *The Microbial World.* Englewood Cliffs, NJ: Prentice-Hall, Inc., 1970.

Stecher, Paul G., ed. *The Merck Index.* 7th ed., Rahway, NJ: Merck and Company, Inc., 1960.

Stevens, Laura J. *The Complete Book of Allergy Control.* New York: Macmillan Company, 1983.

Stoff, Jesse A., and Pellegrino, Charles. *Chronic Fatigue Syndrome.* New York: Random House, 1988.

Stone, Irwin. *The Healing Factor: Vitamin C Against Disease.* New York: Grosset and Dunlap, 1972.

Stortebecker, Patrick. *Mercury Poisoning from Dental Amalgam—A Hazard to the Human Brain.* Orlando, FL: Bio-Probe, Inc., 1985.

Strauss, S. E., and Dale, J. K. "Allergy and the Chronic Fatigue Syndrome." *Journal of Allergy Clinical Immunology* 81:791–95 (1988).

Streltwieser, Andrew Jr., and Heathcock, Clayton. *Introduction to Organic Chemistry.* New York: Macmillan Company, 1976.

Stryer, Lubert. *Biochemistry.* New York: W. H. Freeman and Company, 1988.

Tabor, Robert N. "A Unified Theory of Chemical Hypersensitivity." *Journal of Orthomolecular Psychiatry* XIII(1):6–14 (1984).

Trowbridge, John Parks. *The Yeast Syndrome.* New York: Bantam Books, 1986.

Truss, C. Orian. *The Missing Diagnosis.* Birmingham, AL: C. Orian Truss, 1983.

U.S. Department of Health and Human Services. "The Health Consequences of Smoking—Chronic Obstructive Lung Disease: A Report of the Surgeon General." Public Health Service, Office on Smoking and Health, 1984.

U.S. Department of Health and Human Services. "The Health Consequences of Involuntary Smoking: A Report of the Surgeon General." Public Health Service, Office on Smoking and Health, 1986.

Vander, Arthur J.; Sherman, James H.; and Luciano, Dorothy S. *Human Physiology: The Mechanisms of Body Function.* New York: McGraw-Hill, 1970.

Walczak, Michael, ed. *Nutrition—Applied Personally.* La Habra, CA: International College of Applied Nutrition, 1979.

Wallis, Claudia. "Viruses." *Time* (November 3, 1986):66–78. Reported by Gorman, Chestine; Nash, Madeline; and Thompson, Dick.

Weiss, Linda. *The Kitchen Magician.* Milford, MI: Prosperity Publishing, 1986.

Weiss, Linda, and Weiss, Milton. *How to Live with the New 20th Century Illness.* Milford, MI: Weiss, and X-Press Publishing, 1983.

Wheeler, Margaret F., and Volk, Wesley A. *Basic Microbiology.* Philadelphia: J. B. Lippincott Company, 1969.

Whitney, Eleanor, and Hamilton, Eva. *Understanding Nutrition.* New York: West Publishing Company, 1984.

Williams, Robert Hardin, ed. *Textbook of Endocrinology.* Philadelphia: W. B. Saunders and Company, 1974.

Williams, Roger J. *Biochemical Individuality.* Austin, TX: University of Texas Press, 1956.

Williams, Roger J. *Nutrition Against Disease.* New York: Bantam Books, 1973.

Williams, Roger J., and Kalita, Dwight. *A Physician's Handbook on Orthomolecular Medicine.* New Canaan, CT: Keats Publishing, Inc., 1977.

Williams, Roger J. *Advancement of Nutrition.* Austin, TX: Clayton Foundation, Biochemical Institute of the University of Texas at Austin, 1982.

Windholz, Martha, ed. *The Merck Index.* 10th ed., Rahway, NJ: Merck and Company, Inc., 1983.

Winter, Ruth. *A Consumer's Dictionary of Cosmetic Ingredients.* New York: Crown Publishers, Inc., 1976.

Winter, Ruth. *A Consumer's Dictionary of Food Additives.* New York: Crown Publishers, Inc., 1984.

Wright, Jonathan V. *Dr. Wright's Book of Nutritional Therapy.* Emmaus, PA: Rodale Press, 1979.

Wright, Jonathan V. *Dr. Wright's Guide to Healing With Nutrition.* Emmaus, PA: Rodale Press, 1984.

Yacenda, John. "Your Immune System and Addictions—Any Link?" *Let's Live* (October 1987):20–23.

Yepsen, Roger B., Jr. *The Encyclopedia of Natural Insect and Disease Control.* Emmaus, PA: Rodale Press, 1984.

Zamm, Alfred V. *Why Your House May Endanger Your Health.* New York: Simon and Schuster, 1980.

Index

1. T—The tendency to have allergies is hereditary, but can also be environmentally-induced. Symptoms can be controlled with careful lifestyle management and treatment.
2. F—Formaldehyde, an extremely toxic chemical, is also found in cigarette smoke, fabrics, carpeting, home building materials, and personal hygience products, and has been used as a preservative in flour, poultry, and eggs.
3. T—Gas appliances are among the primary causes of toxic chemical exposure in the home.
4. T—Many women have peeling lips, an allergic reaction to the pigments, flavorings and perfume in lipsticks. Natural lip products made from pure beeswax and oils will heal chapped lips.
5. F—Even non-alcoholic aftershaves may contain chemicals that can cause face irritation, burned or peeling skin, and eye irritation
6. F—Antihistamines only treat symptoms. Allergy extracts, however, relieve symptoms and decrease sensitivity over time.
7. T—But if only the inner corner itches, you may have a food allergy.
8. T—Some women are sensitive to their own secretions of estrogen, estriol, or progesterone, thus contributing to PMS.
9. T—Buffered vitamin C and oxygen, properly administered, are helpful for stopping allergic reactions to many substances.
10. T—Lifestyle changes, biofeedback, relaxation and visualization techniques help many allergy sufferers.

It seems that only a few people do not have allergies/sensitivities of some sort or another. This book by Dr. Jacqueline Krohn will help the reader sort them out. There are positive answers in this well-researched book, so don't give up!

–Lendon H. Smith, **MD**, Portland, Oregon,
Author of *Feed Yourself Right* and *Feed Your Kids Right*

This valuable and important book was written for all of us. It fills a medical need and offers hope and help. In addition, it teaches us coping skills which focus on wellness, and not on the illness—a useful and educational resource for our patients and ourselves.

–Paula G. Davey, **MD**, Ann Arbor, Michigan

Dr. Jacqueline Krohn specializes in pediatrics, and environmental and occupational medicine. She has successfully treated hundreds of allergic adults and children using natural methods at her clinic in Los Alamos. She and her staff have published other medical manuals on the subject of allergies.

Frances Taylor, Dr. Krohn's head allergy technician, holds an advanced degree in microbiology and biochemistry. Nurse-technician **Erla Mae Larson**, a former nutritional therapy instructor, is also on the staff of Dr. Krohn's clinic.